THE LIBRARY

PHARMACEUTICAL SOCIETY OF GREAT BRITAIN

1 Lambeth High Street, London SE1 7JN

Telephone 01 735 9141

This book should be returned not later than the date stamped below.

3 OCT 1982	
26 AUG 1984	
AUG 1986	
31 APR 1987	
17 APR 1988	

The borrower should return the book by the due date without waiting for a notice from the Librarian.
A borrower wishing to retain the book for a longer period must apply for an extension.
[Note: Regulation 3]

Return of books by post. Books must be securely packed to avoid damage in transit. It is advised that Members keep a note of packing and posting details should any claim for loss or damage arise.
[Note: Regulations 4 and 8]

Library Regulations — see overleaf.

TABLET MANUFACTURE

TABLET MANUFACTURE

J.C. Johnson

NOYES DATA CORPORATION
Park Ridge, New Jersey London, England
1974

Library of Congress Catalog Card Number: 74-75898
ISBN: 0-8155-0530-2
Printed in the United States

Published in the United States of America by
Noyes Data Corporation
Noyes Building, Park Ridge, New Jersey 07656

FOREWORD

The detailed, descriptive information in this book is based on U.S. patents since 1967 relating to the manufacture of tablets of all types.

This book serves a double purpose in that it supplies detailed technical information and can be used as a guide to the U.S. patent literature in this field. By indicating all the information that is significant, and eliminating legal jargon and juristic phraseology, this book presents an advanced, commercially oriented review of the art and science of tablet making and the associated technologies.

The U.S. patent literature is the largest and most comprehensive collection of technical information in the world. There is more practical, commercial, timely process information assembled here than is available from any other source. The technical information obtained from a patent is extremely reliable and comprehensive; sufficient information must be included to avoid rejection for "insufficient disclosure."

The patent literature covers a substantial amount of information not available in the journal literature. The patent literature is a prime source of basic commercially useful information. This information is overlooked by those who rely primarily on the periodical journal literature. It is realized that there is a lag between a patent application on a new process development and the granting of a patent, but it is felt that this may roughly parallel or even anticipate the lag in putting that development into commercial practice.

Many of these patents are being utilized commercially. Whether used or not, they offer opportunities for technological transfer. Also, a major purpose of this book is to describe the number of technical possibilities available, which may open up profitable areas of research and development. The information contained in this book will allow you to establish a sound background before launching into research in this field.

Advanced composition and production methods developed by Noyes Data are employed to bring our new durably bound books to you in a minimum of time. Special techniques are used to close the gap between "manuscript" and "completed book." Industrial technology is progressing so rapidly that time-honored, conventional typesetting, binding and shipping methods are no longer suitable. We have bypassed the delays in the conventional book publishing cycle and provide the user with an effective and convenient means of reviewing up-to-date information in depth.

The Table of Contents is organized in such a way as to serve as a subject index. Other indexes by company, inventor and patent number help in providing easy access to the information contained in this book.

15 Reasons Why the U.S. Patent Office Literature Is Important to You –

1. The U.S. patent literature is the largest and most comprehensive collection of technical information in the world. There is more practical commercial process information assembled here than is available from any other source.

2. The technical information obtained from the patent literature is extremely comprehensive; sufficient information must be included to avoid rejection for "insufficient disclosure."

3. The patent literature is a prime source of basic commercially utilizable information. This information is overlooked by those who rely primarily on the periodical journal literature.

4. An important feature of the patent literature is that it can serve to avoid duplication of research and development.

5. Patents, unlike periodical literature, are bound by definition to contain new information, data and ideas.

6. It can serve as a source of new ideas in a different but related field, and may be outside the patent protection offered the original invention.

7. Since claims are narrowly defined, much valuable information is included that may be outside the legal protection afforded by the claims.

8. Patents discuss the difficulties associated with previous research, development or production techniques, and offer a specific method of overcoming problems. This gives clues to current process information that has not been published in periodicals or books.

9. Can aid in process design by providing a selection of alternate techniques. A powerful research and engineering tool.

10. Obtain licenses – many U.S. chemical patents have not been developed commercially.

11. Patents provide an excellent starting point for the next investigator.

12. Frequently, innovations derived from research are first disclosed in the patent literature, prior to coverage in the periodical literature.

13. Patents offer a most valuable method of keeping abreast of latest technologies, serving an individual's own "current awareness" program.

14. Copies of U.S. patents are easily obtained from the U.S. Patent Office at 50¢ a copy.

15. It is a creative source of ideas for those with imagination.

CONTENTS AND SUBJECT INDEX

II. TABLETTING SPECIFIC MATERIALS

INTRODUCTION

Tablets are considered to be formed by compaction of powders, crystals or granulations into small cakes. In this review the definition of tablet has been extended to include other solid forms such as pills, pellets, dragees, lozenges and the like. Although tabletting is frequently considered to be a pharmaceutical process for preparing medicaments in dosage unit forms, it is also used in many other industries for preparing cosmetics, sanitary products, catalysts, fertilizers, and metallurgical materials.

Although a simple tablet might be formed by the mere compaction of the active material in granular form, the tablet of today is often a complex structure. Laminates, core-in-core, multiple layered, and bonded pilules or pellets, are examples of modern tablet structure. The properties of the tablet such as hardness, brittleness, rate of disintegration, rate of dissolution, taste, color, etc., are controlled or modified by the incorporation of diluents, binders, coating materials, flavoring materials, dyes, and stabilizers with the active ingredient.

Many pharmaceutical tablet formulations of today are directed toward the controlled release of the active material. Materials which would be destroyed or inactivated by gastric juices are formulated so that the release of the active ingredient does not take place until the tablet reaches the intestines. Veterinary boluses and implantable tablets with sustained release of hormonal materials are used for fertility control in animals and humans.

This review covers 211 patents issued since January 1967 on the advances made in tabletting techniques and materials. In the first section which covers tablet formation and excipients, the majority of the patents, 99, disclose matrices or binders, coating materials and lubricants used in tablet formation. The remainder cover tablet structure and manufacturing processes.

In the second section, the remaining 67 patents are on the tabletting of specific materials. The majority of these disclosures are on new pharmaceutically active materials or new and improved formulations of long time medicines such as aspirin. Some 19 patents are also reviewed on nonmedical tablets of iron ore, mouthwash, disinfectants, coffee, tea and soap.

I. TABLET FORMATION AND EXCIPIENTS

TABLET STRUCTURE

TABLET SHAPE

Readily Divisible Tablets

A method has been developed by *G.M. Krause and F.C. Ninger; U.S. Patent 3,336,200; August 15, 1967; assigned to Warner-Lambert Pharmaceutical Company* for the preparation of a readily divisible compressed tablet which has a low bulking factor and which is adapted to nest readily in a container on random fill. This structure can be shown in the following Figure 1.1.

FIGURE 1.1: TABLET STRUCTURE

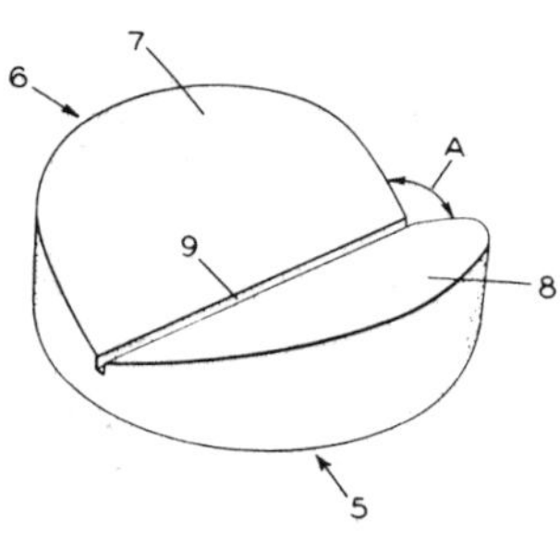

Source: G.M. Krause and F.C. Ninger; U.S. Patent 3,336,200; August 15, 1967

The tablet structure in Figure 1.1 comprises a lower face **5** and an upper face **6** divided into sections **7** and **8**. As shown, each of sections **7** and **8** lie in separate planes which intersect along a line **9** and form an angle **A** intercepting an arc of less than 180° and preferably an arc of 90° to 120°. The material forming the tablet is thicker at the sides than it is at the center and the thinnest portion lies along the line **9** where the surfaces of sections **7** and **8** intersect. Line **9** may be defined merely by the intersection of the surfaces of sections **7** and **8** or it may be defined by providing a somewhat deeper score line, as shown. To subdivide the unitary tablet structure and to separate it into individual dosage units, a moderate manual pressure is applied to the upper and lower faces of the tablet by means of the thumb and forefinger. The leverage exerted on the separate sections of the upper face has its fulcrum along line **9** and since the thinnest portion of the tablet lies along line **9** it is easily broken there thus forming two equal halves. While the tablet structure shown in Figure 1.1 is of unequal thickness from the edges to the center, the tablet may also be of uniform thickness. Multiple units may also be combined linearly so that dosage units can be subdivided into four or more smaller units.

These tablet structures are especially valuable for use where the tablets contain therapeutic agents together with a substantial amount of a wax or similar diluent in order to obtain a timed and sustained release of the active ingredient since a substantial proportion of waxes in the tablet tends to form a very hard and brittle tablet which is difficult to subdivide when formed into the usual shapes.

Example: A granulation is prepared of the following components.

Ingredient	Parts by Weight
Carnauba wax	4
Stearic acid	16
Phenylpropanolamine hydrochloride	10
Lactose	50
Color	0.03

The carnauba wax is melted at 85°C. and the stearic acid added to the molten solution. The phenylpropanolamine hydrochloride and lactose are then added to the molten mixture after which a solution of the color in a small amount of water is also added. The mass is mixed until uniform and allowed to solidify in trays. After solidification, the mix is granulated by being passed through a mill. A second granulation is prepared from the following components.

Ingredient	Parts by Weight
Polyethylene glycol 4000, USP	4
Lactose	30
Phenylpropanolamine hydrochloride	5
Color	0.005
Magnesium stearate	0.2

The polyethylene glycol is heated to 70°C. in a suitable mixer. The lactose and the phenylpropanolamine hydrochloride are then slowly added to the polyethylene glycol. The color is next dissolved in 1.66 parts by weight of water and added as a solution, with mixing, to the other ingredients. After a uniform blend is obtained, the mixture is transferred to trays where it is allowed to solidify. The solidified material is then milled to form a granulation with which the magnesium stearate is uniformly blended.

The separate granulations are then compressed into double layer tablets whose layers are of substantially uniform thickness, each tablet weighing about 705 milligrams, the bottom layer (first granulation) weighing up to about 485 milligrams. The punches employed are shaped to produce a center scored tablet in which the two halves of the tablet which meet along the score line are at an angle of 135° to each other. The tablets obtained even though the bottom layer is of a hard, waxy structure may easily be divided into two halves by exerting manual pressure on the tablet with the forefinger so as to divide it into separate dosage units. The tablets are found to have an average hardness of about 18 Strong-Cobb units.

Multilayer Tablets with Calcium Salt Core

M.G. Grodberg and J.R. Mellberg; U.S. Patent 3,345,265; October 3, 1967; assigned to The Kendall Company have developed multilayered prenatal, prophylactic and therapeutic tablets particularly those in which a nontoxic calcium salt such as calcium carbonate and a soluble nontoxic fluoride such as sodium fluoride are included. Optionally, other ingredients such as vitamins and other minerals may also be included.

In the usual vitamin tablet manufacture the dry vitamins such as B_1, C, B_2, nicotinamide, etc. are mixed and precompressed dry into slugs on a ¾ inch or 1 inch punch. The slugs are then oscillated until they are reduced to approximately #20 mesh granules. Vitamins A and D are usually obtained in dry granular form and these granules are mixed with the other vitamin granules. The minerals including such minerals as sodium fluoride, calcium carbonate, ferrous sulfate and any others are mixed in the usual method with sufficient sucrose syrup to form a coherent mass and are granulated and dried and screened to #20 mesh size.

The vitamins and minerals are combined, the composition mixed well, compressed into tablet form and immediately coated with syrup in several layers, each dusted with a nontoxic material, usually calcium carbonate. This method produces a product wherein the calcium carbonate and the sodium fluoride interact partly while the tablet is being formed and partly after the sugar coating is dissolved in the gastrointestinal tract so that only about 6% of the fluoride is available to the body. By separating the calcium salt core from the fluoride in an outer coating, the production of insoluble calcium fluoride is avoided and maximum availability of both ingredients is provided. The structure of the tablet is shown below in Figure 1.2.

FIGURE 1.2: MULTILAYER TABLET WITH CALCIUM SALT CORE

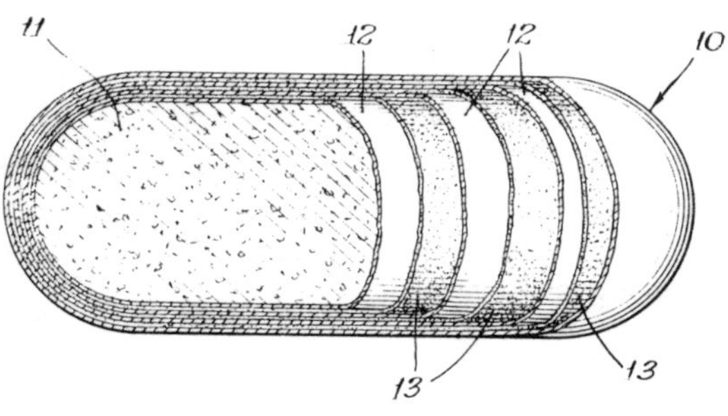

Source: M.G. Grodberg and J.R. Mellberg; U.S. Patent 3,345,265; October 3, 1967

The tablet **10** consists of a matrix **11** which contains all of the vitamins and minerals but not sodium fluoride or other soluble fluoride. The matrix is preferably coated with a plurality of sugar or other readily soluble coatings **12** separated by dusting layers **13** of a mixture of inert dusting material such as talc with a soluble fluoride such as sodium fluoride. But, if desired, the soluble fluoride may be included with the coating syrup preferably excepting the innermost coat but even that coat may have its proportionate share of soluble fluoride without reacting more than 5 to 10% of the fluoride with the calcium of the core.

For making these multilayered tablets, the usual procedure is suitable except for two details. No sodium fluoride or other soluble fluoride is included in the tablet up to the point where the tablet is to receive its sugar or other soluble coating. Usually as many as ten layers of a soluble coating such as sugar are put on in a revolving coating pan. The usual method is to dust each layer of coating deposited and dried from syrup with calcium carbonate. These multilayered tablets have the same sugar or other soluble coatings but they are dusted with a nontoxic material inert to soluble fluoride such as talc, mixed with the proper amount of sodium fluoride or other soluble fluoride. Other usual dusting materials inert to the soluble fluoride such as kaolin or magnesium stearate may be used instead of talc.

This method of manufacturing results in a product in which the calcium salt and the soluble fluoride are kept apart even after the entire tablet has dissolved. The soluble fluoride may start into solution in the mouth but in any event it quickly dissolves in the stomach and upper intestinal tract down to the last coating layer. By the time the first calcium salt goes into solution, the soluble fluoride has already been dissolved and absorbed into the blood stream.

Eyeball Medication Dispensing Tablet

A means has been developed by *R.A. Ness; U.S. Patent 3,416,530; December 17, 1968* for continuously applying medication to the eyeball. This is especially useful in the treatment of glaucoma and other eye diseases. This device conforms to the curvature of the sclera so as to fit comfortably in the cul-de-sac of the conjunctiva between the upper eyelid and the eyeball or globe in radially spaced relation to the cornea, and is disposed in the path of tear flow to the cornea. This device is more clearly illustrated by the following Figure 1.3.

FIGURE 1.3: EYEBALL MEDICATION DISPENSING TABLET

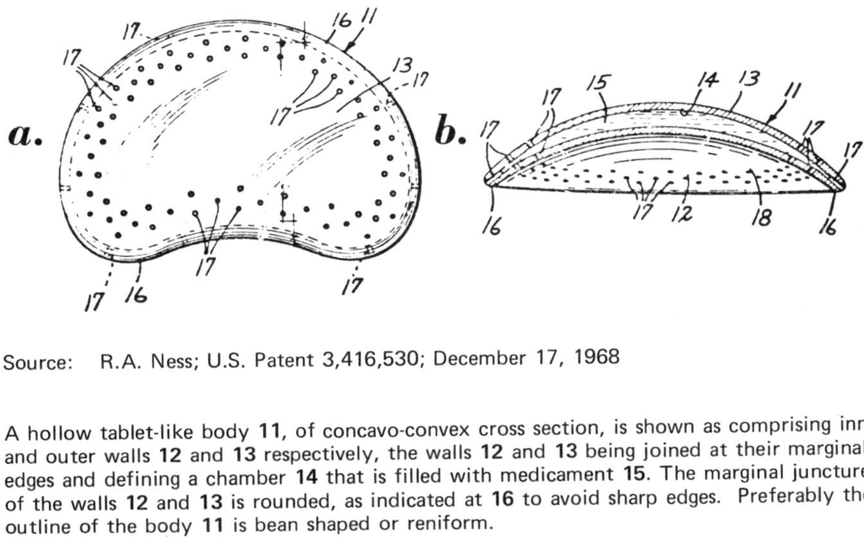

Source: R.A. Ness; U.S. Patent 3,416,530; December 17, 1968

A hollow tablet-like body **11**, of concavo-convex cross section, is shown as comprising inner and outer walls **12** and **13** respectively, the walls **12** and **13** being joined at their marginal edges and defining a chamber **14** that is filled with medicament **15**. The marginal juncture of the walls **12** and **13** is rounded, as indicated at **16** to avoid sharp edges. Preferably the outline of the body **11** is bean shaped or reniform.

Communication between the chamber **14** and the exterior of the body **11** is through a plurality of capillary openings **17** in the walls **12** and **13**, as well as through the joined edges. The marginal edges of the inner and outer walls **12** and **13** may be joined together by any suitable means, such as heat sealing, gluing or the like. Preferably, the capillary openings **17** are disposed in the areas of the walls **12** and **13** adjacent the marginal edges.

In order that the body **11** may comfortably fit in the cul-de-sac of the eye, the overall dimensions of the body **11** are preferably, length fifteen millimeters and width eleven or twelve millimeters. The outer surface **18**, which is adapted to be placed adjacent the sclera, of the inner wall **12** is generally spherical, having a spherical radius of approximately twelve millimeters, corresponding to the radius of the scleral portion of the eyeball.

The tablet-like body **11** may be made from any material that is flexible, biologically inert, nonallergenic, insoluble in tear liquid, and chemically compatible with the medicament in the chamber **14**. The walls **12** and **13** may be made from polyethylene or any other of well-known synthetic plastic materials having the above mentioned characteristics. The medicament **15** in the chamber **14** comprises the desired medication for treatment and a soluble or semisoluble carrier or matrix, the matrix being of any suitable substance such as gum acacia, gum tragacanth, or the like. The matrix serves to hold the medication together during formation of the body **11**, and operates as a diluent during the dispensing operation.

Insertion of the body **11** into the cul-de-sac and removal therefrom is a relatively simple operation. The body **11** may be mounted on or grasped by a suitable holder, which may include a minute suction cup for engaging the outer wall of the body **11**. The upper eyelid is raised upwardly and outwardly adjacent the outer corner portion of the eye to open the cul-de-sac and the body **11** inserted and released from the holder. The holder may be one of several types commonly used to insert and remove present day corneal contact lenses, artificial eyes and the like.

The use of an indicator dye in the medicament to serve as a visual indication as to the supply of medicament within the chamber may also be used. For this purpose, a small amount of methylene blue or any suitable dye material is used. So that the medicament may be easily seen, the outer wall **13** of the body **11** is preferably transparent, the inner wall **12** being preferably opaque and having a color in substantial contrast to the color of the medicament or indicator dye.

Tablets Adhering to Buccal Membranes

A suction or holding feature has been developed by *H.S. Russell; U.S. Patent 3,429,308; February 25, 1969* in tablets, lozenges or pastilles for administering a drug in the buccal cavity. The lozenge is moistened on one side, preferably the concaved side, which side is then pressed firmly onto the gum of the upper jaws above the canine or incisor teeth of the patient to whom the drug is being administered. A suction effect is created when the lozenge is pressed against the gum in this manner. This feature is illustrated in the following Figure 1.4.

FIGURE 1.4: BUCCAL TABLET

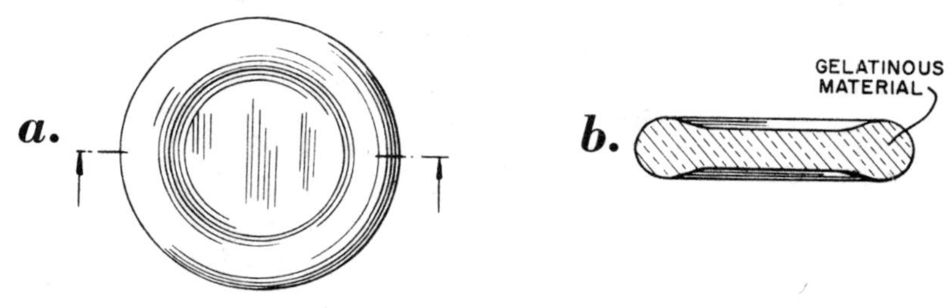

Source: H.S. Russell; U.S. Patent 3,429,308

The drug administering vehicle comprises a substantially thin body of a gelatinous material, e.g., glyco-gelatin, which acts as a diluent for an absorbable drug dissolved in the gelatinous material prior to body formation. In Figures 1.4a and 1.4b, the body is circular and is so formed as to have a generally concave depression in each of its major surfaces. It is of a substantially flexible, but resilient, nature. It can also be of elongate octagonal shape having only one concave depression in one of its major surfaces, the other major surface being substantially planar. These bodies can be made individually, or they can be made as as part of a continuous strip.

The lozenge is formed so as to have a concave depression on one side, to be relatively thin, flexible but resilient, to be shaped so as to become adhered to the mucous membrane of the parabuccal cavity by the suction afforded by the concave depression. The vehicle is made by preparing a liquid solution or melt of a gelatinous material, impregnating the solution or melt with a drug, preferably of hormonal nature, which is effective when absorbed through the mucous membrane of the parabuccal cavity, and forming the impregnated solution of melt into the vehicle. The material, in main part, is a gelatin which acts as a diluent for a water-soluble drug which is dissolved in the gelatin prior to the formation of the lozenge.

During manufacture, the drug is stirred or mixed or otherwise thoroughly dispersed into the batch of glyco-gelatin solution or melt, and the gelatin or analagous material bearing the drug is run into a series of molds and formed and hardened and dried until the requisite solid properties are imparted to each so formed vehicle. Alternatively, the material containing the drug may be cast into sheets or strips from which the vehicles or strips may be punched or pressed, any cutoff material being recirculated into the next melt batch. A small amount of a preservative, e.g., beta-naphthol, and the drug are added to the solution or melt, and therefollowing, any water is removed, e.g., under a reduced pressure, until the gelatinous material is resiliently flexible.

The drugs usually incorporated in these lozenges are of a potent nature such as hormones, anaesthetics, sympathomimetics, etc. and include those which are substantially inactivated in the stomach or intestines when ingested; are active in an unwanted manner upon the stomach or intestines when ingested; are variable in absorption or effect from patient to patient; are slow to act when ingested; or are of local application.

Easily Swallowed Tablets

A. Aufhauser; U.S. Patent 3,536,074; October 27, 1970 has developed a nontoxic, orally administrable pill, tablet, capsule or other medicinal unit to be swallowed whole which is surrounded by a frangible sac containing sufficient water or other liquid to assist in the swallowing of the unit. The frangible sac may be of any convenient size so long as it contains sufficient water or other liquid to assist in swallowing the pill, tablet or capsule. On the other hand, the size of the sac should be consistent with packaging the capsular product in containers that can be conveniently sold and carried. A capsular product whose size is of the order of a large olive contains sufficient water to substantially assist in swallowing a conventional tablet or capsule and may be readily packaged for over-the-counter sales.

Whenever the need arises for oral administration, the capsular product is merely placed in the mouth and the sac is ruptured with the teeth to release the water or other liquid. As soon as the water or other liquid is released it is swallowed along with the pill, tablet or capsule and along with the sac. By making the sac of soft, flexible material it may be readily swallowed and when a nontoxic material such as gelatin is used it merely disintegrates in the stomach or intestine. Alternatively, the sac may be composed of an edible frangible material that is rigid and that is easily broken up in the mouth into pieces that either can be easily swallowed or become dissolved in saliva.

The following Figure 1.5 gives a perspective view on an enlarged scale, portions being broken away to show the constituent elements. This structure may be illustrated with aspirin in the tablet and the use of water to assist in swallowing the tablet. The conventional aspirin tablet containing a normal dosage is a disc-shaped tablet measuring about 1 cm. across and 0.4 to 0.5 cm. in thickness.

FIGURE 1.5: EASILY SWALLOWED TABLETS

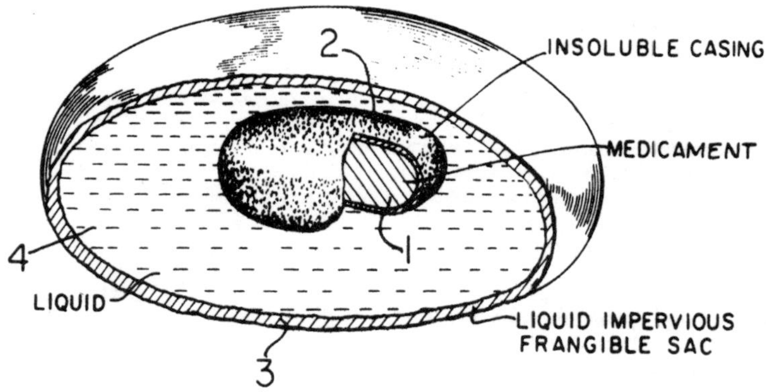

Source: A. Aufhauser; U.S. Patent 3,536,074; October 27, 1970

A conventional aspirin tablet **1**, such as that just described, is encased with a gelatin coating **2**. While gelatin is soluble in hot water to provide a coating solution, it is insoluble in water at ambient temperatures. However, after swallowing, it disintegrates to release the encased medicament. The water-insolubility of the gelatin coating may be enhanced by one or more outer coatings of arsenic-free shellac. If three or more outer coatings of shellac are provided, an enteric coating may be provided in that it acquires the property of resisting solution in the stomach for a period of time sufficiently long to permit entry of the table into the intestinal tract.

The sac **3** which surrounds the pill or tablet is of the soft elastic type and is frangible. Its size is goverened by the amount of liquid **4**, in this case water, to be encased for aiding the swallowing of the pill or tablet. The size of the sac also is selected in relation to that which can be conveniently packaged and sold. While there is considerable latitude in this regard, a sac adapted to contain about 8 cc of water is typical, namely, a sac which, as regards size, may be compared roughly with that of a large olive. Usually, a suitable liquid content ranges between 6 cc and 10 cc.

Soft frangible elastic capsules as such and their production are well-known. The sac or shell is made of gelatin with sufficient glycerin, sorbitol or other plasticizing material to retain permanent flexibility. A blend of approximately equal parts of glycerin and gelatin, with or without about 5% of acacia, is suitable.

The water and the pill or tablet may be introduced into the sac in any desired manner. Known machines of the rotary die type or of the moving die type are especially suitable. When using such machines, two continuous gelatin ribbons are fed into convergence between moving dies and injecting means injects that which is to be placed within the gelatin sac. The machine also cuts out and seals the filled and formed capsules. In the example, each capsule is filled with a predetermined measured quantity of water in conjunction with one pill or tablet. Alternatively, the sac may be produced in empty condition, as by the dipping technique, so as to have an elongated end adapted to be cut off to permit insertion by hand of the pill or tablet and the water. After filling is completed the filling aperture is sealed with hot gelatin solution which, preferably, is a solution of the gelation corresponding with that of the sac.

While aqueous liquids ordinarily are preferred to assist in swallowing the medicinal unit, some other liquid may be used such as a mineral oil, preferably one that is tasteless and is freely fluid. A mineral oil may be especially appropriate in the case of a pill or tablet wherein the medicament is a laxative, for example, cascara. Vegetable oil also could be used. In such case the casing for the unit to be swallowed whole is insoluble in the mineral oil or other nonaqueous liquid and the surrounding sac is impervious to the liquid.

Color Coded Tablets

Tablets with a jigsaw color code design are produced by *C.A. Pazar and J.H. Wiley; U.S. Patent 3,555,144; January 12, 1971; assigned to American Cyanamid Company* using extruded granules. These are therapeutic tablets of improved uniformity, absorbability, size and appearance; increased strength and greater density, as well as elegant appearance; and multicolored surface and cross-section for counterfeit detection and product identification. The medicament, a binder, and a liquid, often water, are compacted, homogenized, and extruded through a high pressure screw extruder as small strands, which are dried, and before or after drying segmented into granules, with the drying giving a surface hardness to the granules. On lubrication and compaction, a denser more uniform tablet is produced, with reduction or elimination of capping and laminating, as compared with conventional procedures.

The process is based upon the discovery that a plasticized mass containing one or more therapeutic materials may be readily converted into an excellent granulation by extruding a blended and moistened mixture of ingredients under high pressure through a die having orifices of critical dimensions so as to produce strands or strings or ribbons of the plasticized mass, of round, elliptical, rectangular, triangular or other cross-section, and then case hardening and drying these strands. The strands may be cut or broken before or after drying, or both, to form rods, not necessarily of circular cross-section. A minimum of hand labor and reworking is required.

The compression involved in extrusion increases the density of the granulation and the resulting granules are of greater density, and hence stronger. The amount of dust produced in comminution of the granules is markedly decreased. Hence, less lubricant is required on the tablet-forming dies, the tablets produced are brighter and shinier, different colors of granules produce tablets with sharper lines of demarkation, and wear on the tablet-forming punches and dies is reduced. The more consistent nature of the granules permits closer tolerances in tablet weight. Various shaped tablets are readily produced, for example triangular shaped tablets. If the cross-section of the granules is triangular for some, and of different colors, very pretty tablets are produced. While ornamental to behold, the varied colors both have trade-identification characteristics and aid in detection of counterfeiting or substitution.

Because the granules are more dense from the extrusion pressure, more pressure may be used in tabletting, and denser tablets produced. This slows the rate of release, so delayed-release products are obtained. The surface of the granules may be sprayed with slowly soluble gums, natural or synthetic, to delay release further. A water-soluble starch may be incorporated in tabletting to give an increased rate of action of the tablets. Hence, the manufacturer has greater control over the characteristics of the tablets as regards solution rates on ingestion by the user. The pressure used in tabletting also affects the rate of solution.

In large scale production as a matter of choice and convenience, the extrusion is from a screw auger type continuous extruder. For smaller batches, the mixing of the granulation mass may be in a power or hand mixer of suitable size, and extrusion may be through orifices at the end of a cylinder, with manual filling of the cylinder and a hydraulic, mechanical or hand operated piston used for extrusion. For small scale operations a hand operated potato dicer gives good results. One such device, is a cylinder about 3" in diameter and 3" long, with a perforated wall and bottom, and piston operated by hand, using a lever for mechanical advantage, with the perforation of appropriate size.

The throughput of a screw extruder is greatly increased by chilling the outer sleeve of the extruder, so that the viscosity is much greater near the auger sleeve, with a consequent increase in extrusion efficiency.

As an example, a dicalcium phosphate white blank from a powder having a size of not less than 99.5% through a 200 U.S. Standard mesh sieve was mixed with water, to form a crumb and placed in the hopper of a jacketed extruder having an auger screw. When the agitated mixture was heated to 33°C., and extruded at the same temperature, a throughput of approximately 72 kg./hr. was obtained. When the hopper was heated to about 60°C. and the jacket cooled to between 18° and 22°C., the extrusion rate was increased to 198 kg./hr. When the jacket temperature was decreased to 10°C., the extrusion rate was increased to 288 kg./hr. The following table is typical of the tablets produced from the screw-extruded compacted granulation and from a conventional wet granulation.

	Convential granulation	Screw-extruded Compacted granulation
Tablet weight (average of 20), gm	1.4849	1.4917
Standard deviation, gm	0.0175 (1.18%)	0.0071 (0.48%)
Tablet thickness (average of 20), in	0.214	0.213
Standard deviation, in	0.00134 (0.63%)	0.00074 (0.35%)
Tablet hardness (average of 20) (crushing stength), kg., Strong-Cobb	11.5	17
Standard deviation, kg	1.28 (11.13%)	1.55 (9.12%)
Tablet friability (run on 10):		
Percent loss in weight after 100 falls	0.97	0.74
Percent loss in weight after 200 falls	2.25	1.61

Rupturable Tablets

Dosage units, i.e., tablets or capsules which rupture in the region of the pyloric sphincter have been developed by *K.-N. Wai; U.S. Patent 3,444,290; May 13, 1969; assigned to Biorex Laboratories Limited, England.* When in contact with gastric juices, these units swell without bursting to such a size that they are ruptured when in the area of the pylorus. The tablet form of the unit comprises an inner medicament surrounded by an outer layer or coating of a nontoxic, film-forming colloid which is resistant to attack by but permeable to gastric juices, the layer or coating being adapted to be ruptured in the region of the pyloric sphincter.

Examples of the colloids which can be used include gelatin (treated as hereinafter detailed), partially or wholly hydrolyzed polyvinyl acetate, copolymers of vinyl alcohol and vinyl acetate, ethers and esters of cellulose, such as ethoxycellulose, carbomethoxycellulose and methylcellulose, and plant mucilages, such as agar agar and alginates, and mixtures thereof. Gelatin capsules which have been hardened or tanned with formaldehyde are liable to aging. This disadvantage is avoided, according to this process, when capsules made from or tablets coated with gelatin or other film-forming colloids, after treatment with formaldehyde, are washed with a solvent, such as industrial methylated spirits (denatured alcohol) or alcohol (methanol, ethanol, etc.) to remove residual formaldehyde and then dried. Alternatively, residual formaldehyde can be removed by neutralization with, for example, gaseous ammonia or a solution of ammonia or an ammonium salt, such as ammonium carbonate, in a nonaqueous or aqueous organic medium.

The formaldehyde treatment has the effect of converting the colloid into a semipermeable membrane which is insoluble in dilute acids, such as are encountered in the stomach, but which swells and permits the passage of small molecules, for example, water, mineral acids and inorganic electrolytes. Disaccharides, such as lactose, do not appear to pass through the semipermeable membrane easily. Capsules and coated tablets treated in this manner appear to provide good protection to their contents when these are known to be hygroscopic and sensitive to moisture. All the capsules and coated tablets appear to be stable for at least 3 months, whether stored, e.g., in well-closed aluminum containers or exposed to the atmosphere.

It is to be understood that the dosage units must be hermetically sealed. This can be achieved by sealing them with a solution of gelatin or of another suitable adhesive, such as a cellulose ether, for example, a methylcellulose, with or without the use of a plasticizer. The sealing can also be accomplished by placing a strip of film-forming colloid over the join in the capsule. In the case of tablets, these can be press-coated with a film-forming colloid and then sealed with a jet of steam. The formaldehyde treatment can be carried out with solutions, of any suitable strength, of formaldehyde in water or in aqueous organic solvents, such as aqueous alcohol. It has been found to be convenient to use, for this treatment, commercial or BP solutions of formaldehyde, commonly referred to as formalin, i.e., 37 to 41% w./v. aqueous solutions of formaldehyde which may contain a variable amount of methanol or ethanol.

The dosage units can also contain one or more components capable of evolving a nontoxic gas, provided that these components and the gas evolved are not incompatible with the active materials in the dosage units. The gas so evolved when the gastric juices permeate into the dosage units will then result in an increase in tension in the interior of the dosage units, thereby preserving their shape and increasing their dimensions, and will also result in an explosion of the dosage units when they are subjected to mechanical stresses in the pylorus with the result that the viscous solution resulting from the disintegration of the dosage units will forcibly impinge on the walls of the neighboring mucosa and adhere thereto for some time.

Laminated Tablets

Laminated, pan-coated tablets are described by *R.O. Fernandez, V.F. Cannito and O. Olsen; U.S. Patent 3,696,188; October 3, 1972; assigned to Schering Corporation* where the various medicament layers are separated by a layer containing 10 to 50% of a silica gel having a specified pore size. This silica gel layer not only substantially reduces the processing time but also aids in preventing migration of the ingredients and in accelerating dissolution. This silica gel-containing coat can be applied to the tablet either as a powder or in slurry form. It is preferred that this silica gel-containing coat additionally be applied directly to the tablet core. This protects against any tendency of the laminated medicaments to migrate into or out of the core.

In a preferred embodiment, the silica gels have an average pore diameter within the range of 125 to 300 Angstrom Units. Examples of commercially available silica gels within this range are Syloid 74 (average pore diameter believed to be about 150 A.) and Syloid 244 (average pore diameter believed to be about 250 A.). The following example of the preparation of decongestant-type cold tablets illustrates a preferred embodiment of the process.

Example: 1,000 cores are prepared in a standard manner by first mixing 162 grams of phenacetin, 32 grams of caffeine and 40 grams of starch and forming a wet granulation with 50 ml. of a 10% gelatin solution. The mixture is passed through a screen, dried in the oven and rescreened. An additional 15 grams of starch and 4 grams of calcium stearate (lubricant) is then added along with 230 grams of aspirin and the mixture compressed into cores. These cores are placed in a coating pan and coated first with Composition A composed of 51.2% sugar, 12.8% acacia, and 36.0% water. The moist coated cores are then dusted prior to hot air drying with Powder B composed of 25% by weight of a silica gel having an average pore diameter of 250 A. (Syloid 244) and 75% by weight of terra alba (dehydrated calcium sulfate).

The dusted cores are dried by hot air and then coated with Suspension C which contains 2 grams of chlorpheniramine maleate and 10 grams of L-phenylephrine base suspended in 50 ml. of Composition A. Dusting Powder B is applied and the coated cores are hot-air dried. This serial application of Suspension C and Dusting Powder B followed by hot-air drying is repeated 5 times. Then follows a sequence of applying a coat of Composition A followed by dusting with Powder B and hot-air drying and this sequence is repeated. Three coats are then applied of a grossing composition composed of 20% Powder B, 3% titanium dioxide, 3% cornstarch, 48% sugar and 26% water. The tablets are then given a white color by coating with a 3% titanium dioxide suspension in sugar syrup. This coating operation can be satisfactorily performed in 1 day. If the specified silica gel is omitted, the coating operation on the moist core requires about 4 days. In addition, the specified silica gel in the above-produced tablets helps prevent the pharmaceutically incompatible aspirin and 1-phenylephrine ingredients from migrating toward each other and additionally accelerated the dissolution of the tablet when ingested.

TABLETS WITH CONTROLLED RELEASE PARTICLES

Tablets Containing Microballs

A process for preparing microballs having controlled release rates has been disclosed by *G. Ross, W. Tillmann and R. Liebenholf; U.S. Patent 3,361,632; January 2, 1968; assigned to Farbwerke Hoechst AG, Germany.* The microballs or pearls prepared by this process have the advantage that they are not easily ruptured or damaged as is the case with known encapsulated products.

In this process, the active substance is dissolved in a liquid carrier and dropped or sprayed through very fine nozzles into a solvent in which the carrier substance is not at all or only sparingly soluble. When operating in this way, nearly round bodies are formed which are removed from the solvent by filtration and then dried. It is likewise possible to drop the solution or a suspension of the active substance in a carrier substance at a temperature above the solidification point of the carrier substance into a gas, whereby the liquid solidifies to microballs. Air, nitrogen, carbon dioxide or noble gases are useful as such gases.

The preparation of the microballs must be adapted in each case to the special properties of the medicament to be encapsulated. Sparingly soluble active substances are, for instance, formed into drops with addition of surface active substances, softening agents, solvents and/or water-soluble auxiliary substances (such as sodium chloride) in order to attain a releasing mechanism in conformity with each individual active substance. As auxiliary agents for the initial active dose there are used, above all, substances capable of forming drops, soluble in water or in gastric juice. Instead of a solution of the medicament in the carrier substance, a suspension of the active substance in the carrier substance may likewise be used.

According to this method, separate operations are carried out for producing pearls containing the same active substance, but different carrier substances. These carrier substances differ from one another as regards solubility and melting points. As carrier substances, there are suitable, for instance, all hydrophobic substances such as fats, waxes, plastics, polymers, cellulose derivative which are capable of forming drops and which release the admixed active substances only slowly. It is likewise possible to use carrier substances which are solid at room temperature, for instance certain fats or waxes, which however, become liquid on being warmed, and which, in this way, can be formed to drops.

Of the various sorts of pearls thus produced certain amounts by weight are mixed at the ratio desired and these mixtures are combined, i.e., they are pressed to tablets which may likewise be cone-shaped or they are filled into capsules.

Compressed tablets may be prepared containing a given quantity of medicament, one third of which is intended to be released within 30 minutes in gastric fluid, a second third of which is intended to be released after about 2 hours in gastric fluid, and the remainder of which is intended to be released after about 8 hours in intestinal fluid. The medicament is uniformly distributed in a homogneous mixture of 3 equal parts by weight of nearly round pearl drops between 0.5 and 3 mm. in diameter, which may be plasticly deformed upon being compressed. One third of the pearl drops are produced by dissolving one third of the medicament in polyethylene glycol 6,000 to form a solution, dropping or spraying the solution through very fine nozzles into liquid paraffin, removing the paraffin by filtration, degreasing and drying. One third of the pearl drops are produced by suspending one third of the medicament in paraffinum solidum, dropping or spraying the resulting suspension through fine nozzles into water, removing the water by filtration, and drying. The final one third of the pearl drops are produced by suspending one third of the drug in cera alba, dropping or spraying the resulting suspension through fine nozzles into a mixture of ethyl alcohol and water, removing this collecting fluid by filtration, and drying.

Tablets with Sustained Release Cores

Mixtures of multicoated cores are incorporated in dosage units, e.g., tablets or capsules, in a process disclosed by *H.H. Berger; U.S. Patent 3,344,029; September 26, 1967; assigned to Ethicals, Inc.* This process provides for sustained release dosage units which do not release large doses of medicament if the dosage unit is accidently crushed in the mouth. Each core consists essentially of a cohesive intimate mixture of a finely divided therapeutically active material and an ingestible material resistant to disintegration in the gastrointestinal tract. The proportion of ingestible material to therapeutically active material in each core varies from 0.1 to 2.0:1 with some variation among the cores to provide varying release rates in the gastrointestinal tract.

In addition, at least a minor proportion of the cores are coated with alternating coatings of therapeutically active material and ingestible material and the proportion of therapeutically active material and ingestible material in the cores and the amount of therapeutically active material in the sum of the coatings is so correlated that the percent of therapeutically active material in the coatings plus the percent of therapeutically active material in the cores released during the first hour in the gastrointestinal tract is less than 50% of the total therapeutically active content of the dosage unit. The therapeutically active materials useful in the dosage units are in general those which are normally administered orally and which are administered in relatively exact dosages.

The ingestible materials useful in the dosage units are those conventionally employed and include methyl- and ethylcellulose, cellulose acetate and phthalate, shellac, castor oil and hydrogenated castor oil, waxes, higher fatty acids, esters of higher fatty acids, higher fatty alcohols and high molecular weight polyethylene glycols. The ingestible material is selected or compounded to provide a core which is resilient and plastic in consistency. Preparation of dosage units falling within the scope of this process is illustrated in detail as follows.

Example: In the first step, 5.4 lbs. of a powder containing 10% by weight of nitroglycerin and 90% by weight of beta-lactose was mixed with 28 lbs. of a mixture of cane and corn sugars and this was mixed with ¼ gallon of a mixture formed from 8 lbs. of pharmaceutical glaze (5 lbs. of shellac per gallon of methyl alcohol) and 10 oz. of castor oil. This damp mixture was partly dried on flat trays and then pressed through a 16 mesh screen to obtain small cores which were then dried.

In the second through fifth steps, 5.4 lbs. of dry mixture as in step one was mixed with 23 lbs. of powdered sugar and 5 lbs. of corn sugar. Using the amounts as shown in the following table for each step, the dry mixture was then intermixed with a liquid mixture of pharmaceutical glaze (5 lbs. of shellac per gallon of methyl alcohol), hydrogenated castor oil and of a polyethylene glycol having an average molecular weight of 4,000. Enough alcohol was sprinkled on the mixture to dampen it. After partial drying the mixture was pressed through a 16 mesh screen to obtain small cores which were dried.

	- - Step 2 - -		- - Step 3 - -		- - Step 4 - -		- - Step 5 - -	
	Lbs.	Oz.	Lbs.	Oz.	Lbs.	Oz.	Lbs.	Oz.
Pharmaceutical glaze	2	6	2	10	2	14	3	4
Hydrogenated castor oil	-	14	1	6	1	12	1	14
Polyethylene glycol	-	14	-	10	-	7	-	6

In step 6, seven-tenths of the total cores weighing about 134 lbs. were placed into a coating pan and moistened with a solution of pharmaceutical glaze and alcohol. One-seventh of the additional active material, 1.83 lbs. of a 10% nitroglycerin-beta lactose mixture was then applied to the seven-tenths of separated cores in 5 coatings alternating with coatings of pharmaceutical glaze. Five additional coatings of pharmaceutical glaze were applied to produce a delayed release effect. The powder was applied in dry form, the intermittent coatings of pharmaceutical glaze were completely dried before the next dusting, and warm air was used for drying.

In step 7, one-seventh of the coated cores were removed from the pan and the above procedure repeated, using another 1.83 lbs. of the 10% nitroglycerine-beta lactose mixture applied in 5 coatings alternating with coatings of pharmaceutical glaze and with 5 additional coatings of pharmaceutical glaze applied. In each of steps 8 through 12, the procedure of step 7 was repeated with one-sixth of the coated cores being removed after step 7, one-fifth after step 8, one-fourth after step 9, one-third after step 10, and one-half after step 11. The three-tenths of the cores of steps 1 through 5 and the coated cores of steps 6 through 12 were then carefully mixed in a pony mixer and assayed for average rate of release of medication which was found to be as follows:

	In Core, %	In Coatings, %	Total, %
After 1 hour	14	–	14
1 to 2 hours	6	8	14
2 to 3 hours	6	7	13
3 to 4 hours	6	6	12
4 to 5 hours	6	5	11
5 to 6 hours	6	3	9
6 to 7 hours	6	2	8
7 to 8 hours	6	1	7
8 to 9 hours	6	–	6
9 to 10 hours	6	–	6
	68	32	100

In case of accidental crushing, the rate of release of medication was found to be 46% after 1 hour, from the 14% in the cores and the 32% in the coatings, and 6% during each additional hour through 10 hours. The intermixed cores were then admixed in calculated amounts with a powder consisting of starch and sugar to provide tabletted dosage units.

Spherical Controlled Release Beads

W.E. Gaunt; U.S. Patent 3,328,256; June 27, 1967 has disclosed a process of making spherical beads containing a medicament which is released in the alimentary fluids at a predetermined controlled rate. These beadlets have the advantage over coated nonpareils in that when compressed into tablets, they do not undergo fracture of the coating material which negates the controlled release feature of the coated granules.

This process incorporates the discovery that when drops of a suitable volatile solvent are permitted to fall from a suitable height onto a bed of very finely divided particles of polymers or copolymers, each separate drop forms as a spherical body a solution of the polymer or copolymer by dissolving and drawing into it particles of the polymeric bed with which the outer surface of the drop is in contact. These spherical beads can be easily separated from the powder phase by screening and remain in discrete form showing no tendency to stick together and their existence as small discrete spherical entities is retained as the volatile solvent is removed as by evaporation and, when dry, the small spherical bodies or beads are firm and hard and capable of withstanding considerable pressure.

Satisfactory spherical bodies or beads have been made, for example, from carboxypolymethylene, cellulose acetate phthalate and carboxylated polyvinyl acetate copolymers, both singly and in combination, but the foregoing are intended as illustrative and not as limitative since other polymers and copolymers can be equally well employed. The solvents that have been used are chiefly the lower alcohols and halogenated hydrocarbons or mixtures of these solvents.

Various types of active ingredients and medicaments can be incorporated into small spherical beads by this process. These include tranquilizing drugs, analgesics, antihistamines, steroids, anorexic drugs, antibiotics, decongestants, antitussive drugs, anticholinergic antispasmodics, the belladonna alkaloids and barbiturates, antibacterials and antifungals. More than one drug can be incorporated into the same bead structure by dissolving all the drugs in the solvent, by blending all the drugs into the powder bed or by dissolving some drugs in the solvent and blending some with the powder bed.

The polymer itself can be exclusively used for bead formation but there is a limit to the proportion of an added substance (cosubstance) which can be used with the polymer to form a bead which, after drying, is hard and firm. In proportions outside these limits the bead is friable and breaks readily under pressure. For example, 5 parts of polymer and 95 parts of cosubstance give a friable bead when using cellulose acetate phthalate and aluminum aspirin, whereas lesser proportions of the cosubstance do not. Thus, when using cellulose acetate phthalate particles as the polymer bed the proportion of cellulose acetate phthalate ranges from 10 to 100%, and the cosubstance such as aluminum aspirin ranges from 90 to 0%.

The ranges under various exemplary circumstances will be apparent from the subjoined examples. The drop size ranges form 1.25 to 15 microliters and the bead size ranges from 0.3 to 3.5 mm. in diameter. The solvent may be a single organic solvent or it may be a solvent mixture composed of a plurality of solvents. A particularly good solvent mixture is 90% methylene chloride and 10% methanol by volume. This process is illustrated by the following examples in which the proportions of solvents in the solvent mixtures are by volume.

Example 1: Drops of a solution of 2 grams of aluminum abietate in a mixture of 9 ml. of methylene chloride and 1 ml. of methanol were permitted to fall on a powder bed of 200 mesh cellulose acetate phthalate. Each drop quickly formed a homogeneous bead of good shape and pleasing appearance. The beads, after separation from the cellulose acetate phthalate powder, were dried to form firm, hard, brittle beads. This example also shows that the powder bed can be 100% cellulose acetate phthalate and that the cosubstance can be in the drops.

Example 2: A solvent mixture composed of 9 parts of methylene chloride and 1 part of methanol was sprayed onto a powder bed composed of 2 parts of 200 mesh cellulose acetate phthalate and 8 parts of 200 mesh aluminum aspirin. The powder was screened through a 200 mesh sieve and the beads which had been formed were collected. These beads were small and well formed and ranged in size from 0.3 mm. to 0.5 mm. in diameter.

The medicament-containing beads may be administered in any suitable dosage form. They may, for example, be used as such or may be sealed into gelatin capsules. In many instances, the beads can also be formed into compressed tablets with or without one of the usual pharmaceutical excipients or carriers.

TABLETTING PROCESSES AND APPARATUS

TABLET FORMING

Feed System for Tablet Press

H.R. Mathison; U.S. Patent 3,411,462; November 19, 1968; assigned to Geigy Chemical Corporation has developed a tablet press overhead feed system in which a wheel supported bin at an upper floor level is movable to align its conically tapered discharge spout with a delivery conduit located at floor level leading to a tablet press at a lower floor level. A fluid pressure operated coupling means is used to couple the discharge spout with the conduit. This process can be shown in Figure 2.1.

Figure 2.1a is a general elevational view of this two-floor system. Figure 2.1b is a side elevation of the lifting and sealing means. This process is used in an industrial plant installation having an upper floor **10** and a lower floor **11**. A conventional tablet press **12** on the lower floor is supplied with tablet composition material gravity fed from the floor above through a delivery conduit **13**. This conduit includes an intermediate expansible and flexible coupling portion **14** which permits the cylindrical upper end portion of the conduit to move axially in and through a complemental opening in the upper floor. The upper end of conduit **13** projects above the floor and is formed as a flat, external, circumferential flange **15** that extends laterally from the conduit in a plane normal to its axis.

The flange **15** seats on and is supported by an axially expansible collar assembly indicated generally as **16** that surrounds the upper end portion of the conduit between the flange **15** and the surface of the floor. Collar assembly **16** is comprised of a flat base ring **17** seated loosely on the floor surface and a movable upper ring **18** on which the conduit flange seats.

The collar rings are connected by fluid expansible chamber means here shown as a plurality of cylinders **19** fixed on the base ring **17** at circumferentially spaced points and provided with fluid actuated pistons **20** that are fixedly attached at their upper ends to the ring **18**. Operating fluid under remote control is supplied to cylinders **19** by inlets **21** leading from a ring manifold **22** that has communication by way of a supply line **23** with a source (not shown) of fluid under pressure. When not in use the pistons **20** normally are retracted so that the upper ring of the collar assembly occupies the lower phantom line position shown in Figure 2.1b.

The collar assembly is a means of connecting the upper end of the conduit **13** to the cone-tapered discharge spout **24** of a portable bin carrier **25** on the upper floor mounted on

FIGURE 2.1: TABLET PRESS OVERHEAD FEED SYSTEM

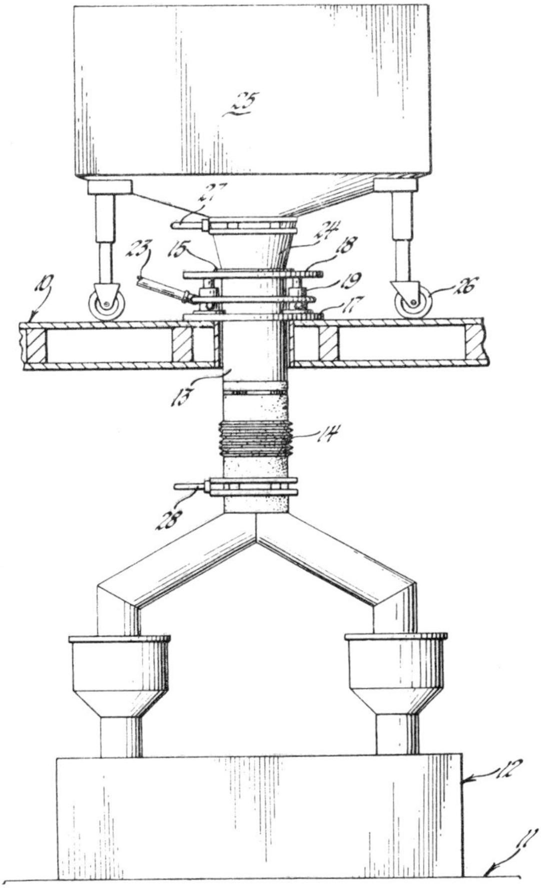

a.

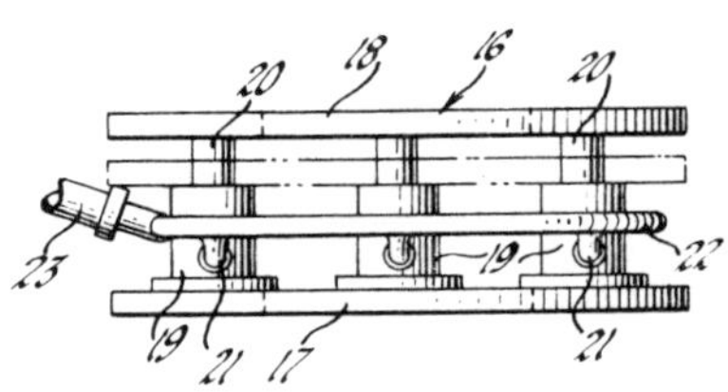

b.

Source: H.R. Mathison; U.S. Patent 3,411,462; November 19, 1968

roller casters **26**. The mouth of spout **24** occupies a plane normal to its axis, and its outer diameter is appreciably less than the internal diameter of conduit **13** at its upper end; so that when the expansible collar assembly elevates the flange **15** the open upper end of the conduit rides up over the tapered surface of the spout into forcible sealing engagement therewith. When the collar is collapsed in the phantom line position of Figure 2.1b the mouth of the spout **24** is spaced above the conduit flange **15** so that it may pass freely thereover.

In operation, a bin **25** carrying a batch of material to be pelleted is rolled into position above the upper end of conduit **13** with its spout **24** registered axially with the conduit. Fluid under pressure then is admitted to the cylinders **19** to elevate the upper ring **18** of the collar and thus lift and hold the upper end of conduit in forced, tight sealed connection with the bin spout. Closure valve means **27** on the bin discharge spout is opened and the contents of the bin flows by gravity down through the delivery conduit to press **12**. Valve means **28** controls delivery from conduit **13** to the press.

Stamping Apparatus

Apparatus for stamping pasty materials into cakes, bars or tablets has been developed by *C. Mazzoni; U.S. Patent 3,574,904; April 13, 1971.* This apparatus eliminates the peripheral contour band as the edges of the mold halves coincide with the equatorial contacting lines of the stamped tablet being produced. This can be shown in Figure 2.2.

Figure 2.2a shows the main portion of the stamping machine as provided with two pairs of mold halves, the rotating disc-shaped box and related molds being applied thereto; Figure 2.2b is a front view showing the rotating disc-shaped box; Figure 2.2c is a sectional view of the disc according to line **3–3** of Figures 2.2a and 2.2b; Figure 2.2d is a sectional view of the disc according to line **4–4** of Figure 2.2b; Figure 2.2e is a sectional view of the disc according to line **5–5** of Figure 2.2b; and Figure 2.2f is a sectional view of the disc according to line **6–6** of Figure 2.2b.

In Figure 2.2b there is shown a portion of the stamping machine and more particularly the device comprising the disc-shaped stamping box **7**, the two pairs of mold halves **8–8'** and **9–9'** carried on plates **10–10'** and **11–11'**, which in turn are fast with two slides **12** and **13**, effecting a horizontal reciprocating motion imparted thereto by a well-known linkage system.

Disc **7**, jerkily rotating about its central axis **18**, has openings **14–14'**, **15–15'** **16–16'**, **17–17'** of a shaped contour for efficient cooperation with mold halves **8** and **9** passing through some of them and meeting mold halves **8'** and **9'** beyond the plane corresponding to the disc face having adjacent the openings a number of projections or lugs **27** and **28** adapted to retain the excess of the paste exiting from the mold halves upon coupling thereof.

Ejectors **19–19'** and **20–20'**, operated by compressed air are accommodated (Figure 2.2d) with mold halves **8–8'** and **9–9'** and attached to plates **10–10'** and **11–11'**. A horizontally reciprocal slide **21** (Figures 2.2a and 2.2d) carries the introducing pushing members **22** and **23** located at the feeding conveyor **24** (Figure 2.2c) terminating with a chute **25** (Figure 2.2d) so as to feed the blocks to be stamped **26–26'** on two parallel rows.

The jerkily rotating movement for the stamping disc **7**, where openings **14–14'**, **15–15'**, **16–16'**, **17–17'** are accommodated, is achieved by a Maltese cross or other kinematic device, not shown, operating in timed relationship with the movement of mold halves **8–8'** and **9–9'**. The eight openings are of the precise form and identical surface of one to three millimeters larger than the median section of the soaps following stamping operation.

Adjacent the two ends of each of the eight openings there are attached projections or lugs **27** having the purpose of retaining the blocks **26–26'** to be stamped adherent to the

FIGURE 2.2: STAMPING APPARATUS

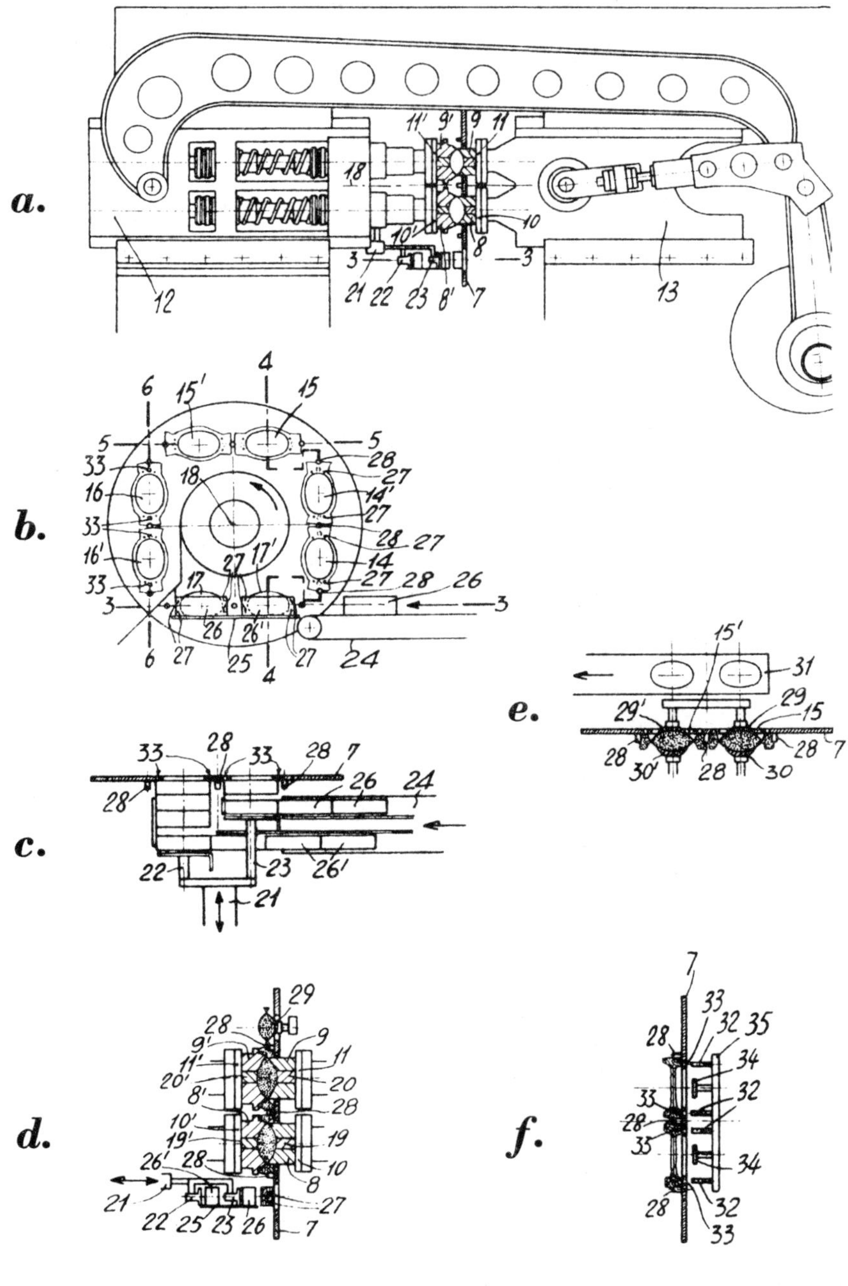

Source: C. Mazzoni; U.S. Patent 3,574,904; April 13, 1971

surface of disc **7** under the thrust of the feeding pushing members **22** and **23**. The projections or lugs are formed of pairs of points **27** on which the blocks **26–26'** are stuck under the thrust of the pushing members **22** and **23**. Thus, the blocks to be stamped are attached to disc **7** just in front of openings **17–17'** and by a rotation jerk they are then brought to face the pairs of mold halves **8–8'** and **9–9'**.

On reciprocating, the pairs of mold halves would gradually approach the blocks to be stamped until joining to provide for the stamping operation, imparting the blocks with the internal shape of the pairs of mold halves and peripherally extruding the excess of material externally of the mold halves.

The outer contour of mold halves **8'** and **9'** is of a conical surface with projections having the function of retaining the material (ejected in surplus from the mold halves during the gradual mutual approaching), as stuck on the points **27**. In order to retain to a larger extent the excess of paste being ejected, further points or pins **28** are attached to disc **7**, the last mentioned points or pins operating on the heads of the ejected paste.

At the maximum approach step, corresponding to the maximum pressure stage, the pairs of mold halves **8–8'** and **9–9'** are spaced apart a few tenths of a millimeter, so that around the stamped tablet there will remain a film connecting the periphery of the stamped tablet with the excess of paste ejected from the molds and which is held adherent to disc **7** by the projections or points **27** and **28**.

After the pairs of mold halves **8–8'** and **9–9'** have moved away from the stamped tablets, disc **7** will jerkily angularly rotate so as to carry the stamped tablets in front of openings **15–15'** (Figure 2.2e) coinciding with the discharge position. At this position, the stamped tablets are detached from the excess of ejected paste through the combination of suitable sucker means **29–29'** (Figure 2.2e) (connected with a vacuum system); pushing members **30–30'** coacting therewith on the opposite side.

Sucker means **29–29'** hold the stamped tablets, cut the film retaining them adherent to the excess of peripheral paste ejected from mold halves **8–8'** and **9–9'** and lay them out onto the discharge or unloading conveyor **31**.

The cutting operation is carried out by causing the stamped tablets to pass through openings **15–15'** in disc **7**. The volumes of excess of paste ejected from the molds are still adherent to disc **7**, as retained by projections or lugs **27** and **28**. Such volumes of paste, generally in the form of a closed loop, are detached from projections or lugs **27** and **28**. (Figure 2.2f) under the actions of a series of pushing members **32** carried on a common plate or cross member **35**, parallel to disc **7** and reciprocally operated so that the pushing members **32**, by passing through the corresponding holes **33** in disc **7**, will move away therefrom the paste remaining attached to the projections **27** and **28** while the members **34** push the stamped tablets from their holes **33**.

Pelletizing Apparatus

W. Eirich and G. Eirich; U.S. Patent 3,698,842; October 17, 1972 have developed an apparatus for pelletizing material of low binding power or low moisture content which includes a conveyor, a spreading and compressing device, and breaking means. The material is fed onto the conveyor belt which in cooperation with the spreading and compressing device forms the material into a layer. As the material travels along on the conveyor belt it is subjected to heat exchange for solidifying the layer. Subsequently the layer is broken up into pellets. This apparatus can be illustrated in Figure 2.3.

Figure 2.3a shows a mixer **1**, below which there is a distributing means **2**, which conveys material onto the apparatus with the aid of deflecting plate **3**. The apparatus comprises a conveyor **4**, a device for conveying a temperature-controlling medium **5**, a breaker **6** in the form of a roller, and a compressing means **17**. The conveyor consists of a belt **8** moving around rollers **7**, and below the upper run of the conveyor belt **8**, supporting members **9**

FIGURE 2.3: PELLETIZING APPARATUS

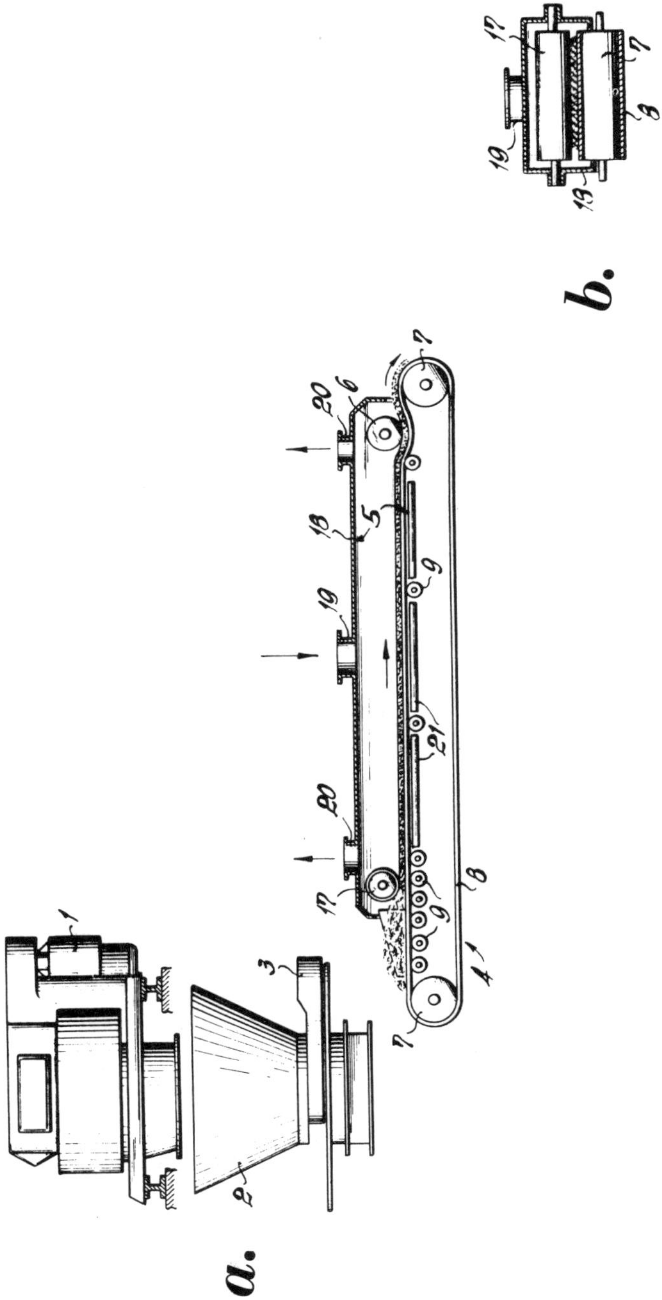

Source: W. Eirich and G. Eirich; U.S. Patent 3,698,842; October 17, 1972

in the form of rollers are mounted with their shafts extending at right-angles to the direction of movement of the belt **8**. This provides a fairly strong support for the conveyor belt and, as shown in Figure 2.3a a compressing means **17** is provided above the upper run of the endless belt, near the distributing device and deflecting plate; the compressing means **17** is in the form of a roller which forms the drawing-in gap or nip together with the supporting rollers **9** and the conveyor belt, so that the loosely poured-on material is spread into a layer and compressed. In the present case the compressing means is shown as a roller. Instead of a roller a pressure plate with a vibrator may be used, working together with a backing plate.

As shown in Figures 2.3a and 2.3b, the endless conveyor belt runs through below a hood **18** which is a component of the device for conveying a temperature-controlling medium. The hood contains an inlet **19** and two outlets **20** to pass through a gaseous temperature-controlling medium, and is constructed so that it also covers the compressing means **17** and the breaker in the form of a roller.

Below the upper run and between individual supporting rollers there are hollow bodies through which, for example, a coolant or steam can be passed. If the material has to be subjected to intensive heat treatment, the hood and hollow bodies **21** may be kept in operation simultaneously. If no strong heat action is desired, one of the two arrangements has to be shut down.

The advantage of the apparatus is that pellets can be formed with it which could not have been produced in conventional machines using the same materials. The apparatus saves processing, for it does not require any finely ground starting materials. Thus, ores, batch, washed sands and similar materials which are not very finely ground can be pelletized. The apparatus also requires smaller quantities of wetting fluid than before, so that great economies in drying are possible.

Pelletizing Molten Materials

Apparatus and method for producing pellets from molten materials have been developed by *U. Storb, H. Kaiser and G. Kaiser; U.S. Patent 3,702,748; November 14, 1972; assigned to Gebr. Kaiser, Maschinenfabrik, Germany*. This comprises using a vessel or ladle provided with one or more nozzles in its bottom which is or are provided with a vertically moving needle leaving an annular gap between it and the nozzle wall into which the molten material flows and then flows on a moving cooling surface for the purpose of solidifying. This can be shown in Figure 2.4.

At the bottom of a ladle **1** as shown in Figure 2.4 at least one nozzle **2** is provided; however, preferably several such nozzles **2** are provided so as to be adjacent to each other. The nozzle bore or hole **10** is provided at its outlet end **11** with a part **6** of reduced diameter which is made up in turn of a cylindrical part **3** of reduced diameter and a transition part **14** of reduced diameter. The whole nozzle **2** can therefore be considered as being made up of three zones, that is to say zone **4** for the flowing-in and sucking-in of the melt **12**, a zone **5** for a relative pressure build up, and a pinched or tapered zone **6**, denoted by the same reference numeral as the pinched part **6**, for flow out of material in a quantity necessary for forming a pellet body **13**.

The diameter of the nozzle bore **10** in the zones **4** and **5** in the flow out zone **6** is arrived at in accordance with the viscosity of the products to be pelletized. The same applies for the lengths of the zones **4, 5, 6** as a function of the diameter of the vertically reciprocating needle **7** in the zones **4** and **5**. Also the stroke **8** and the clearance in the zone **5** between the lower end face of the needle **7** and the pinched part **6** of the nozzle are arrived at in accordance with the viscosities of the products to be processed.

Preferably the diameter of the actual pinched out part is less than the diameter of the needle **7** so that in the nozzle out flow zone **11** there is a defined flow. This leads to an even formation and deposit of the granules on a cooling face.

FIGURE 2.4: APPARATUS FOR THE PRODUCTION OF PELLETS FROM A MELT

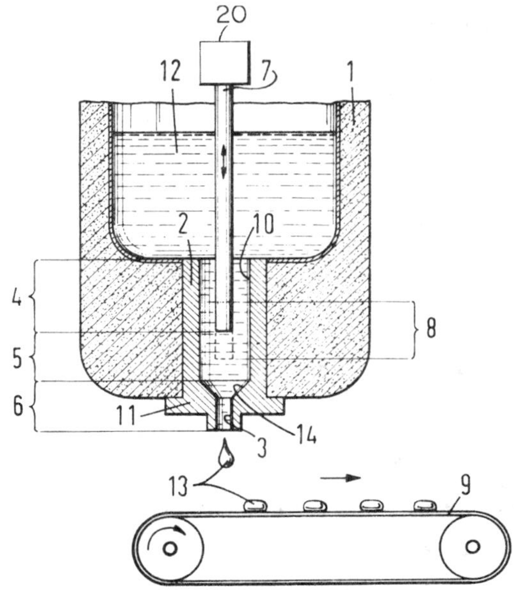

Source: U. Storb, H. Kaiser and G. Kaiser; U.S. Patent 3,702,748; November 14, 1972

Tests have shown that the pinched out part or zone **6** can have a length between 0.5 and 30 mm. depending on the type of product to be pelletized. An important factor for a high rate of granulation and the formation and deposit of well-formed granules on the belt-like cooking face, for example the cooling belt **9**, is however, the tapered part **6** arranged at the nozzle exit end **11**, above which the plunger or needle **7** reciprocates vertically.

The nozzle bore **10** is cylindrical in the zones **4** and **5**. Also the tapering part **3** is circular in cross-section, the transition from the zone **5** to the actual tapering part **3** having the from of a frusto-cone **14**. Furthermore the needle is also cylindrical in construction and its lower circular end face cooperates with tapered part **6**. The needle **7** is caused to reciprocate vertically by any suitable means **20**. Means **20** also permits adjustment of the frequency of movement of needle **7**. The nozzle and needle cross-section can, however, be not only cylindrical but also oval, square, rectangular or be in other shapes.

COATING METHODS AND APPARATUS

Spray Coating Dragees

A dragee product as well as a process of manufacturing them are disclosed by *P. Rieckmann, H. Schalk and E. Theel; U.S. Patents 3,395,213, July 30, 1968 and 3,331,696, July 18, 1967; both assigned to C.F. Boehringer & Soehne GmbH, Germany.* The dragee comprises an inner pill center, i.e., a drug, gum or confectionary core, and an outer encapsulating layer comprising a dried admixture of a liquid carrier and from 1 to 10 weight percent of polyethylene glycol, 40 to 50 weight percent of sugar and 10 to 20 weight percent of solid fillers. In accordance with this process a fully automatic rapid method for the production of dragees having centers formed of gum, candy or medicinal materials characterized by pleasant taste, smoothness of surface, and perfect color has now been found.

When pill centers or cores are coated using an aqueous-sugar coating suspension containing 1 to 10 weight percent of polyethylene glycol in addition to 40 to 50 weight percent of sugar and 10 to 20 weight percent of solid fillers, dragees are obtained characterized by these properties.

In preparing the dragees, the coating suspension is sprayed onto the pills or centers maintained in rotation in a coating kettle, the spraying interrupted and the sprayed dragee centers maintained in rotation for a period of time and thereafter the coated centers dried with a current of warm air. These three steps in the sequence as set out are repeated, if necessary, until the desired total amount of coating suspension has been applied.

In this way and by the incorporation of a small amount of polyethylene glycol in a sugar-containing coating suspension, the tendency to stickiness at the start of the drying of the suspension is overcome, that is the dragees do not stick to one another nor do they adhere to the kettle wall. There is, as a result, made possible a rapid, fully automatic pill center coating process.

The process makes possible the practicability of applying in a single operation the coating suspension onto the pill center and drying the same. The need for handwork is eliminated other than that which is required for adjusting the equipment at the beginning and at the end of the process.

Example: Eight kilograms of dragee centers of 6 mm. diameter (weight of centers 80 mg., number of centers 100,000) are introduced into a kettle having a 60 cm. diameter provided with a powerful exhaust system. The spraying system is adjusted so that about 80 ml. of the coating suspension are sprayed onto the centers within a period of 25 seconds in each of the coating steps. The centers are circulated, i.e., rotated for 1.5 minutes following the spraying without any external interference so that the suspension can be uniformly distributed on the surface of the dragees. The batch is then dried with a current of hot air for two minutes. These three steps are repeated until 8.5 kg. of suspension have been applied.

The coating suspension used is one containing polyethylene glycol in addition to sugar and solid fillers. The dragees which have had smooth coatings from the start of the procedure are now ready for waxing. The total production time amounts to about 6.5 to 7 hours and no supervision of any kind is required in this period. After the coating had been completed, the dragees have a weight of 130 mg. The coating dissolves in the Erweka disintegration tester in about 4 minutes which is comparable with a very good candy coating as formed by the process as used hitherto.

Spray Coating Apparatus

The apparatus as used to prepare the dragees in the previous patents is also disclosed by *P. Rieckmann, H. Schalk and E. Theel; U.S. Patent 3,381,659; May 7, 1968; assigned to C.F. Boehringer & Soehne GmbH, Germany*. This apparatus is shown schematically in Figure 2.5.

As shown in Figure 2.5, as soon as switch **27'** is closed, a certain amount of the coating suspension is fed continuously either from the vessel **21** by means of pump **22** to the spray nozzle **25** via conduits **38** and **37** or is carried back through an over-pressure valve **26** via conduit **36** to the vessel **21**. Depending on the switching position of the electrically controlled three-way valve **23**, the suspension either enters the outer chamber **32** of the three-way valve **23** and leaves it at the middle chamber **33** for introduction into the spray nozzle **25** or returns from the spray nozzle via the middle chamber **33** and the outer chamber **34** to the vessel, releasing the pressure within the conduit **37** via recycle conduits **35** and

FIGURE 2.5: SPRAY COATING APPARATUS

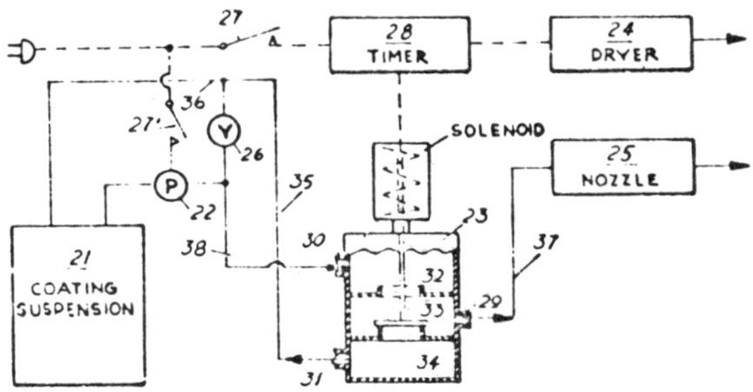

Source: P. Rieckmann, H. Schalk and E. Theel; U.S. Patent 3,381,659; May 7, 1968

36 back toward the vessel **21**. The connection of the three-way valve **23** with the conduits **35**, **37** and **38** is highly unusual, because the outlet **29** of the middle chamber **33** generally is an inlet, whereas the inlet **30** of the outer chamber **32** generally is an outlet. The timer **28** controls: (a) the switching position of the three-way valve by means of a solenoid, and (b) the source of warm air, for example a dryer **24**, as soon as the main switch **27** is closed. Depending on the switching position of the three-way valve **23**, the middle chamber **33** is either connected with the outer chamber **32** or with the outer chamber **34**.

It has proven advantageous to supply the coating suspension at a constant pressure of approximately 10 atmospheres using a gear pump. As shown in Figure 2.5 the coating suspension supplied from vessel **21** is permanently maintained under pressure within conduit **38** and the outer chamber **32** of the three-way valve **23**, as soon as the switch **27'** for the motor of the pump **22** is closed. The safety valve **26** maintains the pressure at 10 atmospheres and releases the rest of the suspension backwards to the vessel **21** via conduit **36**.

If the solenoid has steered the three-way valve **23** as positioned in Figure 2.5, the coating suspension can flow into the middle chamber **33** and from there via conduit **37** to the spray nozzle **25**. As the pressure of 10 atmospheres has already been built up within the system **38** and **32**, the pressure is available at the spray nozzle **25** very quickly, when the timer signals the order to spray. When the timer signals the order for stopping the spraying, the middle chamber **33** is connected with the outer chamber **34**, so that the pressure at the spray nozzle **25** is released immediately via the conduits **37**, **35** and **36** backwards to the vessel **21**. It is only with this specific connection of the valves and the conduits that the pressure at the spray nozzle is available immediately at the beginning and is released immediately at the end of the spraying time.

Tablet Coating Drums

H.M. Gross; U.S. Patent 3,357,398; December 12, 1967; assigned to Abbott Laboratories has developed a coating method and apparatus which has the advantages of low attrition and polishing and smoothening of the tablets as realized in an apparatus having a conventional rotatable coating pan and the highly desirable short drying time as realized in an air suspension coating system.

The coating medium is applied to the tablets evenly and effectively while they are being rolled upon each other, the time required to dry the coating medium on the individual tablets being quite short. It is another feature of the apparatus whereby the flow path of the drying medium which is introduced through the bed of tablets is adjustable to accom-

FIGURE 2.6: APPARATUS FOR COATING TABLETS

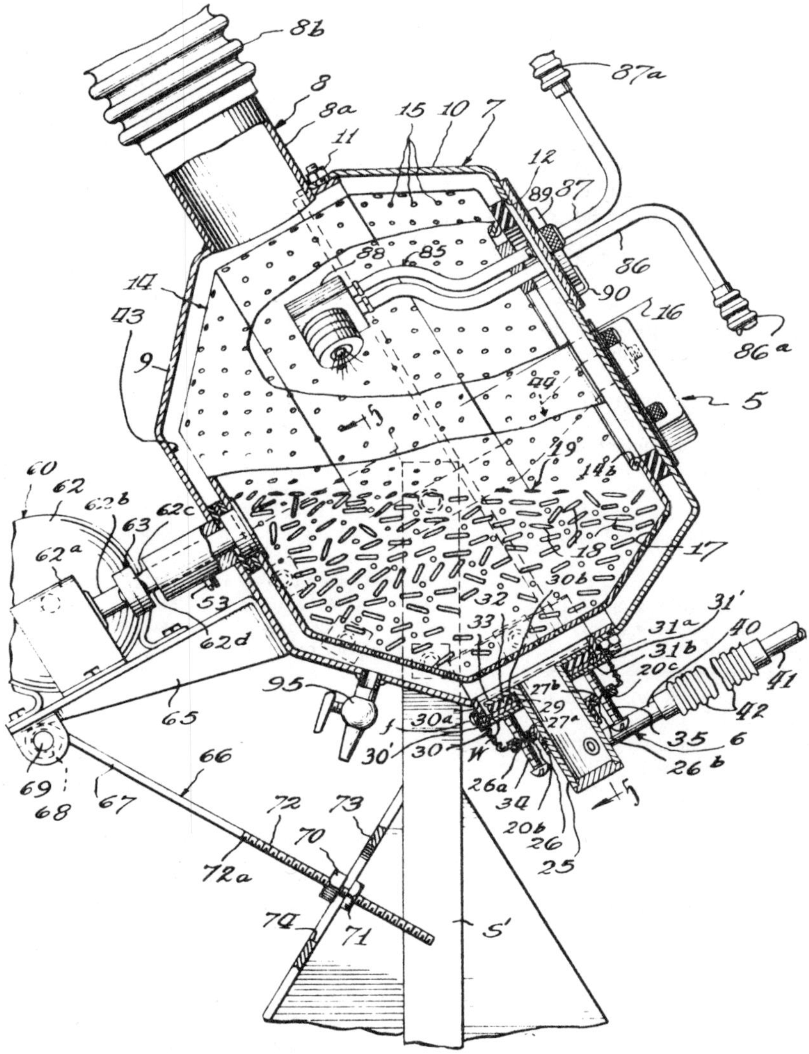

Source: H.M. Gross; U.S. Patent 3,357,398; December 12, 1967

modate for variations of depth and width of the bed of tablets. Referring to Figure 2.6, there is shown a coating apparatus **5** provided with a drying medium inlet **6** which leads into a housing **7** and an outlet **8** which leads from the housing. The housing defines a chamber with a back portion **9** and a front portion **10** removably secured by fasteners **11**. The housing is shown to be pivotally mounted on standard **S'** supported by the floor.

The outlet **8** is shown to include an outlet duct **8a** welded to the housing and a flexible outlet duct **8b** through which the spent drying medium passes to the outside for example. A rotatably mounted coating pan or drum generally indicated at **14** having a plurality of perforations **15** and spaced inwardly from the housing is mounted for rotation about an axis of rotation, **16**. The perforations are substantially smaller than the tablets **18** to be coated so that the tablets will not fall therethrough and so that no sharp edge will be able to present itself to nip the tablets as they contact the coating pan **14**. The coating pan has a smooth, highly polished inner surface **17** which obviates attrition. The smooth inner surface is necessary in the event the tablets are brittle and hence susceptible to attrition.

Since the depth and width of the bed **19** varies as to the speed of rotation of the coating pan, the weight, size and number of tablets, and as the internal configuration and dimensions of the coating pan, it is sometimes desirable to adjust the location of one or both of the dividers **44** and **45** (not shown) along the housing so that the flow path of the drying medium is confined to those perforations in the coating pan which the bed of tablets covers.

In a word, the flow path of the drying medium is able to be adjusted so that all the drying medium will be caused to pass through the bed of tablets. In accordance with the method, a plurality of tablets which form the bed are rolled upon each other while a coating medium is dispensed onto the bed of tablets and while a drying medium is passed through the bed of tablets.

Side Vented Exhaust for Coating Apparatus

A tablet-coating apparatus is provided by *V.B. Hostetler; U.S. Patents 3,601,086, August 24, 1971 and 3,573,966, April 6, 1971; assigned to Eli Lilly and Company* having a vented area about the periphery of a rotary tumbling drum. Exhaust means is removably positioned adjacent a portion of the drum's vented section in a manner which draws air and the coating material through the bed of tumbling tablets.

The exhaust system causes air to flow downwardly through the tumbling bed of tablets and out through the exhaust system, with three direct significant results. First, dust is immediately extracted from the drum and the bed of tablets without having a chance to create problems. Second, the continuous flow of air through the bed of tumbling tablets results in substantially increased ventilation of the tablets and thus faster and more uniform drying of the tablets as they are coated. Third, the current of air moving downwardly through the bed drives the coating material down through the bed of tablets so that instead of just coating the upper surface of the bed there is a much greater and more uniform dispersion of the coating material throughout the bed and consequent greater uniformity of coating application. This apparatus can be illustrated by Figure 2.7.

Referring to Figure 2.7, a rotary tumbling drum or coating pan **11** of a cylindrical configuration is formed from stainless steel or any other rigid and durable material capable of withstanding repeated use in coating tablets and subsequent cleansing operations. The drum is rotatably supported with its axis horizontal by power transmission **13** coupled to a conventional drive unit **14** for rotary motion. Drum **11** has a wide front opening **16** for the introduction of tablets **17** and coating material and for removal of coated tablets.

The drum has a perforate peripheral wall **20** concentric with its horizontal axis of rotation, and generally conical sidewalls tapering axially outward from the surface **20**. A plurality of apertures **19** (shown enlarged for clarity) circumscribe the entire peripheral area or surface **20**. Although these are shown in the form of circular holes, they may also be formed by the use of large mesh screen material or by perforations of other configuration. For convenience the peripheral surface of the drum will sometimes be referred to as being foraminous. Positioned at a lower quadrant of the drum's peripheral apertured area is an exhaust inlet **21**. This inlet has a curved surface which is slightly spaced from the vented peripheral surface **20** of the drum. A number of rollers **25** are positioned on opposite sides of exhaust inlet **21** and are adapted for sliding contact with the drum. The term sliding includes other forms of relative motion contact including rolling contact. It is essential that the exhaust inlet be positioned adjacent to the leading lower quadrant of the drum where the tablets tumble.

The drum or pan rotates at a relatively slow speed of 10 to 30 rpm; and consequently, the tablets are not subjected to a significant centrifugal force. Thus, the tablets tend to remain in a continually tumbling pile or bed on the leading lower quadrant of the drum in the direction of rotation which in this case is clockwise.

The tablet-tumbling action of the pan **11** is enhanced by the outwardly tapered side walls contiguous to its foraminous periphery, whereby the bed of tablets is of varying width throughout its depth. Consequently, as the tablets are tumbled by rotation, they are also caused to move laterally, i.e., axially of the drum, thereby producing composite tablet movement and giving greater assurance of equal exposure of the tablets to the coating material. Also, this accommodates concentration of the exhaust inlet in a limited area without limiting the surface area of the bed for application of coating material to a large surface area.

FIGURE 2.7: SIDE VENTED EXHAUST FOR COATING APPARATUS

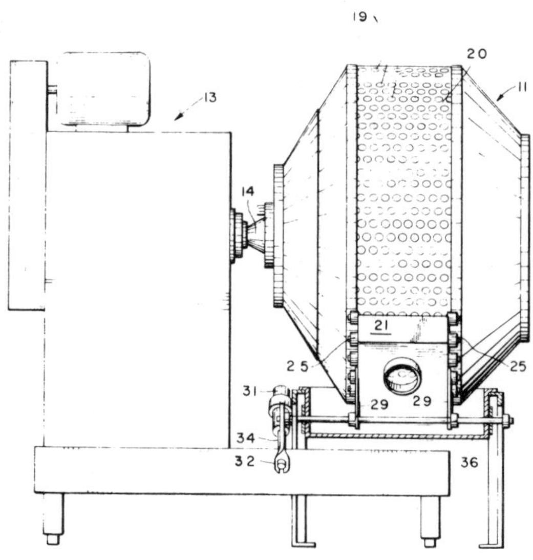

Source: V.B. Hostetler; U.S. Patent 3,601,086; August 24, 1971

In one run a 5% solution of methylcellulose was used to coat tablets. The coating solution was introduced into the drum by an airborne type spray system under 25 pounds pressure. Drum speed was 22 to 24 rpm. In the conventional apparatus an exhaust line was associated with the opening of the drum. The amount of time required for satisfactorily coating the tablets with this conventional apparatus was 45 minutes.

This apparatus in which a side exhaust was utilized, substantially reduced the amount of time for coating tablets with an identical solution. The time was reduced from 45 to 15 minutes. There was no abrasion of the methylcellulose film on the tablets; and, in fact, it was noted that the apertures in the pan tended to aid in the rolling action of the tablets. It is believed that the coating time required for these tablets was reduced primarily due to the exhaust system which simultaneously pulled the coating solution and drying air downwardly through the bed of tumbling tablets.

Horizontal Coating Drum

F. Martin; U.S. Patent 3,390,648; July 2, 1968; assigned to Dr. A. Wander, SA, Switzerland has developed a procedure for coating particles, such as tablets of, for instance, bi-convex shape, and in particular those produced by the pharmaceutical industry, by spraying on a lacquer solution, and revolving the particles while being coated in the interior of a drum rotating round its horizontal axis.

The inner surface of the drum is of such a nature that the particles slide considerably better among themselves than against it, the particles forming a revolving layer occupying considerably less than 10% of the internal volume of the drum. The maximum height of the revolving layer is between three times the smallest and ten times the largest diameter of the particles.

The adhesion of the particles to the inner surface of the drum, which is necessary in this procedure, can be achieved by cladding the surface with a profiled rubber lining or something similar. The essential point is that the particles resting on the surface and those immediately next to them are drawn along by the ascending drum wall, so that the desired revolving motion can actually develop and that the load in its entirety does not slide down along the ascending drum surface, as would be the case with the thin layer if no special measures were taken to increase adhesion. The apparatus is shown in Figure 2.8.

FIGURE 2.8: HORIZONTAL COATING DRUM

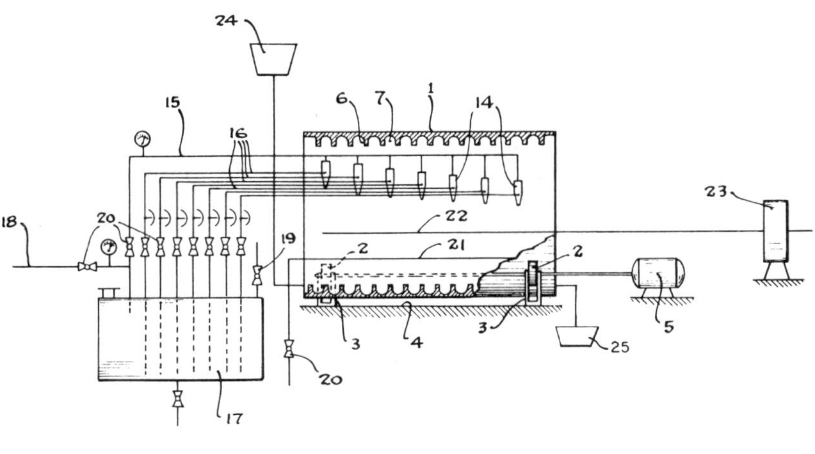

Source: F. Martin; U.S. Patent 3,390,648; July 2, 1968

A horizontal drum **1** rests at both ends on pairs of rollers **2** which turn in bearings **3** mounted on a base **4**. One or more of these rollers can be set turning by means of an electromotor **5** to rotate the drum slowly and regularly. On the inner surface of the drum and at right angles to its axis is a continuous helicoidal rib or lamella **6** broadened at its base to form a helical groove **7** which in cross-section has a concave bottom lined with profiled rubber **8**.

In the groove are the tablet batches **9** which when the drum rotates take the shape and dynamics of a revolving layer with a lower turning point **10**, an upper turning point **11**, a forward acceleration stretch **12** and a backward acceleration stretch **13**.

Along the interior of the drum are several sprayers **14** aimed at the backward acceleration stretch of the revolving layers formed by the tablet batches. These sprayers are connected to a common compressed-air duct **15** and to individual solution supply ducts **16** fed from a container **17** (or fed individually or in groups from several such containers). This container is put under pressure by means of a compressed-air duct **18** which also feeds the duct **15**, and during filling the air can be let out by opening a valve **19**. In the ducts **15**, **16** and **18** there are regulating valves **20** as well as pressure gauges, flow meters etc.

A duct **21** extending horizontally through the interior of the drum, and also equipped with a regulating valve **20**, has side nozzles (not shown) pointing downwards, through which hot air is blown. Above this extends through the interior of the drum a suction duct **22** connected to a suction pump **23** and having a large number of openings to remove solvent vapors from the drum.

Numeral **24** represents a device for feeding tablets to the one end of the helical groove **7**, and numeral **25** represents a device for removing the coated tablets. For example, the tablet feeding device **24** can be a simple mechanical means for discharging at regular intervals into the grooves a weighed amount of the tablets or, if preferred, a continuous stream of tablets can be fed to the groove by means of a vibratory feed means.

The process for coating tablets or other particles is carried out by this continuously operating equipment as follows. A small quantity of the cores is fed continuously into the slowly rotating drum by the device **24**. These quantities move from one end of the drum to the other through the drum's rotation and the force of gravity, and are coated in the way already described. Each quantity of tablets contained in a lower section of the helical groove goes through a revolving motion, the tablets lying on the surface of the revolving layer being especially exposed to the spray from the nozzles **14**. The particles sprayed on dry almost immediately with the aid of the hot air blown on to them.

Example:

Rotating drum **1**:	
Length	140 cm.
Diameter	80 cm.
Revolution speed of the drum	5 rpm
Width of the helical groove	3.5 cm.
Height of the helical groove	6 cm.
Number of turns of the helical groove	35
Hot air directed on the upper turning point of the tablets	40-60°C.
Quantity of tablets fed per drum revolution	300 g.
Weight of a single bi-convex tablet	0.5 g.
Maximum diameter of a tablet	1.1 cm.
Minimum diameter of a tablet	0.6 cm.
Maximum height of the revolving layer	4-5 cm.

This gives for travelling through the 35 turns of the helical groove an operating time of seven minutes and a capacity of 1.5 kg. of tablets per minute or 90 kg. of tablets per hour.

Fluidized Coating

A method of coating fragile bodies has been disclosed by *H. Nack; U.S. Patent 3,382,093; May 7, 1968; assigned to The Battelle Development Corporation.* The fragile bodies are introduced into a fluidized bed of particles having a greater density than the fragile bodies and an average particle size that is smaller than the fragile bodies. Coating is then effected by spray coating a solution onto the bed that consists of the coating material and a volatile liquid. The volatile liquid readily volatilizes leaving the coated bodies. A preferred embodiment of the process is the use of a fluidized bed of particles that are no greater in size than 1/5 the size of the fragile bodies.

Figure 2.9 is an illustrative cross-sectional schematic view of a fluidized-bed spray coating apparatus containing a fluidized bed of particulate solids and fragile bodies being spray coated in accordance with this method.

In a specific embodiment a gas, such as air, is employed to fluidize finely divided solids, such as an inert powdered material; fragile articles to be coated, for example, in the form of pills, pellets, lozenges, tablets, and the like, are added to the fluidized particulate solids so that there is provided a fluidized bed made up primarily of fluidized solids having suspended and dispersed therein the fragile articles to be coated; and then a liquid coating composition is introduced, such as by spraying a solution of the coating composition into the fluidized bed. In such a process, the introduced liquid coating composition coats the fragile articles and the fluidizing gas evaporates liquid constituents of the coating composition to leave a solid coating on the fragile articles.

A prime feature of the process is that, while being coated, the fragile articles are suspended in a primary fluidized bed of particulate solids which serves to cushion and prevent breakage and attrition of the fragile articles. Following buildup of a desired coating on the fragile articles, the coated articles are separated from the particulate solids with which they were fluidized during the coating.

Through a solid feeding inlet **10**, particles **11** to be coated and inert bed particles **12** are fed into a fluid bed column **13**. These particles **11** and **12** are fluidized by fluidizing gas **14** which enters below the fluidized bed **15** and is uniformly distributed into the fluid-bed area **16** by an air distributor plate **17**. A rotameter **18** in fluidizing air line **19** measures the amount of air that passes into the fluidized bed **16**. A heater **20** heats this air.

The coating solution **21** is metered **22** at a fixed rate into coating solution spray nozzle **23** where the solution is well mixed with the spraying air **26** which also enters into the nozzle **23**. From the coating solution spray nozzle a very fine mist of coating material **21** is directed downward into the bed of fluidized particles where uniform coating is accomplished on the fluidized particles.

Uniformly coated particles **11** are removed from the bed through bed emptying line **24**. The coated particles **11** are screened in a screener **25** to separate the larger coated particles **11** from the small inert bed particles **12** which fall through the screen. In the following example which serves to illustrate the process, all parts, percents, and amounts are by weight unless stated otherwise.

Example: A liquid coating composition is prepared by dissolving 450 grams of granulated sugar, 18 grams of a finely divided acacia gum and 18 grams of granular gelatin in 300 grams of water. At 20°C., the resulting composition is a thick dark liquid mixture. This mixture is admixed in a 1:2 parts ratio with ethyl alcohol, and 3 drops of a red certified-pure food color added to provide the liquid coating composition.

The fragile articles are commercially available 5 grain aspirin tablets, each weighing about 4 grams and each being about 1/8 inch thick. These aspirin tablets, if fluidized by themselves in an air stream, require such a violent air current for fluidization that , within several minutes of fluidization, a significant proportion (greater than 25%) of the fluidized

FIGURE 2.9: FLUIDIZED BED COATING OF FRAGILE BODIES

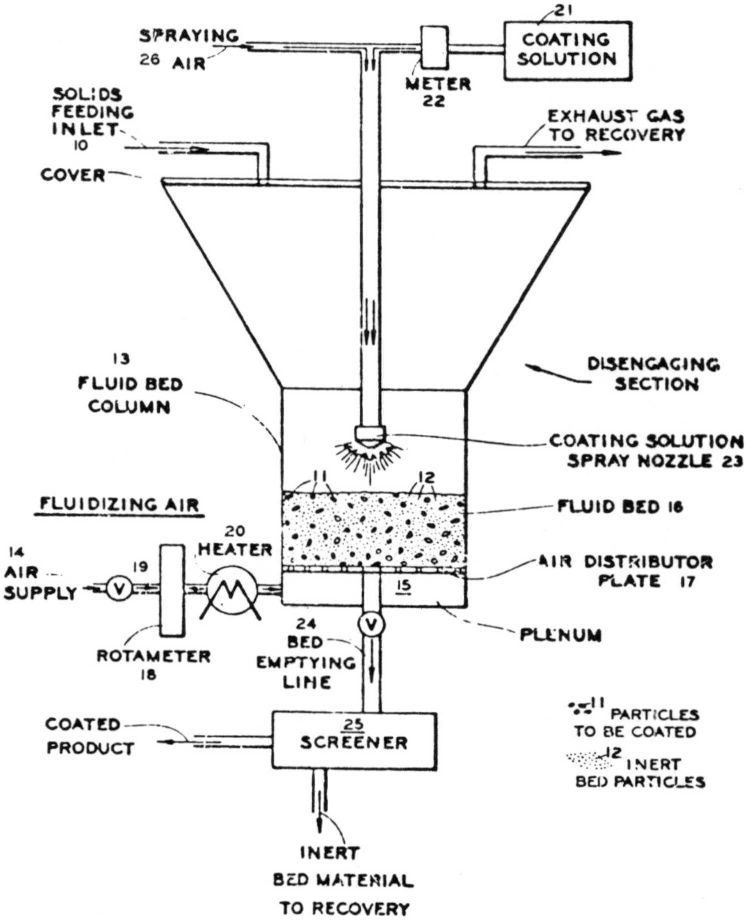

Source: H. Nack; U.S. Patent 3,382,093; May 7, 1968.

aspirin tablets show attrition. About one pound of granulated sodium chloride, table salt grade, averaging about 40 mesh size and ranging from +150 to -20 mesh size, are placed in a vertically positioned, 4" i.d., tubular gas-fluidization apparatus and air of 20°C. is introduced through a porous distributor plate of the apparatus at 10 scfm to fluidize the granulated sodium chloride. About 100 of the aspirin tablets are then added to the fluidized sodium chloride granules and a concurrently fluidized bed of aspirin tablets and sodium chloride granules results.

A very fine spray of the coating composition is sprayed on the upper free surface of this concurrently fluidized bed at an average rate of 3.3 ml. per minute for 15 minutes. At this time fluidization is discontinued, and the contents of the apparatus are removed.

These contents are gently screened into two portions, one consisting essentially of sodium chloride granules and a portion of the introduced coating composition, and a second consisting essentially of the aspirin tablets which now are coated with a thin, hard, red, surface coating. Examination of the coated aspirin tablets reveals less than 4% show any attrition as apparent from chipped edges or other portions of the tablet being broken off.

Foamed Coating Methods

An improvement over prior spraying, pouring or dipping methods for coating tablets has been disclosed by *B. Lopez and S.S. Kornblum; U.S. Patent 3,607,364; September 21, 1971.* This comprises applying a foamed coating medium to the solid form surface, and then destroying the foam to produce an even coat of the coating medium on the solid surface. The foamed coating medium may conveniently be applied to the solid form surface, by atomizing the foamed coating medium and spraying onto the solid form surface.

Foaming of coating medium may be carried out by any convenient means. For example, a gaseous medium, such as air, may be mechanically dispersed in the coating medium. Alternatively, a gaseous medium may be introduced under pressure into the coating medium, and the pressure then reduced to allow the gaseous medium to expand in discrete volumes within the coating medium. Further, a gaseous medium may be injected into the coating medium, which gaseous medium may be injected at high speed to cause a state of turbulence in the coating medium.

Urging of the coating medium against the solid form surface may be effected by tumbling the solid on a tumbler surface, such as in a conventional coating pan. The high standard of coating achieved in this conventional apparatus is attributed to a simultaneous spreading and breaking down of the foamed coating medium as the solid form tumbles on the tumbler surface.

This process has a great number of practical advantages, particularly the shortening of dwelling and drying times required in conventional coating processes.

Example: Components of the coating medium were as follows, and in the percentages by weight indicated;

Components	% w./w.
F.D. & C. Dye, q.s.	
Sugar	35.0
Gelatin	0.3
Acacia Gum	0.9
Talc	15.0
Terra Alba	25.0
SDA 30 Alcohol	1.0
Distilled Water	21.3
Pluronic F-68	1.5

The pluronic F-68, gelatin, acacia gum, sugar, F.D. & C dye and alcohol were dissolved in the water. The terra alba and talc were suspended in the so-formed syrup and the resulting slurry was homogenized by means of a suitable colloid mill.

The homogenized slurry was poured into a modified DeVilbiss QMR-530 pressurized tank. A known amount of carbon dioxide gas was then sparged through the slurry until a 80 to 90 psi pressure was reached inside the tank. During saturation of the slurry, the baffled mixer of the pressurized vessel was employed constantly. The temperature of the slurry was maintained at about 50° to 55°C.

100,000 placebo tablet cores, 7 mm. in diameter and having an average weight of 180 mg., were placed in a CP-2 Manesty coating bench, provided with an automatic system as described by D.S. Mody [Mody, D.S. Scott, M.W. & Liebermann, H.S., *J. Pharm. Sci.* 53,

949 (1964)], which regulates the spraying, dwelling and drying cycles of the coating process. The foamed slurry was sprayed using automatic De Vilbiss AGB-504 spray guns equipped with an internal mixing nozzle 0491. Information concerning the coating operation is shown below.

Spraying time	45 seconds
Dwelling time	4 minutes
Drying time	5 minutes
Liquid pressure	80 to 90 psi
Air pressure	10 psi

Fifteen coats were applied to the tablets which was sufficient to produce elegant coated tablets which were then finished and polished. Only 90 minutes were necessary to produce the elegant coat.

HARDNESS TESTER FOR TABLETS

A testing method having high dependability and high operator safety has been developed by *K.A. Flury; U.S. Patent 3,757,566; September 11, 1973; assigned to Heberlein & Co., Switzerland.*

This hardness tester for tablets comprises a power-driven pressure slide supporting the tablets and a measuring slide mechanically connected to a weight. The slides and the weight constitute a pendulum weight to which a cord is fastened. The cord is trained about guide rolls and carries between two of the rolls an engaging means actuating a drag pointer fastened to a second cord parallel to the first cord. The force acting on the tablet is indicated on a linear scale. This is shown in Figure 2.10.

FIGURE 2.10: HARDNESS TESTER FOR TABLETS

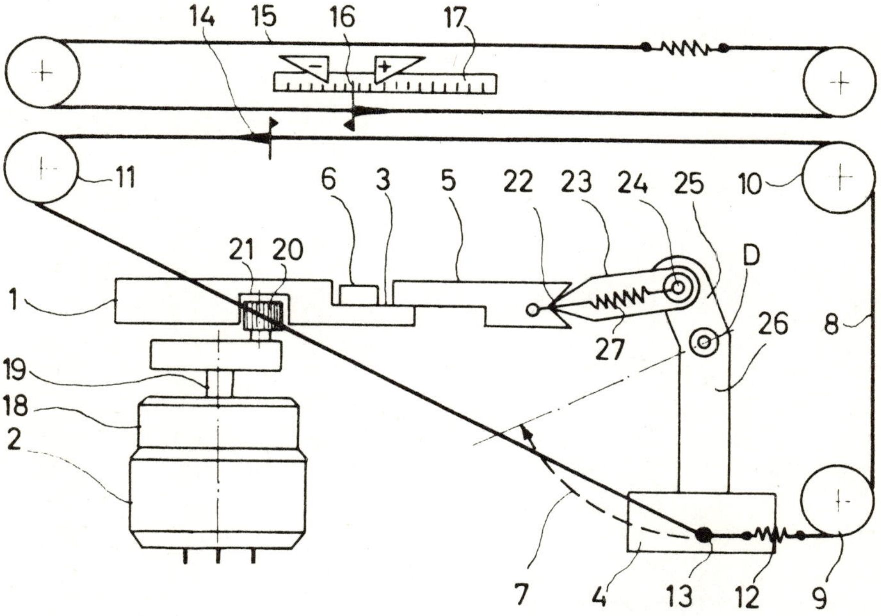

Source: K.A. Flury; U.S. Patent 3,757,566; September 11, 1973

The tester as shown in Figure 2.10 comprises a pressure slide **1** driven by an electric motor **2** and provided with a tablet support **3**. A measuring slide **5** provided with a pendulum weight **4** cooperates with the pressure slide, so that a tablet **6** can be clamped between two jaws displaceable relatively to each other, one jaw belonging to the pressure slide, the other to the measuring slide, with the effect that the tablet is stressed by a diametrically acting force.

During this process, the pendulum weight is swung out from a fixed pivot D in the direction of the arrow **7**. The swinging motion is converted into a linear motion by a cord which is fastened to the pendulum weight and carried around guide rolls **9**, **10**, **11** with the aid of a spring **12**. The cord **8** is fastened to the pendulum weight at point **13**.

The representation of the linear motion is effected by an engaging means **14** arranged in the zone between the two guide rolls **10** and **11**. A second cord **15** is arranged parallel to the first cord **8** in the zone of the engaging means **14** in the form of a closed loop. This second cord is provided with a drag pointer **16** sweeping the zone of a linear scale **17**.

The pressure slide is driven by the motor acting through gearing **18** and an eccentric assembly fitted to the output shaft **19** of the gearing. The eccentric assembly comprises a roll **20** which is eccentric with respect to the output shaft and which engages a groove **21** in the pressure slide at right angles to the movement direction of the slide.

The transmission of the motion from the measuring slide to the pendulum weight is by a knife-edge **22** fitted to the measuring slide and by an intermediate piece **23** which engages the knife-edge and is connected by a needle bearing **24** to an extension **25** of a pendulum weight support **26**. To ensure a uniform rest for the knife-edge, a tension spring **27** is arranged between measuring slide and needle bearing **24**.

In operation, the force exerted by the pressure slide on the specimen tablet is transmitted by the measuring slide to the pendulum weight, so that the latter swings out of its home position in the direction of the arrow, against the action of gravity. The cord **8** fastened to the pendulum weight **4** transmits the movement of the pendulum to the drag pointer **16** fastened to the second cord **15**. The drag pointer indicates on the linear scale the force acting on the tablet.

On failure of the tablet, the pendulum weight briefly falls back a certain distance, so that contact with the engaging means **14** and the drag pointer **16** is briefly interrupted. This interruption is used to reverse the gearing **18**, so that the pressure slide returns to its home position.

The function of the tension spring **27** arranged between the measuring slide and the journal of the needle bearing **24** is to suppress the play in the system transmitting the force to the pendulum weight **4**. For this, the angles of attack of the connecting elements are such that the measuring slide is subjected to a force which is approximately proportional to the deflection angle of the pendulum weight.

TOOL FOR FEEDING PILLS TO ANIMALS

R.F. Smart; U.S. Patent 3,757,781; September 11, 1973 has devised a tool for administering medicines to felines so the person administering the medicines may maintain his hands out of reach of the fangs or front claws of the felines.

This tool comprises an elongated hollow sleeve having a split sleeve member constructed of resilient material telescoped over one end and including a plunger insertable in the other end of the sleeve. The other end of the sleeve and the plunger include coacting portions for support of the tool in one hand and manipulation of the plunger for projecting the latter through the sleeve and into the sleeve member whereby a tablet or capsule frictionally supported within the split sleeve member may be ejected therefrom by the plunger when the tool has been positioned with the split sleeve member disposed in the back of the mouth of an animal to which a medicant is to be administered. In addition, the tool further includes a squeeze bulb removably engageable with the end of the sleeve remote from the sleeve member after removal of the plunger in order that the tool may also be used in the manner of an eye dropper for administering liquid medicants. This tool can be shown in Figure 2.11.

FIGURE 2.11: TOOL FOR FEEDING PILLS TO ANIMALS

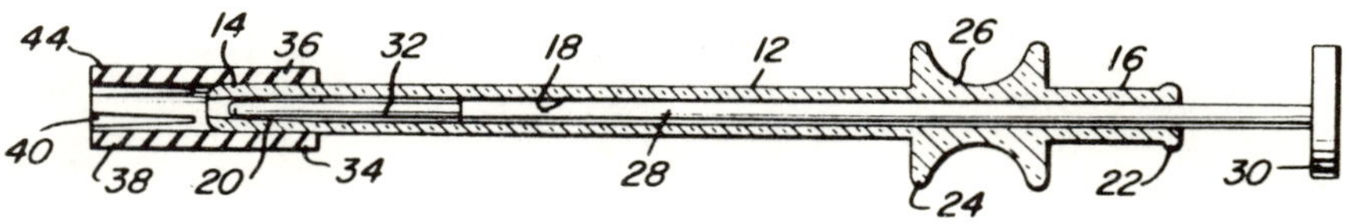

Source: R.F. Smart; U.S. Patent 3,757,781; September 11, 1973

The tool includes an elongated tubular body **12** including first and second ends **14** and **16** and provided with a longitudinal bore **18**. The bore **18** extends through the body and is of substantially constant diameter, except in the first end **14** of the body where the bore is slightly tapered as at **20**.

The second end **16** of the body includes a circumferentially extending and slightly radially outwardly projecting retaining flange **22** and also a considerably diametrically enlarged portion **24** spaced slightly toward the first end **14** from the retaining flange. The diametrically enlarged portion includes a wide and relatively deep circumferentially extending semicircular groove **26**.

An elongated plunger **28** is reciprocal through the bore and includes a diametrically enlarged head **30** on its end projecting outwardly of the second end **16** of the body. The head is circular in cross-sectional shape and the end of the plunger remote from the head includes a diametrically reduced terminal end **32** for reciprocation through the tapered end of the bore formed in the first end of the body **12**.

A resilient and slightly radially expandable sleeve **34** is provided and has a first end **36** thereof telescoped over and frictionally retained on the end **14** of the body. The second or other end **38** of the sleeve is provided with circumferentially spaced and longitudinally extending tapered slots **40** which render the second end **38** of the sleeve **34** more readily expandable than the end **36** of the sleeve. The slots taper in width inwardly of the terminal end of the second end **38** of the sleeve **34**. In operation, a pill or capsule is frictionally retained between the fingers **44**. In manipulating the tool, the first and second fingers of the hand holding the tool are seated in diametrically opposite portions of the groove in order to firmly support the tool from the hand. Then, firm pressure is applied to the head to advance the plunger to the left whereby the diametrically reduced terminal end of the plunger will forcibly eject the pill or capsule from the slotted end of the sleeve.

SYNTHETIC POLYMER MATRIX MATERIALS

CARBOPOL MATRIX BLENDS

Carbopol-Basic Hydroxide Blends

Many delayed release pharmaceutical tablets use a matrix containing a cross-linked polymer of acrylic acid, also known as a carboxyvinyl polymer or carboxypolymethylene. Briefly stated, the material is a polymer of acrylic acid which is cross-linked with from 0.75 to 2% by weight of the polymer, preferably about 1%, of a copolymerized polyalkenyl polyether.

The polymerization of the monomers ordinarily is carried out in an inert hydrocarbon with a free radical catalyst. The preferred cross-linking polyalkenyl polyether monomers are polyallyl sucrose and polyallyl pentaerythritol, desirably containing an average of at least 3 allyl groups for each molecule of sucrose or pentaerythritol. The preferred polyallyl sucrose contains an average of 5 to 6 allyl groups per molecule of sucrose (theoretical maximum is 8 allyl groups) and the preferred polyallyl pentaerythritol contains 4 allyl ether groups per molecule (the theoretical maximum).

The carboxypolymethylenes used in this process described by *C.H. Johnson, Jr.; U.S. Patent 3,330,729; July 11, 1967; assigned to The B.F. Goodrich Company* are high molecular weight polymers, e.g., usually having a molecular weight greater than 200,000 and preferably greater than 300,000. Specifically, this process relates to compressed tablets having delayed or sustained release characteristics which contain, in addition to the medicinal agent, a water-insoluble, cross-linked polymer of acrylic acid and a particular, very slightly water-soluble, basic magnesium or calcium compound.

The pharmaceutically acceptable basic diluents which are used in these compositions are limited to three compounds, specifically, magnesium oxide, calcium hydroxide and magnesium hydroxide. These compounds are only slightly soluble in water, e.g., 0.0086 gram per 100 ml. of water at 30°C., 0.158 gram per 100 ml. at 25°C. and 0.0009 gram per 100 milliliters at 18°C., respectively. Despite this slight solubility, these compounds impart an alkaline reaction to water.

The weight ratio of the carboxyvinyl polymer to the basic diluent in the tablets may be within the range of 0.3:1 to 10:1. The preferred weight ratio is from 0.5:1 to 2.5:1. As the weight ratio of polymer to basic diluent is increased (less basic diluent in the tablet), the diluent is less effective in magnifying the efficacy of the delayed release characteristic which the polymer imparts to the tablet. Sustained release of the drug over an extended period, e.g., at least about four hours, is obtained with tablets containing as little as about 5% by weight of carboxyvinyl polymer. A series of tablets were prepared having the following formulation, the amounts of the ingredients being in percent by weight of total tablet weight.

Riboflavin-5-phosphate	1.67
Magnesium stearate (lubricant)	1.00
Carbopol 934* (carboxyvinyl polymer)	25.00
Diluent	72.33

*Carbopol 934 is a polymer of acrylic acid cross-linked with 1% of a polyallyl ether of sucrose having an average of about 5.8 allyl groups per each sucrose molecule.

The composition of the diluent portions of the tablets are given below in Table 1. The weight ratio of the carboxyvinyl polymer to the magnesium and calcium compound is also given.

TABLE 1

Sample No.	Diluents, Weight Percent of Tablet	Weight Ratio of Carbopol to Basic Diluent
A	Lactose, 72.33	*
B	Lactose, 62.33	
	$Ca(OH)_2$, 10.00	2.5:1
C	Lactose, 47.33	
	$Ca(OH)_2$, 25.00	1:1
D	$Ca(OH)_2$, 72.33	0.35:1
E	Lactose, 47.33	
	MgO, 25.00	1:1
F	Lactose, 22.33	
	MgO, 50.00	0.5:1
G	MgO, 72.33	0.35:1
H	Lactose, 47.33	
	$CaCO_3$, 25.00	1:1
I	Lactose, 22.33	
	$CaCO_3$, 50.00	0.5:1
J	$CaCO_3$, 72.33	0.35:1

*Control.

An additional control tablet, sample K, had the following formulation:

	Weight Percent
Riboflavin-5-phosphate	1.67
Magnesium stearate	1.00
Carbopol 934	35.00
Lactose	62.33

These tablets were prepared by mixing the powdered ingredients and compressing the dry blends on a Stokes single punch tabletting machine using 0.625 inch concave dies. Tablet size and tablet weight were uniform. Each tablet weighed 0.225 gram and had a Strong-Cobb Hardness of 20 to 25 units. The drug release rates of the tablets were determined by the standard USP method using the conventional Stoll-Gershberg disintegration apparatus.

Six tablets of each formulation were placed in the basket of the apparatus and the basket was immersed into a 1,000 ml. beaker containing 600 ml. of a simulated gastric juice (1 liter of hydrochloric acid-water solution of pH 1.2 containing 2 grams of dissolved sodium chloride). After 30 minutes, half of the simulated gastric fluid in the test beaker was replaced by a simulated intestinal fluid (1 liter of sodium hydroxide solution of pH 7.5 containing 6.8 grams of dissolved monobasic potassium phosphate). Every hour thereafter, half of the contents of the beaker was again replaced by simulated intestinal fluid. The temperature of the simulated fluid was maintained at 37° ± 2°C. At regular intervals, small samples of the fluid were taken from the beaker and analyzed to calculate the cumulative amount of the drug released. The determinations were made by means of a spectrophotometric analysis which measured the concentration of dissolved riboflavin-5-phosphate. The results of the disintegration tests are tabulated in Table 2. The symbol (-) in the table indicates that the measurement was not made.

TABLE 2: CUMULATIVE PERCENT OF DRUG RELEASED VERSUS TIME OF IMMERSION IN GASTROINTESTINAL FLUID

Time, Hours	Sample No. A	B	C	D	E	F	G	H	I	J	K
0.5	11.9	5.6	9.1	2.4	6.4	3.5	3.1	9.0	6.3	2.7	7.9
1.5	25.5	22.8	15.7	5.1	13.8	7.8	8.1	26.1	13.1	7.1	21.6
2.5	39.2	31.6	19.8	5.6	17.4	9.8	8.1	39.3	17.6	9.7	31.3
3.5	51.2	37.6	21.0	5.7	21.6	10.8	9.2	54.0	27.0	15.1	42.2
4.5	-	43.7	21.0	-	24.8	12.6	9.2	65.4	55.5	22.5	51.1
20.7	-	-	-	-	57.8	-	-	-	-	-	-

Polyvinylpyrrolidone-Carbopol Blends

A controlled release medicament described by *J.A. Hill; U.S. Patent 3,458,622; July 29, 1969; assigned to E.R. Squibb & Sons, Inc.* comprises a blend of polymeric vinylpyrrolidone together with a carboxyvinyl hydrophilic polymer. The medicament is mixed with the dry polymer and the blend is then granulated, dried and compressed into tablet form. When the resulting tablet is placed in water or gastric fluid, the two polymeric substances react to form a complex of low solubility which is gum-like in consistency and the reaction mass thus alters and retards the diffusion of the active material from the tablet. There is practically no swelling of the polymer complex as differentiated from the usual behavior of a hydrophilic colloid.

The vinyl polymer which constitutes one member of the blend is polyvinylpyrrolidone, e.g., having a molecular weight of 5,000 to 80,000, preferably about 40,000. The second component of the polymer blend is a carboxypolymethylene hydrocolloid polymer as described in U.S. Patent 2,909,462 being a polymer of acrylic acid cross-linked with polyallyl sucrose marketed under the trade name Carbopol, with designations 934, 940, 941. The proportions, i.e., the ratio (by weight) of the vinyl polymer to carboxypolymethylene polymer is about 1:10 to 10:1. Preferably, however, they are used in a ratio of about 1:1 by weight. The following example is illustrative of the process.

Example: The following ingredients are used.

	Per tablet (mg.)	Per batch 600 tablets (gm.)
Polyvinyl Pyrrolidone K-30	185.0	111.0
Carbopol 934	185.0	111.0
Procaine amide hydrochloride, micropulverized	500.0	300.0
Ethyl cellulose	15.0	9.0
Triethyl citrate	7.5	4.5
Piccolyte resin Type S-115-L	12.5	7.5
Stearic acid	9.0	5.4
Magnesium stearate	2.27	1.36
Total	916.27	549.76

The procainamide hydrochloride, polyvinylpyrrolidone and Carbopol are admixed in a planetary type mixer. While mixing, the powders are wet with 150 ml. of a 6% w./v. solution of ethylcellulose also containing 3% w./v. of triethyl citrate and 5% w./v. of Piccolyte resin in methylene chloride solvent. The moist mass is granulated by forcing through a No. 16 mesh screen and allowed to air dry. After drying the powder is passed through a

No. 20 mesh screen. Stearic acid and magnesium stearate are added to the dried granulate, and the mixture is tumbled. The release rates of the active ingredient determined by the procedure of Souder et al., *Drug Standards* 26, 77 to 83, 1958 are shown below. Theoretical procainamide content is 500 mg./tablet, GF and IF are simulated gastric and intestinal fluid.

Time period	Mg. procainamide assay residual	Mg. procainamide corrected to 500 mg.	Mg. procainamide released	Percent of total procainamide released
Initial	494.6	500.0		
1 hr. GF	331.4	335.0	165.0	33.0
1 hr. GF and 1 hr. IF	299.4	302.7	197.3	39.5
1 hr. GF and 3 hr. IF	233.9	236.5	263.5	52.7
1 hr. GF and 7 hr. IF	115.4	116.7	383.3	76.7

Carbopol-Caseinate Blends

Long lasting troches are prepared by *G.L. Christenson and H.E. Huber; U.S. Patent 3,594,467; July 20, 1971; assigned to Richardson-Merrell Inc.* having from 4 to 17% of carboxypolymethylene and from 15 to 70% of sodium caseinate, preferably 4 to 10% of carboxypolymethylene and 30 to 70% of sodium caseinate. The remainder of the troche can be a conventional water-soluble tablet diluent or base. Additionally, minor quantities of conventional pharmaceutical tabletting excipients such as lubricants, dyes and flavoring agents can be employed in the troche composition.

The compressed troches can be made by either wet or dry granulation methods maintained at 3% or less moisture. Heat or moisture labile compounds can thus be included in the formulations and handled in a manner to maintain the compounds' integrity. The bland powders used as the troche matrix are readily flavored with a wide variety of fragrances to meet the widely varying products' needs.

The drugs or medicaments used in the troche are those which are useful in treating the oral cavity or which have utility by sublingual or transbuccal administration. The medicament can be in powdered form or it can be absorbed on the various powdered ingredients of the troche. Examples of drug substances for use in these troches are as follows: thymol, cresols, creosote, eugenol, hexachlorophene, cetylpyridinium chloride, tetracyclines, nystatin, penicillins, amphotericin B, erythromycin, neomycin, diphenhydramine HCl, doxylamine succinate, chlorpheniramine maleate, pyrrobutamine phosphate, dexchlorpheniramine maleate, butacaine sulfate, dyclonine HCl, benzocaine, sodium fluoride, stannous fluoride, potassium peroxymonosulfate, and vitamin A. The quantity of medicament in the troche can vary from 0.05 to 15% of the troche and preferably from 0.2 to 5%. Unless otherwise described, percentages are given on a weight basis in the following examples.

Example 1:

	500 Troches, (grams)
Carbopol 934 (5%)	12.50
Sodium caseinate (70%)	175.00
Mannitol	53.87
Sodium fluoride	1.13
Zinc stearate	5.00
Flavor	2.50

Blend the Carbopol 934, sodium caseinate, mannitol, and sodium fluoride in a suitable mixer and add sufficient deionized water to make a wet granulation. Dry the granulation in an oven at 120°F. to between 2 and 6% moisture. Pass the dried granulation through a 12 or 14 mesh oscillator screen, add the flavor powder and zinc stearate lubricant. Compress the mixture into 500 mg. troches on a Stokes tabletting machine at approximately 4,000 psi and with 7/16 inch flat beveled punches.

Example 2:

	500 Troches, (grams)
Carbopol 934 (8½%)	85.00
Sodium caseinate (34%)	340.00
Mannitol	496.40
Cetylpyridinium chloride	2.50
Benzocaine	0.75
Menthol	0.35
Talc	37.50
Carbowax 6000	37.50

Blend the Carbopol 934, sodium caseinate, mannitol, cetylpyridinium chloride, benzocaine, menthol, 18.75 grams of talc, and 18.75 grams of Carbowax 6000. Compress the mixture into ¾ inch flat faced slugs at approximately 4,000 psi on a Stokes tabletting machine. Grind the slugs through 12 or 14 mesh oscillator screen. Add the remaining talc and Carbowax 6000 to the granules and mix well. Compress the mixture into ¾ inch flat beveled troches at approximately 4,000 psi and to a weight of 2 grams each.

Polyacrylic Acid-Polyethylene Glycol Complex

It has been found by *J.W. Poole; U.S. Patent 3,634,584; January 11, 1972; assigned to American Home Products Corporation* that the release of a drug from a therapeutic composition may be made independent of pH where the composition includes a carboxyvinyl polymer and a polyethylene glycol. The drug preferably is utilizable in powdered form. The drug comprises 1 to 90%, preferably 5 to 20% by weight, of the tablet composition. The total of the carboxyvinyl polymer and polyethylene glycol comprises 10 to 60%, preferably 20 to 50% by weight, of the composition. The remainder may be a fast release drug, extenders, lubricants, flavoring agents, coloring agents and the like, as is known in the art.

The carboxyvinyl polymers used in this process are described in U.S. Patent 2,909,462, of particular interest being the preparation produced in acid form. A particularly effective embodiment of the high molecular weight carboxyvinyl polymer is a water-soluble polymer of acrylic acid cross-linked with 1% of a polyallyl ether of sucrose having an average of about 5.8 allyl groups for each molecule of sucrose (Carbopol 934, formerly known as Good-rite K-934). The following examples illustrate the effect on the dissolution rate of a relatively insoluble compound.

Example 1: Tablets were prepared from the following control formula which does not contain polyethylene glycol.

Formula (A)

Ingredient	Milligrams	Weight percent
Oxazepam	30	9.7
Carbopol 934 (2.5% Carbosil)	62	20.0
Lactose	211	68.1
Magnesium stearate	7	2.2
Total	310	100.0

The ingredients were weighed, screened, and blended, then densified by compacting in a tabletting machine. Dissolution tests on the tablets were performed using a low agitation procedure. In such a procedure one tablet is placed in a two liter, round bottom flask containing 1,750 milliliters of a solvent, and agitated. Agitation is accomplished by rotating a 7.5 cm. Teflon paddle located 2.5 cm. from the bottom of the flask at 50 rpm. One group of Formula (A) tablets were placed in one-tenth normal hydrochloric acid (0.1 N HCl). The pH of 0.1 N HCl is about 1.5. The amount of oxazepam in solution at various time intervals was recorded. A second group of Formula (A) tablets was placed in 0.2 molar solution of disodium phosphate and monosodium phosphate buffered to a pH of 7.5.

Samples were withdrawn at the times indicated by the dots in Figure 3.1, either 1, 2, 3, 3½, 4, 5 or 6 hours. The samples were filtered and assayed for drug content. The results are shown in Figure 3.1 where the percent of drug in solution is recorded.

FIGURE 3.1: VARIATION OF OXAZEPAM CONCENTRATION WITH TIME

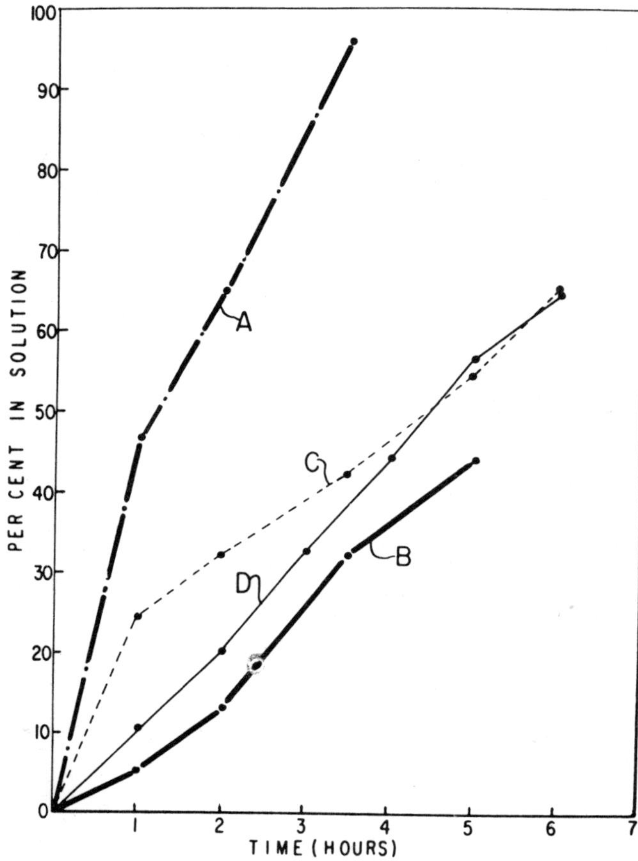

Source: J.W. Poole; U.S. Patent 3,634,584; January 11, 1972

Example 2: Tablets were prepared as in Example 1 in which the delayed release portion had the following formula which includes polyethylene glycol.

Formula (B)

Ingredient	Milli-grams	Weight percent
Oxazepam	30	7.8
Carbopol 934 (2.5% Carbosil)	93	24.2
PEG 4000	75	19.5
Lactose	180	46.7
Magnesium stearate	7	1.8

Following the procedure of Example 1, one group of Formula (B) tablets was placed in 0.1 N HCl and another group of Formula (B) tablets was placed in a phosphate solution buffered to a pH of 7.5. The amount of oxazepam in solution was determined at various time intervals as indicated by the dots in Figure 3.1. The results are shown in Figure 3.1.

In Figure 3.1, Curve **A** shows the amount of oxazepam from Formula (A) in solution in a pH 1.5 medium at various times after immersion. Curve **B** shows the amount of oxazepam from Formula (A) in solution in a pH 7.5 medium at various times after immersion. Curve **C** shows the amount of oxazepam from Formula (B) in solution in a pH 1.5 medium at various times after immersion. Curve **D** shows the amount of oxazepam from Formula (B) in solution in a pH 7.5 medium at various times after immersion.

As may be seen from a comparison of curves **A** and **B** with curves **C** and **D**, the oxazepam in tablets containing both Carbopol 934 and PEG 4000 was released at a rate independent of pH. The oxazepam in tablets without PEG 4000 was released more quickly in a pH 1.5 solution than in a pH 7.5 solution. The oxazepam in tablets containing both Carbopol 934 and PEG 4000 was released at a rate that was substantially independent of pH. Also, there is a substantially lower release rate in an acidic medium such as gastric juices, so that the oxazepam will not be totally released in the stomach, but will continue to be released in the intestines and at a substantially uniform rate.

ACRYLATE POLYMER MATRIX MATERIALS

Hydroxyalkyl Acrylate Polymers

T.H. Shepherd and F.E. Gould; U.S. Patent 3,577,512; May 4, 1971; assigned to National Patent Development Corporation have developed a hydrophilic polymer system which may be used as a coating or as a matrix for sustained release medicament. This is a dosage combination of a hydrophilic polymer which is insoluble and nonassimilable in a biological system and a therapeutic substance which can be leached from the combination to provide an intended effect on the system. The hydrophilic polymer can be mixed with the therapeutic and/or employed as a coating. Preferably, it is employed as a coating, whether or not it is also mixed with the therapeutic.

The hydrophilic monomer used is a hydroxy lower alkyl acrylate or methacrylate, or hydroxy lower alkoxy lower alkyl acrylate or methacrylate, e.g., 2-hydroxyethyl acrylate, diethylene glycol monomethacrylate, 2-hydroxypropyl acrylate, 3-hydroxypropyl methacrylate and dipropylene glycol monomethacrylate. The preferred monomers are the hydroxyalkyl acrylates and methacrylates, most preferably 2-hydroxyethyl methacrylates.

While homopolymers can be employed, for best results a cross-linked copolymer is used. Preferably, the cross-linking agent is present in an amount of 0.1 to 2.5%, most preferably not over 2.0%. Care should be taken that cross-linking agents are not used in an amount which renders the product toxic. Typical examples of cross-linking agents include ethylene glycol diacrylate, 1,3-butylene dimethacrylate, 1,4-butylene dimethacrylate, propylene glycol diacrylate, dipropylene glycol dimethacrylate, diethylene glycol diacrylate, dipropylene glycol diacrylate, divinyl benzene, divinyl toluene, diallyl tartrate, allyl pyruvate, allyl malate, and the like. The following examples will further illustrate the process.

Example 1: Purified 2-hydroxyethyl methacrylate (100 grams) is stirred with 0.15 gram isopropyl percarbonate in an anaerobic atmosphere at ambient temperature. Ethylene glycol dimethacrylate in the concentration of 0.1 g./100 grams 2-hydroxyethyl methacrylate is added. Phenoxymethyl penicillin is dissolved in ethyl alcohol and added to the mixed methacrylate solution in an amount to provide for gradual release of 1,200,000 units per gram of casting syrup. The resulting casting syrup is set aside as a stock solution for later casting or other use. The casting syrup and the resulting cast product either in shaped or powdered form are used as a pharmaceutical carrier for the antibiotic. The use of the casting syrup or resulting shaped or powdered preparation has the advantage that it prevents deterioration and loss of potency to which the antibiotic is subject in conventional pharmaceutical carriers. In addition, the hydrophilic polymer has the desirable characteristics, whether dry or solvent filled, of preventing the imbibition with microbial and fungal contaminants, such as gram negative and gram positive microorganisms, yeast, molds and viruses. This is of particular importance in the presence of contaminants, such as preventing contamination of penicillin with various yeast forms. The polymerization of the casting syrup to a solid can then be completed, e.g., by adding 0.3 gram of further isopropyl percarbonate and heating to 40°C. The product can serve as the core of the tablet and a similar casting syrup omitting the phenoxymethyl penicillin can serve as the outer coating.

Example 2: Distilled 2-hydroxyethyl methacrylate (100 grams) is stirred with 0.1 gram tertiary butyl peroctoate in an anaerobic atmosphere at 25° to 70°C. for 15 to 40 minutes. The resultant mixture is cooled to 25°C. and tertiary butyl peroctoate added to make a concentration of tertiary butyl peroctoate in the system of 0.2/100 grams of 2-hydroxyethyl methacrylate. Ethylene glycol dimethacrylate, in a concentration of 0.2 gram/100 grams of 2-hydroxyethyl methacrylate is added at the same time as the catalyst concentration is brought up to the theoretical content.

100 grams of the resulting syrup was added to three times its volume of water with vigorous agitation. The white precipitate was isolated by filtration and dried to yield 9.0 grams of polymer showing an intrinsic viscosity of 1.03 when dissolved in absolute methanol.

Discs of hydrophilic polymer, prepared as shaped articles from this solution, measuring ¼ in. in diameter and 0.05 mm. in thickness, were saturated with an antibiotic solution of lincomycin hydrochloride monohydrate (Lincocin) and tested against standard staphylococcic strains on agar plates. The zones of inhibition were compared with standardized 1 mg. discs obtained from the manufacturer. Multiple transfers of the hydrophilic polymer also were made on blood agar to determine how long the elution of the antibiotic from the gel would take place.

It was observed that inhibition of the standard bacterial strain occurred up to 22 days. Comparable paper discs with the same antibiotic exhibited zones of inhibition only for 48 hours. In some cases 6 transfers of the discs, each to a fresh blood agar plate, were carried out. From the results, it was apparent that the elution of the agent from the hydrophilic polymer disc is a gradual process and extends over a significant period of time. Moreover, it appears that it is possible to heavily saturate the gel with the desired agent.

Polymer Hydrogel Carriers

K. Kliment, J. Vacik, Z. Ott, V. Majkus, M. Stol, V. Stoy and O. Wichterle; U.S. Patent 3,689,634; September 5, 1972; and U.S. Patent 3,551,556; Dec. 29, 1970; both assigned to Ceskoslovenska Akademie ved, Czechoslovakia have developed polymeric carriers for biologically active substances which are fully insoluble in the liquids of the body, but strongly swell therein. Biologically active substances are not bound chemically to the carrier and enter the organism by dissolution or diffusion.

The carriers are three dimensional hydrophilic polymers, either homogenous or heterogeneous, physiologically inert and innocuous. A typical example is copolymer of glycol methacrylate, cross-linked with from 0.1 to 5% of glycol dimethacrylate, where glycol means not only ethylene glycol, but also polyglycols, copolymers of ethylene or polyethylene glycols with propylene glycol, and other water-soluble dihydric alcohols. Glycol monomethacrylate or glycol monoacrylate can be partly or fully replaced by other neutral hydrophilic, physiologically inert monomers such as methacrylamide or acrylamide.

Glycols can be partly or fully replaced by other polyols such as glycerol, mannite, or pentaerythritol. Glycol dimethacrylate can be replaced by any other suitable cross-linking agent such as a low molecular polyester of an unsaturated dicarboxylic acid, e.g., maleic or itaconic acid, or by N,N'-methylene-bis-methacrylamide. Biologically active substances can be absorbed by the carrier or freely deposited therein, e.g., in its center, either as a solid or as a dispersion, or in the form of a solution. In contact with living tissue, a mucous membrane or skin, the biologically active substances diffuse gradually into the body. The diffusion rate is influenced by the structure of the polymer, particularly by the cross-linking degree and the presence or absence of visible pores (macroporosity). The structure can be changed by choosing the conditions of polymerization. The carriers can be taken orally, implanted subcutaneously, can constitute a part of a prosthesis or be inserted in a cavity of the human body. A planary carrier may be placed in contact with skin, with a mucous membrane or with surface wounds.

If an implant is readily accessible, the physiologically active substance, when exhausted, can be replenished by using a hypodermic needle. In this way it is also possible to use two or more different active substances sequentially. Physiologically active substances which can be applied with the carriers include antibiotics, disinfectants, chemotherapeutics, hemostatics, cytostatics, hormones and other preparations for external or internal use.

The rate at which active substances are released depends, under otherwise constant conditions, on the ratio between the surface and the volume of the particle. Small grains release the sorbed substance sooner than the large ones.

It is important to introduce the hydrophilic cross-linked carrier into the gastrointestinal tract or into a muscle in a state in which it is still capable of swelling so that the concentration of the released drug decreases slowly or if the swelling capacity is great enough, increases from an initial comparatively low value to a maximum. By choosing the distribution according to a predetermined schedule it is possible to obtain any desired change of concentration with time.

For intramuscular application granular gels may be suspended in oil or in glycerol, or even in aqueous solutions, if the carrier is previously saturated with, e.g., glycerol and the aqueous suspension is prepared immediately before the application. For applications in which the carrier makes direct contact with living tissue or mucous membranes other than those of the gastrointestinal tract, it is advantageous to provide an outer layer of a neutral, nonionogenic hydrogel such as the copolymer of a glycol methacrylate or acrylate with a small amount of a neutral cross-linking agent such as glycol bismethacrylate. Neutral, inert hydrogels are easily tolerated by the organism.

Example 1: A mixture of 70% distilled water and 30% ethylene glycol monomethacrylate, containing 0.24% of ethylene glycol bismethacrylate, was mixed with 0.5% of a 2% aqueous solution of ammonium persulfate and 0.1% dimethylaminoethyl acetate. Then 1.5% of an aqueous dispersion of chloramphenicol was added, the mixture was well stirred and poured into a flat glass mold blanketed with carbon dioxide. The mold was left for 3 hours at room temperature. The microporous sponge thus formed could be used for treating burns.

Example 2: A spongy hydrogel was prepared according to Example 1, squeezed out and soaked in a concentrated aqueous solution of tetracycline hydrochloride. Then a cut and weighed piece of impregnated sponge is coated with a thin polyvinyl alcohol layer and suspended by means of a thread of carboxymethylcellulose in a glass mold, which is then filled with a mixture of 55% ethylene glycol monomethacrylate, 20% diethylene glycol monomethacrylate, 0.3% ethylene glycol bismethacrylate, 0.8% of a 2% aqueous potassium persulfate solution, 0.5% of a 2% aqueous solution of potassium pyrosulfite, 0.01% of 0.1% aqueous copper sulfate (pentahydrate) solution and 23.39% of distilled water.

The mixture polymerized readily under an inert atmosphere at room temperature. The mold with the polymerized mixture is then immersed in ethanol whereby the polymer is released from the mold and the residual catalyst is washed out. Ethanol is removed either by evaporation or by immersion of the hydrogel in cold water. Prior to subcutaneous implantation, the hydrogel body is immersed in physiological salt solution. The entire procedure is carried out under sterile conditions. The diffusion rate of the antibiotic depends on the thickness of the surface layer of transparent hydrogel.

Example 3: A copolymer is prepared from 97 parts of ethylene glycol monomethacrylate,

2 parts of methacrylic acid and 1% of ethylene glycol bismethacrylate by suspension polymerization in a concentrated, aqueous solution of sodium chloride, using 0.05 parts of diisopropyl percarbonate as a polymerization initiator. The copolymer beads, 0.1 to 2.0 mm. in size, are thoroughly washed and then soaked in a saturated aqueous solution to tetracycline hydrochloride.

After a week, when even the largest particles have reached equilibrium with the solution, the surplus solution is centrifuged or sucked off and the polymer is dried at low pressure and 40°C. The polymer is then divided by means of calibrated sleeves into three fractions: (1) 0.1 to 0.5 mm.; (2) 0.5 to 1 mm.; and (3) 1 to 2 mm. To obtain protracted activity through the entire gastrointestinal tract after oral application, a mixture of 1 part of (1), 0.5 part of (2) and 3 parts of (3) is used.

OTHER POLYMERIC MATRIX MATERIALS

Thermoplastic Matrix Materials

According to *L.-E. Fryklof, E. Sandell and J.I.G. Ostholm; U.S. Patent 3,317,394; May 2, 1967; assigned to Aktiebolaget Hassle, Apotekare Paul Nordstroms Fabriker, Sweden* a tablet having a delayed and sustained action is prepared by mixing a powder which is substantially insoluble in the fluids that the tablet contacts, with a powder which contains the medicinal substance and is soluble in those fluids, and then compressing the resulting powder mixture to form tablets.

The properties and the amount of the insoluble material are so chosen that, upon compressing that powder mixture, the insoluble material forms a firmly coherent, skeleton structure, the interstices of which form pore-like interconnecting continuous ducts and canals in which the soluble material is compactly contained. The ratio of the soluble to the insoluble material forms a united but porous or sponge-like structure in which the pores have the form of continuous or interconnecting ducts or tubular canals serving as the holders or repositories for the soluble material.

The soluble and insoluble materials are mixed in weight ratios of 1 part of the soluble one to from 1 to 5 parts of the other. The most practical content of insoluble material may be determined readily in each case by a simple routine test. Thus, the insoluble material is mixed with the soluble substance in different ratios, e.g., 40 to 60, 50 to 50, 60 to 40, 70 to 30, 80 to 20, 90 to 10 and 95 to 5; these various mixtures then are compressed into tablets, and the mechanical strength and the course of releasing of the soluble substance is determined for each such test tablet. The test sample giving the desired behavior as to strength, firmness of structure and release of soluble content indicates the proportion of soluble to insoluble ingredients to use in the operating batch.

When preparing medicinal tablets, it is suitable to prepare tablets having a strength of from 6 to 15 kg. However, a strength of from 10 to 12 kg., measured by the Strong-Cobb Hardness Tester, is preferred generally. The specific range of pressures to use in the compression of the final tablets cannot be given as applicable to all the various possible compositions and tablets having retarding layers and/or overall coatings.

In principle, the insoluble material may consist of any powdered or granular nontoxic material substantially insoluble in digestive juice and of such consistency that it will form a coherent porous skeleton structure when compressed together with the soluble pulverulent material. It is preferred to use thermoplastic synthetic materials, such as polyvinyl chloride, polyethylene, acrylic resins such as polymethyl methacrylate, polystyrene, polyvinyl acetate, cellulose derivative materials such as cellulose acetate, and copolymers of these substances, e.g., a polyvinyl chloride-acetate copolymer.

Example: 14 mg. of ephedrine hydrochloride having a grain size of about 100 microns was mixed with 74 mg. of sodium chloride and 110 mg. of polyvinyl chloride, the two latter substances having a grain size of about 500 microns. The mixture was compressed to form a tablet having a diameter of 8 mm. and a height of 2.7 mm. That tablet was placed as a core in a die of a tablet machine and was covered on all sides with a powder mixture containing 9 mg. of ephedrine hydrochloride, 36 mg. of sodium chloride and 180 mg. of polyvinyl chloride, all substances having the same grain size as the respective substances of the core.

The aggregate was compressed to form a composite tablet, having a diameter of 10 mm. and height of 4.7 mm. After about 1 hour of leaching in water, the soluble material in the coating had been dissolved, and the medicament contained in the core then began to penetrate the coating at such a constant rate that all of the medicament was released from the tablet after the lapse of about 8 hours.

Injection Molded Resin Matrix

A process for preparing injection molded medicaments has been developed by *P. Speiser; U.S. Patent 3,432,592; March 11, 1969; assigned to Ciba Corporation.* These tablets, which may be used for peroral administration, contain the active substances or mixtures of active substances embedded in a thermoplastic synthetic resin or synthetic resin mixture which is capable of being injection molded, physiologically tolerable and at least partially soluble in the digestion juices.

Synthetic resins which can be used are those which have a low softening point, e.g., below 160°C., preferably within the range of 80° to 140°C. Furthermore, they should be inert to the active substances and be soluble or at least partially soluble in artificial gastric and/or intestinal juice, so that release of the active substances is ensured, and also be resistant to a high relative atmospheric moisture content and to tropical temperatures.

Synthetic resins which can be used are, for example, linear polycondensation or, polyaddition resins, such as polyamides, and furthermore preferably polyaddition products obtained from diepoxide compounds and primary alkanolamines, for example, 2-amino-2-ethyl-1:3-propanediol. Also included are the condensation products of glycerin with phthalic anhydrides, polyurethanes, polymers, such as polyvinyl resins, and polymers with end-position, free or esterified carboxyl or carboxamide groups, or cellulose derivatives. The mixing ratio of active substance and synthetic resin in the medicaments is determined by the dosage of the active substance and the desired rate of release of the latter.

The tablets may also contain fillers or swelling substances, such as lactose, starch derivatives, talc, bole, kaolin, Aerosil, as well as electrolytes. To hydrophilize lipophilic substances, surface-active substances, such as fatty alcohols, or fatty acids, may also be included. In order to obtain a retarded effect, the active substance or substances or portions thereof may also be previously encased in thermoplasts which are difficultly soluble in digestion juices, such as acrylic resin combinations, preferably a copolymer of methyl methacrylate and acrylic acid, or waxes or fats. It is also possible to employ a mixture of such more difficultly soluble thermoplasts with more readily soluble synthetic resins, such as polyvinylpyrrolidone, cellulose derivatives or polyvinyl alcohols as starting materials. The process is illustrated in the following examples.

Example 1: A pulverulent mixture of 60 parts by weight of a synthetic resin consisting of 4 parts of an epoxide compound and 5 parts of 2-amino-2-ethyl-1:3-propanediol and 40 parts by weight of 5-(1-cyclohexenyl)-5-ethylcalcium barbiturate of an average particle size of 200μ is injection molded in an apparatus at about 140°C. in cylindrical tablet molds, the variable plunger of which is adjusted to a gross weight of 200 mg.

The plastic used in this example can be obtained as follows. 4 parts of a polyglycidyl ether obtained by condensation from epichlorohydrin with bis(p-hydroxyphenyl)dimethylmethane in the presence of alkali and which is liquid at room temperature and has an epoxide content of 5.2 epoxide equivalents per kilo, and 5 parts of 2-amino-2-ethyl-1:3-propanediol are mixed at room temperature and heated to about 60°C.

Example 2: A pulverulent mixture of 7.5 parts by weight of 1-methyl-2-phenylethylamine sulfate, 10 parts by weight of D-sorbitol and 82.5 parts by weight of the synthetic resin described in Example 1 is worked up in an injection molding apparatus into octahedral tablets with a gross weight of 300 mg. and having an active substance content of 22.5 mg.

Example 3: A pulverulent mixture of 10 parts by weight of 1-methyl-2-phenylethylamine sulfate, 20 parts by weight of D-sorbitol and 70 parts by weight of a synthetic resin obtained from 95% polyvinyl alcohol and 5% polyvinyl acetate (Movilith D) is worked up in an injection molding apparatus into moldings having a gross weight of 200 mg. and with an active substance content of 20 mg. at a temperature of 135°C.

Storable Polymer Matrix

P.M. Hill; U.S. Patent 3,453,360; July 1, 1969; assigned to Abbott Laboratories has developed a dry, powdered or granulated component for sustained release pharmaceutical tablets consisting of 10 to 100 parts of finely divided, insoluble, nontoxic, inert, nonhygroscopic, inorganic salt particles coated with 1 part of a nontoxic, insoluble, high-melting, film-forming polymeric material.

The method of preparing this universally applicable sustained release medium comprises intimately dispersing 10 to 100 parts of the inorganic salt in a solution of 1 part of the polymeric material dissolved in a volatile solvent for the polymeric material, evaporating the organic solvent and breaking up any agglomerates of the resulting dry powder into finely divided particles. If desired, the particles so prepared can be used in that form and stored until needed or they may be converted into granules by passing the still moist mixture through a screen or similar known methods. The new medium does not require a water-soluble component. This discovery enables the preparation of a medium devoid of any waxy or low-melting polymer which ultimately makes tabletting considerably easier.

In a simple form, calcium sulfate is placed in a mixing device and a solution of a film-forming polymer in a volatile organic solvent is added to the calcium sulfate. The mixture is homogenized while permitting the organic solvent to evaporate. The resulting mixture is dried thoroughly and subsequently passed through a screen to break up any lumps. This material may be used in the finely divided form so obtained or it may be converted into granules by known techniques.

The amount of the film-forming polymer may be between 1 and 10% of the inorganic salt; a preferred range is between 1 and 3%. No advantage is gained by using larger amounts of the usually more costly polymeric binder. The amount of the polymer does not affect the sustained release pattern when this mixture is compressed with granules of an active drug. However, a minimum of about 1% of the polymer should be used to provide sufficient coherence in the tabletting process.

Suitable film-forming polymers include polypropylene, polyvinyl acetate, carboxylated copolymer of vinyl acetate and crotonic or acrylic acid, polyacrylonitrile, cellulose acetate phthalate, ethylcellulose, cellulose acetate or butyrate, copolymers of maleic anhydride and ethylene, copolymers of methyl methacrylate and methacrylic acid, copolymers of methyl acrylate and methyl methacrylate, polymethylstyrene, methyl methacrylate, polyvinyl chloride and polymethylstyrene modified with acrylonitrile and mixtures of copolymers.

Suitable inorganic salts are calcium carbonate, hydrous calcium phosphate, dibasic calcium phosphate, calcium sulfate, talcum powder, bentonite, alumina, magnesium trisilicate, silicic acid, terra alba, etc. Calcium sulfate is preferred since it provides an excellent release pattern, is inexpensive, white and easily available in pharmaceutically pure form.

Example 1:

Ingredients	
Calcium sulfate	100 grams
Carboxylated copolymer of vinyl acetate and a minor amount of crotonic acid (Gelva C3-V30)	2 grams
Methylene chloride	40 ml.

The copolymer is dissolved in methylene chloride and the solution is slowly added to the calcium sulfate under agitation. Agitation is continued until the material becomes a flowable powder again. The thus obtained polymer coated calcium sulfate is dried at 50°C. to strip all remains of the solvent. After passing the mixture through a 20 mesh screen to break up any lumps it is ready as a universally applicable medium for the preparation of sustained release tablets. It can be stored as each until needed or it can be granulated.

Example 2: This example illustrates a tablet of desoxyephedrine hydrochloride with the release sustained over a period of 7 hours.

Ingredients	Mg./Tablet
Desoxyephedrine HCl	10.0
Calcium sulfate (sustained release matrix prepared according to Example 1)	188.0
Magnesium stearate	2.0

The three items are passed through a 40 mesh screen, blended and compressed into $^9/_{32}$ inch tablets, each tablet weighing 200 mg. Twelve of these tablets are put into each of three bottles containing 300 ml. of water at pH 7, 7.5 and 1.2 and the bottles are rolled for 7 hours at room temperature. An additional test is run in the same manner in water of 40°C. and pH 7. A 10 ml. sample is withdrawn from each bottle at periodic intervals and assayed for content of desoxyephedrine HCl. The results shown in the following table indicate the total percentage of drug found in the liquid.

Time, Hours	25°C., pH 7, Percent	40°C., pH 7, Percent	25°C., pH 7.5, Percent	25°C., pH 1.2, 1 Percent
½	27.1	27.9	17.7	29.4
1	37.1	41.8	24.8	43.1
4	61.2	84.9	53.6	77.5
7	75.2	98.8	68.6	91.6

The corresponding values obtained by following the procedure involving the disintegration basket described in the U.S.P. are 30.3, 42.8, 70.7 and 86.2% respectively.

Matrix from Polymer Latices

G.S. Banker and H. Goodman; U.S. Patent 3,629,292; December 21, 1971 have disclosed a process for preparing controlled release drugs wherein an aqueous latex of a polymer having acidic and/or basic groups is contacted with a pharmaceutically active material or drug having basic and/or acidic groups. In a preferred form, the water is then removed and the product formulated into a suitable dosage form. It is believed that the drug molecules are chemically or physicochemically bonded to the polymer chains. In addition, the extremely high surface area presented by the polymer due to the colloidal size of the polymer particles is believed to result in adsorption of drug molecules on the surface of the polymer particles.

The polymers useful in the process are commercially produced by conventional emulsion polymerization and contain one or more monomers having either basic or acidic groups. Suitable monomers having acidic radicals include acrylic acid, methacrylic acid, crotonic acid, itaconic acid, maleic acid, half esters of maleic acid, maleic anhydride, sulfonated styrene, phosphonated styrene, etc. Suitable monomers containing basic functionality include, for example, polyvinyl amine, the aminoalkyl esters of any of the aforementioned acids such as aminoethyl methacrylate, etc.

The latices of dispersed colloid of the polymer emulsions useful in the process present a highly concentrated dispersed polymer system of high molecular weight material, (20 to 60% solids) which is impossible to match in high concentration in solution due to solubility and viscosity limitations. For example, it has been estimated that such a typical polymer emulsion contains in the order of 10^{14} or 100 trillion polymer particles per cubic centimeter of dispersion. This process permits easy and precise control of drug dispersion and more uniform drug distribution which is predicated on physicochemical principles rather than mechanical factors. This is accomplished by contacting an aqueous solution of the drug with a considerable excess of polymer. The drug, being in solution, will be distributed throughout the emulsion as separate molecules or ions randomly distributed throughout the polymer.

Thus, instead of dividing 1 gram of drug into 100,000 approximately equal particles by fine milling, the process permits highly uniform distribution of the drug as 6×10^{23} molecules/mol throughout the polymer, e.g., at a level of 1 gram of drug/kg. of polymer, thus simplifying the problem for the formulator, greatly improving the reliability of mixing, and reducing the mass of dispersed drug by many orders of magnitude. A typical drug with a molecular weight of 300 would produce 2×10^{21} molecules or ions for every gram in solution as compared to 1×10^5 to 1×10^7 milled particles per gram. The following example is illustrative of the process. All reactions are at room temperature.

Example: The methapyrilene hydrochloride (200.0 grams) is dissolved in 1,000.0 ml. distilled water, and is continuously mixed with the air of a power stirrer as 1,250 ml. of Latex A. Latex A is an acrylic copolymer containing about 35% carboxylic acid functionality. It is available from the Rohm and Haas Co. under the trademark Acrysol ASE-75. The latex contains 40% solids.

Immediate flocculation and coagulation of the latex occurs on addition to the drug solution. After addition of the latex is completed, stirring of the resultant slurry is continued for an additional five minutes. The mixture is then vacuum filtered through a coarse sintered glass filter. The collected solid material is placed in flat glass trays and is dried at 50°C. for approximately four hours. The resultant granular dried material is then comminuted or ground to appropriate size, and is then screened through 60 mesh screens. Reproducibility of the entrapment procedure, utilizing the formula and procedure of the example is demonstrated in the table below.

Batch number	Mg. of methapyrilene HCl [1]	Average of two assays
1	135.28 134.59	134.94
2	133.05 139.11	136.08
3	133.94 133.87	133.91
	130.99 129.77	130.38
5	132.95 131.69	132.32
6	127.22 131.98	129.60

[1] Per gm. of collected solid.

A similar matrix material is disclosed by *G.S. Banker; U.S. Patent 3,608,063; September 21, 1971* wherein a carboxylic acid is added to the matrix formulation disclosed in U.S. Patent 3,629,392. Carboxylic acids have been found to promote sorption of drug during the process by which the drug is trapped, as well as to provide a further mechanism by which subsequent drug release may be controlled. The acids may act as counter or protective ions, retarding polymer flocculation or coagulation and/or as bridging moieties, facilitating surface sorption of drug to polymer.

The acids useful in this process comprise monocarboxylic acids as well as polycarboxylic acids provided they are sufficiently soluble in the reaction system to form salts with the drugs. Even acids which are only slightly water-soluble can be used since as dissolved acid is used up in the reaction, more will go into solution.

Typical useful monocarboxylic acids are acetic acid and aminoacetic acid (glycine). Useful polycarboxylic acids include saturated aliphatic acids such as oxalic acid, malonic acid, succinic acid, glutaric acid and adipic acid; unsaturated aliphatic acids such as maleic acid and fumaric acid; hydroxy acids such as citric acid and tartaric acid; acids of a more complex functionality such as ascorbic acid; and carboxylic acids such as the phthalic acids. The carboxylic acid additives can be added directly to the polymer drug system or can be reacted and added as a carboxylate. Thus, the acid can be mixed with a solution of drug hydrochloride salt and the polymer added thereto and flocculated. Alternatively, the acid can be added to a solution of the drug and reacted therewith, and the drug acid carboxylate crystallized from solution; typically, the carboxylates are recrystallized from one to three times from an isopropanol/ether solution, and vacuum dried.

The crystallized carboxylates are then mixed in solution with the polymers for the sorption flocculation step. In general, the acid and drug are mixed and/or reacted in approximately equimolar concentrations. However, the carboxylic acid, e.g., a dicarboxylic acid, may be added in less than equimolar concentration but the resulting sorption increase will be something less than the possible maximum, albeit, greater than if no carboxylic acid were utilized.

Example: Aqueous drug solutions were prepared from methapyrilene salts. To 50 ml. portions were added 50 ml. of Latex A (Rohm and Haas Co.) with constant stirring. The resulting mixtures were suction filtered, the filtrates were assayed and the amount of drug in the filtrate and flocculant were determined. The tests are summarized in the table below.

- - - - - Initial Drug Solution - - - - -		- - - - % of Initial Drug - - -	
		In Filtrate	In Flocculant
Methapyrilene HCl	0.07 Molar	45.8	54.2
Methapyrilene HCl	0.08 Molar	36	64
Succinic acid	0.08 Molar		
Methapyrilene HCl	0.08 Molar	9	91
Succinic acid	0.08 Molar		
NaOH	0.08 Molar		
Methapyrilene succinate	0.08 Molar	9	91

The effect of the dicarboxylic acid or of the dicarboxylate drug salt on the concentration of drug entrapped by the polymer in the presence of the dicarboxylate or dicarboxylic acid compound is apparent. Only about 54% of the drug in the 0.07 molar drug hydrochloride solution was sorbed and swept from solution, while over 90% of the drug carboxylate (succinate) was sorbed under the same conditions, except at a higher drug solution concentration (0.08 molar vs. 0.07 molar). It should be recognized that the proportion of the initial drug found in the flocculant generally decreases with an increase in the initial drug concentration.

Low Melting Polymeric Materials

Tablets containing delayed action coated granules and having good cohesion and porosity are prepared by *K.G. Eriksson and A. Mangen; U.S. Patent 3,670,065; June 13, 1972* using polymeric matrix or carrier substance. The carrier is used in the molten state and permits the formation of tablets by casting.

The carrier substance should have a melting point above 37°C.; preferably a melting point above 40°C., it being undesirable that the dosage unit melts at body temperature. A carrier substance having a melting point above 43°C. is most preferred. For obtaining good casting properties, the carrier substance should be present in 20% of the weight of the dosage unit, although in exceptional cases good shaping properties can be obtained with as little as 10% of carrier substance.

A wide range of substances and mixtures thereof may be used as carrier substance, the only limitation being that the carrier substance must be of a pharmaceutically acceptable kind and should have a melting point preferably not below 43°C. and not higher than 150°C. because heat sensitive medicinal components may be affected undesirably at higher temperatures. Furthermore, the carrier substance should be acted upon by the gastrointestinal fluids so as to be dissolved or softened so that under slight pressure it will decompose within the time period during which the dosage unit is to be effective. Substances of water-soluble as well as of fat-soluble types may be employed. Examples of water-soluble substances are condensation products of ethylene glycol such as, for instance, substances of the formula $H(OCH_2CH_2)_nOH$ where n is a number of from 5 to 400, preferably within the range of 60 to 200, and condensation polymers of propylene glycol, propylene oxide and ethylene oxide in which the polyoxyethylene portion amounts to at least 50% by weight.

Examples of fat-soluble substances that are suitable as carrier substance either alone or in admixtures with one another are condensation polymers of propylene glycol, propylene oxide and ethylene oxide in which the polyoxyethylene portion amounts to less than 50% by weight, paraffin, hydrogenated vegetable oils, stearic acid, cetyl alcohol, stearyl alcohol, and fatty acid esters such as for instance, glycerol monostearate.

The active medicinal ingredient in the dosage unit may be incorporated in the carrier substance in the form of granules produced, for instance, by spraying and cooling a mass obtained by dissolving and/or slurrying the medicinal substances in a melt of, for instance, polyethylene-containing paraffin, or may be incorporated in the carrier in the form of such granules that have been produced by granulation in a fluidized bed or in some conventional manner in mixing vessels. The auxiliary substances employed for delaying dissolution of the medicinal component must be pharmaceutically acceptable and should be such that they remain unaffected or substantially unaffected when the granules are worked into the warm or hot mass which is to be cast.

A suitable size of the granules is within the range of 80 microns to 2.5 mm., preferably 500 to 800 microns. The medicine particles present in the granules and also any such free medicine particles that may be incorporated in the carrier substance and/or in a surface layer applied after the casting will preferably have a size of 1 to 50 microns, although they may be larger, but preferably they should have a size of less than 1 mm.

The number of granules in the dosage unit may vary within wide ranges; the lower range limit is determined by the dosing accuracy required. For instance, it is possible to introduce into each dosage unit as few as 10 granules, but greater numbers, up to several thousands, may be used. However, the dosage unit as a whole should not weigh more than 1 gram. The casting may be in molds of any suitable type, e.g., it may be done with a pair of rollers having surface mold cavities as described in U.S. Patent 3,874,417. Examples of medicines that may be used in the process and are stable under the conditions employed are penicillin, acetyl salicylic acid, lithium sulfate, potassium chloride, ferrous sulfate, ascorbic acid, ephedrin chloride, N-[2-(diphenylmethoxy)ethyl]-N,N-dimethylammonium chloride, caffein, papaverin chloride and mixtures thereof. The process is further illustrated by the following example. All percentages are by weight.

Example:

Components	Percent
Ferrous sulfate, dried powder	25
Polyethylene glycol (average molecular weight 6,000)	61.5
Hydrogenated castor oil	13.5

The hydrogenated castor oil is melted at 90°C. and mixed with the ferrous sulfate. The warm melt is run through a three roller mill and then sprayed into cold air with a spray gun of the paint sprayer type, having an opening of about 2 mm. The powder obtained is slurried in a melt of the polyethylene glycol heated to 65°C. and maintained at this temperature while being fed into the nip between a pair of rollers having mold cavities in their peripheries, the melt being maintained agitated so as to ensure homogeneousness. The rollers are cooled to a temperature of between -2 and +2°C. The dosage units thus produced weighed 1 gram. These dosage units were tested by the so-called cup method which involves the following procedure: 20 dosage units are placed into a 600 cc cup into which 500 cc extraction liquid at 37°C. is introduced. The contents of the cup are stirred, and the percentage of the medicine content dissolved out from the dosage units is recorded at successive time intervals. The temperature is maintained at 37°C. In the present case, a 1% Tween 80 solution was employed as extracting agent, and the rate of stirring was 50 rpm. (Tween 80 is polyoxyethylene sorbitan monooleate.) 93% of the ferrous sulfate was found to have been extracted after 6 hours, so on an average 15.5% of the ferrous sulfate was extracted per hour. In the samples taken each hour it was found that each hour 15.5% ± 4.5% of the ferrous sulfate had been extracted.

CARBOHYDRATE MATRIX MATERIALS

SUGAR BASED MATRIX MATERIALS

Reinforced Lactose Matrix

A process has been developed by *R.T. Stevens and M. Hersh; U.S. Patent 3,344,030; September 26, 1967; assigned to American Home Products Corporation* whereby medicinal tablets can be prepared using conventional crystalline lactose as an excipient by direct compression on conventional automatic tabletting equipment.

By direct compression is meant the direct compaction between two punches and without previous processing beyond simple mixing, of a powder into tablets in a die cavity filled loosely with a large number of small crystals. As the upper punch descends and makes contact with the surface crystals, a densification of the bed occurs through particle movement, void spaces being filled by migrating or elastically deformed crystals. Cold bonding may occur at those contact points where two lattices are correctly aligned. When maximum pressure is applied, a compact aggregate approaching the density of the original crystals is obtained. The primary purpose of such direct compression is to reduce manufacturing cost and to improve or promote such necessary properties as tablet strength, appearance and disintegration.

This process is based on the discovery for tabletting pharmaceuticals by the use of crystalline lactose combined with a fibrous reinforcing agent. Suitable reinforcing agents such as, methylcellulose, orange flour, alpha-cellulose or carboxymethylcellulose in the range of 2 to 30% by weight and preferably 5 to 15% by weight will permit the use of the crystalline lactose.

The following tabular comparison of conventionally processed lactose versus spray dried lactose shows the improved tablet characteristics obtained with the use of this process with fibrous reinforced conventionally processed lactose.

	Conventionally Processed Lactose, Percent of Methylcellulose						Spray Dried Lactose, Percent of Methylcellulose					
	0.0	5.0	10.0	15.0	20.0	30.0	0.0	5.0	10.0	15.0	20.0	30.0
Hardness, kg.	15	19	22	23	25	30	22	25	26	26	25	23
Thickness, inch	0.143	0.144	0.145	0.146	0.147	0.148	0.143	0.145	0.146	0.148	0.150	0.150
Friability, k.	1.00	0.02	0.02	0.01	0.01	0.01	0.10	0.20	0.30	0.30	0.50	0.50
Disintegration (minutes)	1.45	0.90	1.60	1.77	3.00	6.00	28.0	20.0	18.8	18.8	18.5	29.3

Mixed powders were dry blended for 7 minutes and compressed on a standard rotary tablet press using conventional force feed techniques and using a ⅜" diameter, flat beveled, scored top punch.

Example 1:

	Percent
Phenobarbital powder	37.00
Conventionally processed lactose	47.70
Alpha-cellulose	13.00
Suitable lubricant	2.30
	100.00

Sieve lubricant through a #60 screen, add remaining ingredients, mix 7 minutes, compress.

Example 2: Tranquilizer tablets having the following composition and intended to contain 10 mg. each of active ingredient were prepared by direct compression in the following manner:

Ingredient	Per Tablet, mg.	Per 100,000 Tablets, kg.
7-chloro-1,3-dihydro-3-hydroxy-5-phenyl-2H-1,4-benzodiazepin-2-one	10.0	1.00
Methylcellulose, USP, 400 cp.	30.0	3.00
Amberlite XE-88	3.0	0.30
FD&C Yellow #5 Lake	0.4	0.04
Magnesium Stearate, USP	1.5	0.15
Lactose, USP	145.1	14.51
Total Weight	190.0	19.00

Sorbitol-Gum Acacia Blends

Sublingual tablets are prepared by *H. Lowey; U.S. Patent 3,428,728; February 18, 1969,* which tablets can last, i.e., distribute the medicament, for as long as one hour. Conventional sublingual tablets are prepared for acute relief and are very rapid acting and immediately absorbed. This, for example is characteristic of sublingual nitroglycerin tablets taken for angina pectoris or related heart conditions. Ordinary oral tablets to be taken several times per day are also well known and some medication is prepared in special sustained release dosage form wherein the active ingredient is released according to a desired pattern, for example, over a period of 6 to 12 hours.

According to this method, sublingual tablets are produced from which the active ingredient is released gradually and continuously over a short period of time of the order of 15 to 60 minutes from administration. It has been found that this is important and has unpredictable advantages. For example, notroglycerin tablets in sublingual form and which act rapidly over a very short period of time cause serious or unpleasant side effects, such as flushing, headache, tachycardia and dizziness. Tablets embodying this binder lack these drawbacks and have slower and continuous release without the side effects.

These pharmaceutical tablets are prepared by cooking a mixture of sorbitol and gum acacia until the solids content is 65%, adding at least one artificial sweetener for sweetening and absorption regulation, cooling to 90°F., adding the active ingredient, converting the mixture into sublingual oral unit dosage form and administering the product sublingually while being able to discontinue medication at will.

Example 1: The formula for 20,000 pieces of ¹⁄₁₀₀ grain Prolinguals of Nitroglyn molded to weigh 17.5 grains each is shown on the following page.

Liquid sorbitol	37 lb. 8 oz.
Powdered gum acacia	7 lb. 8 oz.
Nitroglycerin beta-lactose mixture	5 oz.
Color	30 gr.
Flavor	2 oz.
Calcium cyclamate	5 oz. 313 gr.
Soluble saccharin	250 gr.

Example 2: The formula for 20,000 pieces of 1½ grain glyceryl guaiacolate tablets molded to weigh 19 grains per piece is as follows. This formula is used as a cough preparation.

Liquid sorbitol	37 lb. 8 oz.
Powdered gum acacia	7 lb. 8 oz.
Glyceryl guaiacolate	4 lb. 5 oz.
Color	30 gr.
Flavor	2 oz.
Calcium cyclamate	5 oz. 313 gr.
Soluble saccharin	250 gr.

Example 3: The formula for 20,000 pieces of an enzyme preparation molded to weigh 22½ grains each is as follows. This preparation contains 2,000 units each of amylase and protease, but can be varied to contain from 1,000 to 10,000 units each. The product is used as a tooth-cleaning agent and in periodontures.

Liquid sorbitol	37 lb. 8 oz.
Powdered gum acacia	7 lb. 8 oz.
Amylase	7 lb.
Protease	7 lb.
Color	30 gr.
Flavor	2 oz.
Calcium cyclamate	5 oz. 313 gr.
Soluble saccharin	250 gr.

Massecuite Aggregated Total Sugar Granules

R.E. Brouillard and C.L. Griffith; U.S. Patent 3,619,292; November 9, 1971; assigned to Penick & Ford, Limited have found that a new physical form of Total Sugar, which is referred to as "Massecuite Aggregated Total Sugar" granules (or as MATS granules) has remarkable tabletting properties, which make it highly advantageous as a binder or binder-filler in the formation of compression tablets, especially by the method of direct compression. MATS granules can also be used as a binder in known granulation processes, and it provides a considerable advantage in the precompression or dry-granulation method of tabletting, but its advantages are maximized in the direct compression process.

In the formation of tablets by direct compression from a particulate mixture, the MATS granules can be blended into the mixture as a partial or complete substitute for spray dried lactose or spray dried mannitol, resulting in a tabletting composition which is free-flowing, compressible, and which produces tablets having excellent cohesive properties.

The resulting tablets can therefore provide other advantages of dextrose as a binder or filler, such as taste or organoleptic properties. For example, dextrose hydrate produces a cooling effect when dissolved in the mouth, which can be highly desirable for tabletted food or pharmaceutical products, which are to be chewed or sucked. The dextrose hydrate can also enhance other flavors in the tablets, which may be particularly desirable for tabletted food or candy products, such as candy drops or lozenges containing fruit or spice flavoring agents.

The term Total Sugar is applied to starch hydrolyzate sugar mixtures of relatively high

DE (dextrose equivalent) which are produced in solid form, and which are usually composed largely of crystalline or anhydrous dextrose, but which also contain residual oligosaccharides of the hydrolysis, which are essentially, noncrystallizable, and are present in the form of a solid solution. Some of the dextrose may also be present as a "glass" or solid solution.

MATS, the granular binder or binder-filler for use in this method can be produced by the process described in U.S. Patent 3,540,927. Specifically, a water solution of a crystallizable sugar is subjected to partial crystallization to form a pumpable massecuite composed essentially of microcrystals of sugar dispersed in a water solution of sugar. This massecuite, which may contain from 40 to 60% of the sugar in crystalline form, is sprayed into a drying air stream to form atomized droplets and to remove part of the water from the droplets in the air stream to form granular aggregates of the microcrystals containing residual crystallizable sugar solution.

Essentially each droplet forms a single aggregate of generally spherical shape. This step is preferably carried out in a spray dried tower where the massecuite droplets are formed at the top and fall downwardly with the evaporation of water. Where the hydrate crystal form is desired, the spray drier is operated at a sufficiently low temperature to avoid formation of anhydrous dextrose or other unstable crystal forms. For example, the massecuite droplets during spray drying of a starch hydrolyzate can be kept below 50°C. With sucrose and other sugars, the spray drying temperature can be varied over a wider range, especially where the sugar has only one crystalline form, such as with sucrose which only forms anhydrous crystals. This process is illustrated by the following examples in which the tablets were all made by direct compression without slugging or regranulation.

Example 1: Spray Dried Aggregated, microcrystalline Total Corn Sugar (92 to 93% dextrose) was blended with 0.1% by weight of magnesium stearate powder. The latter was added as a lubricant to prevent adhering to the die wall or sticking to punch face. The mixture was placed in a Colton Type Tablet Press and tablets were formed. The tablets were smooth, uniform, sharp-edged and there was no evidence of sticking, splitting or capping.

Example 2: Two parts of citric acid were dissolved in 30 parts of a 70° Brix concentrated grape juice and the mixture was blended into 100 parts of SDA corn sugar (prepared by the process of U.S. Patent application # 674,168). After air drying the free-flowing granular product, it was blended with 0.5 part of powdered magnesium stearate and tabletted in a four pocket Colton tablet press. No sticking to the dies was observed and the tablets showed no splitting or capping. They were smooth, sharp-edged and had excellent strength characterisitcs. When added to cold water, they dissolved readily to form a clear solution suitable as a fruit drink.

Example 3: A uniform dry blend of the following was prepared: 0.5% Prednisone, 0.5% powdered magnesium stearate, and 99.0% SDA Total Sugar granules (which contained about 0.5% free moisture). The free-flowing mixture was then readily made into 5 grain (total weight) tablets which were hard, smooth, and sharp-edged. They had the desirable feature of dissolving completely in cold water in less than four minutes, whereas, tablets using conventional formulations frequently take several times that long to dissolve.

Sugar Matrices for Direct Compression Tabletting

Direct compression vehicles for preparing tablets have been developed by *J.P. Troy, A. Monti, F.J. Lynch and C.B. Broeg; U.S. Patent 3,627,583; December 14, 1971; assigned to SuCrest Corporation*. This material comprises generally spherical, firm, porous agglomerates of sugar particles in a cementum or matrix. The agglomerates are dry (from about 0.1 to about 3% moisture), free-flowing particles having particle size from 325 to 12 mesh. Tablets formed using such sugar agglomerates as the direct compression vehicle are uniform, possess good physical properties, do not discolor on aging, and readily dissolve in aqueous media.

These sugar agglomerates are obtained by: spraying a particulate solid sugar with an aqueous solution of binder; providing the resulting mixture with sufficient high intensity agitation to uniformly intermingle the sugar and binder and to build up agglomerates of a desired size; "snowballing" the agglomerates to impart a general spherical shape thereto and to firm or densify the agglomerate; drying; and if necessary, separating over- and undersized agglomerates.

The particulate sugar can be a mono-, di- or trisaccharide, such as arabinose, xylose, ribose, fructose, mannose, galactose, glucose, sucrose, maltose, lactose and the like, including mixtures of two or more of such sugars, with sucrose being preferred. The particulate sugar can be obtained synthetically, or it can be a refined natural product, such as corn syrup solids, molasses solids, honey solids, maple syrup solids and the like.

The second component which is used to form the agglomerate is a noncrystallizing aqueous solution of a polyhydroxy compound as a binder. Illustrative polyhydroxy compounds include propylene glycol, glycerol, erythritol, arabitol, xylitol, adonitol, mannitol, dulcitol, sorbitol, sugars, such as arabinose, xylose, ribose, glucose, mannose, fructose, sucrose, maltose and lactose, dextrin and the like, with polyols of the formula $HOCH_2(CHOH)_xCH_2OH$, where x is 1 to 4. Propylene glycol, glycerol, mannitol, sorbitol, glucose, fructose and invert sugar are of particular interest, with invert sugar being most preferred.

The concentration of binder in the aqueous medium is not critical provided that it is not so high as to cause crystallization or provide solutions so viscous as to prevent spraying and intimate intermingling and uniform distribution of binder and solids.

The mixing is ordinarily conducted at about room temperature (65° to 75°F.). Higher and lower temperatures can be employed, if desired, provided the properties of the aqueous medium and the agglomerate product are not adversely affected.

Simultaneously with the spraying, the mixture is agitated to thoroughly intermingle the solid sugar and the aqueous binder medium and to effect agglomeration. This requires high intensity mixing, such as is obtained with a Patterson-Kelley blender or a Lodige mixer.

The resulting agglomerate is admixed with the active material and the resulting mixture compressed without granulation or slugging to form a tablet. The amount of the agglomerate obviously will depend upon the properties of the active and any other additives which are to be incorporated into the finished tablet, for it is well known that the compactibility of tablet compounds and mixtures are subject to wide variation. In general, however, the agglomerate will comprise at least 10% of the tabletting mixture and, therefore, at least 10% of the tablet. In most cases, however, the agglomerate will comprise from about 70 to about 95% of the tabletting mixture and the tablet. The following examples are illustrative. All parts and percentages are by weight unless otherwise stated.

Example 1: To 90 parts of finely pulverized sucrose is rapidly added over 5 minutes by spraying at room temperature and while agitating the pulverized sugar, 14 parts of an aqueous invert sugar solution (72% total solids) in a Patterson-Kelley liquids-solids blender. After continuing agitation for an additional 10 minutes, the agglomerated material is screened through a vibrating 16-mesh screen and the screened material is dried to a moisture content of 1.5% or less. To 97 parts of dry agglomerated product is added, under agitation, 1 part of dry citric acid, 0.25 part of dry flavoring material and 1.75 parts of magnesium stearate. The properly blended material is fed to a tabletting press and wafers are formed from it.

Example 2: Employing procedures similar to those in Example 1, 98 parts of finely pulverized sucrose is mixed with about 6.7 parts of an aqueous invert sugar solution (30% total solids). The agglomerated material is screened through a vibrating mesh screen and the screened material is dried to a moisture content of 1.5% or less. Equal parts of the agglomerate and vitamin C are blended. This blend can be further mixed with other dry ingredients such as minerals or other nutritionally active ingredients before being compressed into tablets.

Direct Compression Binders

A. Monti, J.P. Troy and C.B. Broeg; U.S. Patent 3,639,168; February 1, 1972; assigned to SuCrest Corporation have developed similar vehicle where a solid hydratable polymer is blended with a diluent such as sugar for use in forming tablets. These direct compression vehicles comprise minute particles of a dispersion of certain water-soluble or dispersible inert diluents in a matrix of a hydratable high polymer.

The diluent can be any normally solid material provided it is inert, edible and permissible in the table formed from the direct compression vehicle. Thus, it can be water-soluble or insoluble in water. If insoluble, however, it must be capable of reduction to a size which is useful in a direct compression vehicle, i.e., a size below 200 mesh, and preferably below 10 microns.

Preferred diluents include normally saccharine materials, i.e., a mono- or disaccharide such as glucose, mannose, galactose, fructose, arabinose, xylose, sucrose, maltose and lactose; as well as certain polyols of the formula $HOCH_2(CHOH)_xCH_2OH$ where x is 1 to 4, such as glycerol, erythritol, arabitol, xylitol, adonitol, mannitol, dulcitol and sorbitol. In addition, certain salts may be employed, including sodium chloride, sodium citrate, calcium carbonate, calcium sulfate and tricalcium phosphate. The diluent may be one or a mixture of two or more of these substances. In the event the diluent is a sugar, it may be of synthetic or natural origin, and may be supplied to the mixing step in the form of a solution or syrup, such as molasses, affination syrup, invert syrup and the like.

The hydrated polymer includes hydrophilic polysaccharides, hydrocolloids or proteinaceous materials which, although not soluble in water, are hydrated upon admixture with water, and when substantially fully hydrated form a clear aqueous sol of swollen polymer and water. Illustrative examples of these high polymers include starch, agar, locust bean gum, carrageen, dextrin, cereal flour and the like.

The polymer, diluent and water are admixed in any convenient manner and in proportions such that there is obtained a substantially clear fluid mixture comprising an aqueous solution or dispersion of diluent dispersed throughout the swollen hydrated polymer. The precise conditions and proportions will vary widely, depending upon the polymer employed, and the amount of and additive employed.

The ratio of water-soluble additive to hydratable polymer can vary widely, depending upon the materials employed and the characteristics desired in the direct compression vehicle. In general, ratios of preferably from 2 to 50 parts additive per part of polymer are useful. Ratios of from 20 to 30 parts additive per part of polymer are most preferred.

Drying of the resulting dispersion may be effected by a variety of techniques, such as spray drying, tray drying, drum drying and the like. In a preferred technique, the dispersion is dried by deposition on a heated surface to effect evaporation and convert the dispersion into a dry, hot, plastic film, removing the film from the heated surface and attenuating the film while simultaneously cooling it, to convert the plastic film to a brittle or frangible condition. After the film has been cooled, it is fragmented and ground to a desired particle size and the ground product is employed. In this technique, the mixture of hydratable polymer and diluent should, of course, have the property of being plastic when in a hot, dry state.

The granular direct compression vehicle is admixed with the active material which it is desired to incorporate into tablet form and, if necessary, a lubricant, and the mixture tabletted by known compression procedures. The proportions of vehicle, active material and lubricant are not critical, and depend upon the active material and the unit dose desired in the tablet. In general, however, the direct compression vehicle will comprise at least 10% of the tabletting mixture and the resulting tablet, although amounts from 70 to 95% are most common. The following examples are illustrative. Unless otherwise specified, all parts and percentages are by weight.

Example 1: A mixture of 182 pounds of sucrose, 35 pounds of tapioca flour, 300 pounds of starch and 400 gallons of water was heated to 180°F., and 714 pounds of a 70% invert syrup was added. The resulting mixture was drum dried to a moisture content of about 2.13%, and then broken up into flakes of about one-half inch. The resulting particulate flake material was admixed with calcium stearate in a ratio of 99 parts to 1 part and after pulverization to yield a product having a particle size of below about 200 mesh (95% through 200 mesh), compressed to form 13/32-inch, 0.5-gram tablets at 1,000 and 3,000. The resulting tablets had Stokes hardnesses of 3.25 and 4.1 kilograms, respectively, and evidenced no capping.

Example 2: The direct compression vehicles of the foregoing example can be blended in accordance with the following recipe and compressed to form tablets or wafers. In preparing a lemon-flavored confectionery tablet, 100.0 parts direct compression vehicle, 1.0 part dry citric acid, 0.25 part encapsulated lemon flavor, 0.10 part yellow color #5 and 1.0 part magnesium stearate are combined.

C.B. Broeg, A. Monti and J.P. Troy; U.S. Patent 3,639,169; February 1, 1972; assigned to SuCrest Corporation have also developed similar multicomponent direct compression vehicles having sugar as the predominant component plus a compaction aid.

Illustrative compacting aids include high molecular weight ethylene oxide polymers, i.e., polyethylene glycols having molecular weights in the range of from about 2,000 to about 10,000 such as the "Carbowaxes," especially Carbowax 6,000; glycerol monostearate; sorbitol; lactose; mannitol; microcrystalline cellulose such as "Avicel"; fatty acids such as palmitic; instantized gums such as those disclosed in U.S. Patents 2,963,373 and 3,042,668; proteins; starch and hydrolyzed polysaccharide derivatives such as hydrolyzed cereal starch and dextrin; and certain sugar agglomerates.

One suitable sugar agglomerate is one comprising generally spherical, firm porous agglomerates of sugar particles in a cementum or matrix of a noncrystalline sugar. These agglomerates are dry (from about 0.1 to about 3% moisture), free-flowing particles having particle sizes within the range of from about 325 to about 12 mesh, and are obtained as disclosed in U.S. Patent 3,627,583.

Preferred direct compression vehicles are those where a sugar, especially sucrose, is mixed with one of the above compaction aids. In such compositions, the sugar comprises from 50 to 90% of the direct compression vehicle.

Although not essential to the process, it is desirable that the compacting aid and the remaining components have substantially similar particle sizes to minimize segregation by size on handling before compacting. As a general rule, the particle sizes of the components should not vary more than ±50% from the mean particle size of the entire mixture. It should be noted, however, that at small mean particle sizes, deviations of larger than 50% may be tolerated because at lower overall dimensions, small absolute variations in particle size represent larger percentages of the mean size. The various components are then mixed by suitable means, such as ribbons blenders, Lodige mixers, Patterson-Kelley mixers and the like to produce a uniform blend of the several particulate components.

The resulting blend is fed to a compactor which converts the particulate mixture into a compact, nonfriable sheet. The degree of compaction will vary widely, depending upon the nature and proportions of the compacting aid and the remaining components, but it is essential that the sheet does not disintegrate under slight pressure. More particularly, the sheet should not, upon granulation, form more than about 40, preferably about 20% dust upon granulation. The next step of the process is granulation, i.e., reduction of the compacted sheet to particles of a desired average size, preferably within the range of from about 16 to about 325. This size reduction is effected with conventional equipment and may be accomplished in one or more steps. The final, and optional, step of the process is screening of the particulate product to a desired size range. Illustrative size ranges include 16 to 100 mesh; 100 to 200 mesh; and 200 to 325 mesh. The following examples are illustrative. Unless otherwise specified, all parts and percentages are by weight. In the examples, the following products were employed.

Flake A – A flake containing 34% starch, 27% sucrose and 39% invert (sucrose and invert dispersed throughout a starch matrix) prepared by mixing 3,750 parts water, 350 parts starch and 284 parts powdered sucrose, cooking the resulting mixture at 180°F. to hydrate the starch and dissolve the sucrose, and adding 571 parts of a 70% invert syrup, followed by drum drying to about 2% moisture and granulating to about one-half inch.

Agglomerate A – A product comprising generally spherical agglomerates of about 8.5% invert, 91.5% sucrose and less than 1% water prepared by spraying a 72° Brix full invert syrup on sucrose in a Patterson-Kelley blender, drying and screening to a fraction having a size of from 20 to 80 mesh.

Agglomerate B – A product comprising generally spherical, uniform agglomerates containing about 2.5% invert, 97.5% sucrose and less than about 1% moisture produced in a manner similar to Agglomerate A, except that the syrup comprised 20% invert and 52% sucrose.

Example 1: A mixture of 1,125 parts of Agglomerate B, 37 parts of Flake A, 5 parts of magnesium stearate and 83 parts sugar was charged at a rate of 3,000 parts per hour to a Chilsonator at a roll speed of 16 rpm and a hydraulic pressure of 1,200 psi, and the resulting compacted sheet was fed to a Fitzmill equipped with 225 K blades and a No. 1 screen operating at 1,590 rpm. The resulting granular product contained 3.95% invert, 0.5% magnesium stearate, 0.35% moisture, 0.7% starch and 94% sucrose and had the following sieve analyses:

Particle Size	Parts by Weight
+20 mesh	0
20 to 40 mesh	2.8
40 to 100 mesh	14.8
100 to 200 mesh	21.0
-200 mesh	61.4

Example 2: A mixture of 250 parts of the -200 mesh fraction of Example 1, 930 parts of Agglomerate A, 30 parts of Flake A and 40 parts of sucrose was blended, pulverized by a Mikro pulverizer to a particle size of less than about 800 mesh (95% through 200 mesh), and fed to a Chilsonator under essentially the conditions described in Example 1. The product, after granulation on the Fitzmill, was screened through 40-, 100- and 200-mesh screens to yield three products (coarse, plus 40 mesh; medium, 40 to 100 mesh; fine, 100 to 200 mesh). The yields and analyses of these products, based upon the dry blend fed to the Chilsonator, is as follows:

Product	Coarse	Medium	Fine
Yield, %	21.6	16.8	26.4
Density, g./cc.	0.796	0.811	0.756
Sieve Analyses:			
+20 mesh	0.8%	Tr	Tr
20 to 40 mesh	93.3%	0.2%	Tr
40 to 60 mesh	Tr	60.5%	Tr
60 to 80 mesh	Tr	22.3%	8.8%
80 to 100 mesh	Tr	8.0%	41.3%
100 to 140 mesh	Tr	5.2%	25.6%
140 to 200 mesh	Tr	1.0%	20.3%
-200 mesh	Tr	Tr	

These vehicles can be used to form confectionery tablets, pharmaceutical formulations and specialty materials.

STARCH BASED MATRIX MATERIALS

Dialdehyde Starch Blends

Insoluble matrix sustained release medicinal compositions adapted for peroral administration are described by *S.J. Merabi and S.B. Prussin; U.S. Patent 3,495,000; February 10, 1970; assigned to Dart Industries Inc.* The medicinal agent is distributed in a matrix comprising a mixture of a dialdehyde starch and polyvinylpyrrolidone, polyvinyl chloride or ethylcellulose.

Starch can be selectively oxidized under influence of periodate ion, resulting in the oxidation of the two adjacent hydroxyl groups in the anhydroglucose units of the starch molecule to the aldehyde form. The selectively oxidized starch, commonly known as dialdehyde starch, is described in *Journal of the American Chemical Society*, 73, 4484 (1951) and in U.S. Patents 2,648,629 and 2,713,553.

It has been found that a dialdehyde number of at least 90 is required for dialdehyde starches useful in the preparation of the matrix of the sustained release medicinal preparations. Such dialdehyde starches have been found to be substantially free of toxicity and useful in preparations intended for oral administration. The process is shown in the following examples.

Example 1: Three granulations were prepared containing aspirin; one with dialdehyde starch and ethylcellulose, one with dialdehyde starch but without the ethylcellulose, and one with ethylcellulose but without dialdehyde starch.

(a) Aspirin-dialdehyde starch-ethylcellulose:

Acetylsalicylic acid, powdered	184.0 g.
Dialdehyde starch (dialdehyde number = 90)	15.0 g.
Mix well and granulate with a solution of ethylcellulose (1.0 gram) in absolute ethanol (49 ml.)	

(b) Aspirin-ethylcellulose:

Acetylsalicylic acid, powdered	199.0 g.
Granulate with a solution of ethylcellulose (1.0 gram) in absolute ethanol (49 ml.)	

(c) Aspirin-dialdehyde starch:

Acetylsalicylic acid, powdered	185.0 g.
Dialdehyde starch (dialdehyde number = 90)	15.0 g.
Mix well and granulate with absolute ethanol (45 ml.). Dry overnight with forced room temperature air.	

Dried granules prepared from these granulations were tested for their sustained release characteristics by the rotating bottle method. In this procedure, a 2 gram sample of granules, or a sample equivalent to 3 tablets, is accurately weighed into an 80 ml. glass vial fitted with a plastic lined screw cap. 60 ml. of digestive fluid is added and the vial mounted in the apparatus which is maintained at 37°C. (plus or minus 1°C.). The following schedule is used:

(1) 1 hr.; Simulated Gastric Fluid; 1.5 pH
(2) 1 hr.; Simulated Intestinal Fluid; 4.5 pH
(3) 2 hrs.; Simulated Intestinal Fluid; 6.9 pH
(4) 1 hr.; Simulated Intestinal Fluid; 6.9 pH
(5) 2 hrs.; Simulated Intestinal Fluid; 7.2 pH
(6) 1 hr.; Simulated Intestinal Fluid; 7.5 pH

The digestive fluids used are made according to USP XV. The residues are removed at desired intervals by emptying the vials through a 40 mesh screen. The residue on the screen is then rinsed with distilled water. It is then drained from excess water by pressing the screen to a towel or paper towel. The residue is then put on a watch glass and dried in a 45°C. oven overnight. The residue is then weighed and the percentage weight loss is plotted.

Granulation composition	Percent released			
	1 hr.	2 hrs.	3 hrs.	6 hrs.
Aspirin-dialdehyde starch-ethyl cellulose	29.0	36.3	49.8	93.3
Aspirin-ethyl cellulose	100.0			
Aspirin-dialdehyde starch	93.0	99.7		

Example 2: Two granulations were prepared containing aspirin as the active ingredient; one with the admixture of dialdehyde starch and polyvinyl chloride and one with polyvinyl chloride but without dialdehyde starch.

(a) Aspirin-dialdehyde starch-polyvinyl chloride:

Acetylsalicylic acid, powdered	160 g.
Dialdehyde starch (dialdehyde number = 90)	10.0 g.
Polyvinyl chloride	10.0 g.

Mix well and granulate with absolute ethanol (50 ml.).

(b) Aspirin-polyvinyl chloride:

Acetylsalicylic acid, powdered	170.0 g.
Polyvinyl chloride	10.0 g.

Mix well and granulate with absolute ethanol (50 ml.).

Employing the technique described in Example 1, dried granules prepared from these two granulations were tested for their sustained release characteristics. The results are as follows:

Granulation composition	Percent released			
	1 hr.	2 hrs.	4 hrs.	6 hrs.
Aspirin-dialdehyde starch-polyvinyl chloride	35.0	49.5	75.8	80.6
Aspirin-polyvinyl chloride	100.0			

Water Swellable Starch Binders

R.W.P. Short and F. Verbanac; U.S. Patent 3,622,677; November 23, 1971; assigned to A.E. Staley Manufacturing Company have developed the process for preparing directly compressed tablets containing as a binder-disintegrant ingredient, a partially cold-water-soluble, cold-water swelling starch material derived from compacted granular starch, e.g., compacted native cornstarch.

The compacted granular starch is a superficially dry, free-flowing powder in which the starch is in the form of a mixture of birefringent granules and nonbirefringent fragments of granules, in which some aggregates of granules and fragments are present. The use of the starch binder-disintegrant ingredient allows active ingredients, e.g., pharmaceuticals, to be tabletted by direct compression.

The more desirable tablets are prepared from superficially dry formulations containing from 5 to 15% moisture based on the formulation total weight. Accordingly, appropriate adjustment of the moisture content may be made, where necessary or desirable, during the formulation operation to improve the tabletting characteristics of the mixture. It may also be desirable, after mixing the ingredients, to screen the formulation to remove any oversize particles introduced in the active ingredient or tabletting aids and thereby to improve tabletting efficiency. In this respect, removal of +40 mesh particles by screening generally is desirable. The process can be illustrated by the following example.

Example: This illustrates the preparation of suitable tablet binder-disintegrant starches from an unmodified cornstarch and the use of the binder-disintegrant starches in the preparation of tablets by direct compression. Three samples of ground hypochlorite-bleached native cornstarch (starch A) having the properties set forth in Table 1 were converted to compacted starch powders by three different techniques.

Pelletizing — One sample of the hypochlorite-bleached native cornstarch was moistened to a water content of 24 to 25% by weight and the moistened starch was pelletized at a rate of about 960 pounds/hour on a California Process Series CM-FB Master pellet mill having dies 3⁄16 inch in diameter and 1½ inches in length and operated at about 130 rpm. The resultant pellets (¼ inch length) were then dried in a rotary drier to 7.4% by weight moisture.

The dried pellets were then ground to -10 mesh in a Model DS-6 Series 1606 stainless steel Fitzmill grinder, and the -10 mesh material was further ground to -100 mesh in a Model PC 20 Strong-Scott Pulvocron grinder operated at 3,500 rpm with the classifier at 1,000 rpm and the tailings return at 100%. The resultant powder was remoistened to 11.5 to 12.5% by weight water in a horizontal ribbon blender, and the moistened material was screened to -40 mesh. The properties of the resultant compacted starch powder (starch A_p) are set forth in Table 1.

Differential Roll-Milling — The second sample of the ground hypochlorite-bleached native cornstarch was compacted, after being moistened to a water content of about 25.2% by weight, in an EEMCO Laboratory differential roll mill having 12-inch length rolls of 6 inches diameter. The mill was operated with a mill gap of 12 mils, and roll speeds of 50 and 70 linear feet/min. on the respective rolls. Roll temperature was maintained at about 23°C. by cooling water circulating through the rolls.

The compacted starch sheet stripped from the rolls was then subjected to three additional passes through the mill. The resultant compact was then dried to a moisture content of 6 to 9% by weight. The dried compact was ground first to less than about 1.0 mm. in a Wiley mill and then to less than about 0.5 mm. in a Raymond hammermill. The ground material was then remoistened with water to a moisture content of 11.8% by weight, and screened to -80 mesh. The resultant compacted starch powder (starch A_{DRM}) had the properties set forth in Table 1.

Compaction in Allis-Chalmers Compacter — The third sample of the ground hypochlorite-bleached native cornstarch was adjusted to a moisture content of 21.6% by weight and then treated using force feeding in a compacter having rolls 24 inches in diameter and 8 inches in length. The compacter was operated with the rolls at ambient temperatures, a roll gap of 0.05 inch, a roll speed of 2.5 rpm, a force feeder speed of 15 rpm and a starting bearing pressure of 1,000 psig.

The ribbonlike compact obtained was dried to 7% by weight water and then ground as in the milling above. The ground material was then adjusted to a moisture content of about 12.0% by weight, and then finally screened to -80 mesh. The properties of the resultant compacted starch powder (starch A_{AC}) are set forth in Table 1.

TABLE 1

Starch	Description	H_2O content, percent	Cold-water solubility, percent	Swelling power	Loose bulk density, gm./ml.	Flowability, angle of repose
A	Hypochlorite bleached native corn starch	10.0	0.2-0.5	1.9-2.1	0.52-0.56	44-45
A_p	Pelletized Starch A	12.4	9.2	6.6	0.57	33
A_{DRM}	Differential roll-milled starch A	11.8	13.1	6.8	0.60	31
$A_{A.C.}$	Roll mill compacted starch A	12.0	11.6	7.2	0.59	31

The data in Table 1 indicate that the three different compaction methods can each produce compacted starch powders essentially equivalent in these properties.

Superficially dry tabletting formulations were prepared by thoroughly blending the resultant compacted starch powders, each in turn, with separate powdered preparations of ascorbic acid, phenacetin, sodium p-aminosalicylate dihydrate (NaPAS) and N-acetyl-p-aminophenol (APAP) in the proportions set forth below in Table 2, incorporating talc and/or colloidal silica (Cab-o-Sil) as tabletting aids into the formulations, and screening the resultant mixtures to -40 mesh. The free-flowing powders obtained were then directly tabletted on a Colton No. 204 four-punch press.

A set of ⅜ inch diameter standard cap punches and dies was employed, and the press was operated at 35 rpm to produce 140 tablets/min. The pressure setting of the press was increased in each run to a value consistent with good press operation as indicated by a "thump" in the tabletting. A sample of each of the compacted starch powders also was tabletted using the same tabletting procedure. The properties of the tablets obtained also are set forth in Table 2.

TABLE 2

	Formulation composition					Tablet properties			
				Adjuvants, percent by weight total formulation			Average—		
	Starch binder	Drug	Drug/binder weight ratio [1]	Talc	Colloidal silica	H_2O content, percent	Hardness, kg.	Friability percent weight loss	Disintegration time, minutes
Tablet Number:									
1	A_P	....	0:100	....	....	12.4	13.7	0.08	4.5–5.0
2	A_P	Ascorbic acid	40:60	7.5	0.0128	7.3	5.9	0.19	1.5
3	A_P	Phenacetin	35:65	....	0.0092	8.4	5.9	0.44	2.5
4	A_P	APAP	40:60	6.0	0.0087	7.4	5.7	0.23	1.5
5	A_P	NaPAS	50:50	7.0	0.0096	13.3	6.4	0.39	70–80
6	A_{DRM}	....	0:100	....	....	11.8	14.0	0.12	6.5–7.0
7	A_{DRM}	Ascorbic acid	35:65	5.0	0.0082	7.7	4.5	0.37	2.0–2.5
8	A_{DRM}	Phenacetin	25:75	....	0.0091	9.1	5.4	0.35	4.0
9	A_{DRM}	APAP	25:75	3.0	0.0082	8.4	6.6	0.20	2.5–3.0
10	A_{DRM}	NaPAS	40:60	5.0	0.0082	13.3	5.8	0.51	60–90
11	A_{AC}	....	0:100	....	....	12.0	14.7	0.1	9.0–9.5
12	A_{AC}	Ascorbic acid	30:70	5.0	0.0092	8.2	6.3	0.16	3.0
13	A_{AC}	Phenacetin	30:70	....	0.0091	8.6	6.7	0.42	3.0–3.5
14	A_{AC}	APAP	30:70	3.00	0.0093	8.4	7.2	0.43	2.0
15	A_{AC}	NaPAS	35:65	3.5	0.0076	12.7	6.4	0.31	90–105

[1] Based on binder dry substance weight.

Rice Endosperm as Matrix

Good tasting, chewable tablets have been prepared by *W.E. Gaunt and M.C. Gaunt; U.S. Patent 3,629,394; December 21, 1971* from water-soluble, bad tasting drugs and vitamins. A water solution or water-alcohol solution of the bad-tasting substance is absorbed into rice endosperm using about enough solution for complete hydration or slightly less, followed by drying.

The drugs include phenothiazine tranquilizers and barbiturates and the vitamins include thiamin, niacinamide and pyridoxine. The water-soluble substance may constitute up to 60% of the finished product, with the rice endosperms, which may be previously comminuted, making up the balance. The pleasant tasting chewable tablets contain the bad tasting substance with the bad taste masked, conventional chewable tablet base constituents for the tabletting of the rice endosperm-drug particles being combined with the treated rice endosperms.

By using precooked rice, the so-called "minute" rice, the process of hydration of the rice endosperm with a water solution of a water-soluble substance can be accomplished without the application of heat, a great advantage if the water-soluble substance used is heat-sensitive. The rate of hydration of such precooked rice at room temperature is quite rapid and complete and if the proper proportion of water is used the hydrated precooked rice endosperms remain discrete entities which may be readily dried retaining within their structure the water-soluble substance, there being no migration of the water-soluble substance to the surface of the precooked rice endosperm.

Whether the regular rice endosperm or the precooked rice endosperm is used they both on fracture exhibit the same appearance under moderate magnification: the fractured surface appears glass-like and homogeneous with no evidence of crystallization of the water-soluble substance within the structure of the rice endosperm when the water-soluble substance with which the rice endosperm is loaded is a crystalline chemical entity. The rice endosperm loaded with the water-soluble substance can be easily reduced to smaller particles by suitable milling equipment to give firm, hard particles which under moderate magnification appear to be of homogeneous glass-like structure.

It has also been observed that the loading of the endosperm of precooked rice with a water-soluble substance is appreciably hastened when the temperature of the water solution is raised above room temperature. Furthermore, the rate of hydration can be hastened by milling the precooked rice into smaller particles before exposing them to the water solution of the water-soluble substance.

In addition, it has been found that aqueous-alcoholic solutions containing up to 40% (volume by volume) of methanol, ethanol or isopropanol can be used to hydrate the rice endosperm, a factor which is of advantage when the solubility of the water-soluble substance in water is limited and is greater in a water-alcohol mixture.

Particles of rice endosperm loaded with a water-soluble solid substance by the procedures described above are quite hard and resilient and cannot readily be compressed in admixture with a basic chewable tablet granulation into acceptable nongritty tablets.

It has, however, been found that the rice endosperm will admit into its structure aqueous solutions of glycerin, propylene glycol, or the lower polyethylene glycols, and on removal of the water by evaporation the glycerin, propylene glycol or lower polyethylene glycol is retained within the structure of the endosperm and imparts to it a degree of softness and flexibility. The following examples are cited to illustrate the preparation of the tablets.

Example 1: Ten grams of chlorpheniramine maleate are dissolved in 120 ml. of water to which is added 20 grams of glycerin and 60 grams of rice endosperms. The mixture is heated with gentle stirring to the boiling point, loosely covered, until all of the aqueous solution has entered into the structure of the rice endosperms (approximately 15 minutes). The loaded endosperms are removed from the container, spread on trays, dried at 60° to 65°C., ground, and screened through a 30 mesh sieve.

The dry 30 mesh granules are placed in a jacketed vessel and warmed by hot water to 60°C. Ten grams of molten acetylated monoglyceride are added with stirring. Stirring is continued as the mixture is allowed to cool, the particles of loaded rice endosperm remaining discrete, each acquiring a thin film of acetylated monoglycerides on its surface. The resulting product is again screened to remove any adventitious lumps. It contains 10% of chlorpheniramine maleate on the dry basis.

Twenty grams of the chlorpheniramine maleate preparation are blended with 400 grams of a conventional basic granulation for chewable tablets, suitably flavored and sweetened, and compressed on conventional tablet making equipment, into pleasant tasting chewable tablets of 420 mg. weight and containing in each tablet 2 mg. of chlorpheniramine maleate.

Example 2: Twenty grams of phenylephrine hydrochloride are dissolved in 100 ml. of water to which 20 grams of propylene glycol are added. The solution is stirred and to it are added 50 grams of precooked rice endosperms (minute rice). The mixture is stirred at intervals at room temperature as the solution hydrates the precooked rice endosperm.

When all of the aqueous solution has been absorbed the endosperms are spread on a drying tray at 65°C. The dry endosperms are ground in a suitable mill and screened to 30 mesh. The dry 30 mesh granules are placed in a jacketed vessel and heated to 65°C. with stirring. Ten grams of molten hydrogenated vegetable oils are added with stirring continuing as the mixture cools. The resultant product is screened to remove adventitious agglomerates and contains 20% of phenylephrine hydrochloride.

Fifty grams of the phenylephrine hydrochloride granulation are blended with 400 grams of a conventional basic granulation for chewable tablets, suitably flavored and sweetened, and compressed on conventional tablet equipment into pleasant tasting chewable tablets of 450 mg. weight and containing in each tablet 10 mg. of phenylephrine hydrochloride.

Spray Dried Starch Binder

Carrier ingredients which give rapidly disintegrating tablets formed by direct compression have also been developed by *D. Hanssen and A. Knecht; U.S. Patent 3,725,556; April 3, 1973.* The process consists of

(1) spray drying, after inert gas foaming, a suspension of
   (A) 1 to 20% by weight of very finely divided silicon dioxide or aluminum oxide and
   (B) 60 to 98% by weight of at least one fine-grained, inert filler material chosen from the group consisting of starches selected from the group consisting of substantially water-insoluble rice starch and cornstarch, and alkaline earth metal phosphates, in an aqueous solution of
   (C) 1 to 20% of a water-soluble binder,
(2) adding the active ingredient to the resulting spray dried, ungranulated tablet premix, and
(3) compressing the resulting composition, together with the active agent and a tablet lubricant, into pharmaceutical tablets.

The disintegration properties of pharmaceutical tablets prepared by this method may be further improved by using the spray dried three-component mixture described in the preceding paragraph in combination with a spray dried two-component mixture obtained by spray drying a suspension of component (A) in an aqueous solution of component (C). The quantity of the spray dried two-component mixture may amount to between 5 and 50% by weight, based on the total weight of the finished pharmaceutical tablet inclusive of the active ingredient.

The silicon dioxide or aluminum oxide used as component (A) should be in highly dispersed to colloidal form with a particle size of 10 to 100 mμ or a surface area of 10 to 500 m^2/g. Colloidal silicic acid (Aerosil) is a particularly suitable example. Component (B) is preferably provided in fine-grained form with a particle size between 10 and 20 μ.

Examples of water-soluble binders suitable for use as component (C) are water-soluble cellulose derivatives, such as hydroxyethylcellulose or carboxymethylcellulose, water-soluble starches such as amylum pectinum soluble, water-soluble plant gums such as gum arabic or tragacanth, alginates, gelatin and polyvinylpyrrolidone. The process will be further illustrated in the following example where all parts are by weight.

Example: Rapidly disintegrating pharmaceutical tablets were prepared from the following ingredients:

	Parts
Penicillin V potassium	145
Sulfadimethoxine	150
Spray dried composition (1)	558
Talcum	40
Colloidal silicic acid	20
Magnesium stearate	12

The spray dried composition (1) was prepared in the following manner from the following ingredients:

	Parts
Substantially water-insoluble rice starch	70
Colloidal silicic acid	15
Soluble starch	15

The soluble starch was dissolved in hot water, the resulting solution was cooled to about 40°C., and then the silicic acid and the rice starch were stirred in. The suspension thus obtained was spray dried in a convespray-drying tower with an entrance temperature of about 200°C. and an exit temperature of about 75°C. The tablets were made in the following manner:

The penicillin V potassium and the sulfadimethoxine were passed through a fine screen, thoroughly admixed with the other ingredients, and the resulting mixture was pressed into 925 mg. tablets with a diameter of 15 mm. with the aid of a conventional tablet making machine. Each tablet contained 145 mg. of penicillin V potassium and 150 mg. of sulfadimethoxine and completely disintegrated within 2 to 3 minutes after coming in contact with water or an aqueous liquid.

CELLULOSE BASED MATRIX MATERIAL

Rapidly Disintegrating CMC Matrix

S.A.R. Bentholm and W.E. Koenen; U.S. Patent Reissue 27,679; June 19, 1973; assigned to Akzona Incorporated have found that a very rapidly disintegrating solid dosage unit form is obtained when there is incorporated as a disintegrating agent, an alkali metal salt of carboxymethylcellulose (CMC) having a degree of polymerization between 100 and 2,000 and having a degree of substitution between 0.02 and 0.17 at polymerization degree 100, and between 0.02 and 0.57 at polymerization degree 2,000.

When these disintegrating agents are mixed with an active ingredient, together with conventional tabletting excipient binders and/or lubricants, and compressed at high pressure, they yield tablets or pills which retain their hardness and stability when stored at high relative humidities, but nevertheless disintegrate rapidly in presence of moisture. The small amount of the disintegrating required leaves additional space in the dosage unit for greater amounts of active ingredient and other substances.

The term "alkali metal salt" as used here includes the sodium, potassium, and ammonium salts of the carboxymethylcellulose. These alkali metal salts when employed as disintegrating agents in accordance with this process are especially effective in very low concentrations, ranging from 0.3 to 3% by weight, preferably 0.5 to 2%. They are far superior to all other known disintegrating agents in the same range of concentration. In the following examples a number of compositions are given, in which CMC salts have been incorporated as disintegrating agents.

Example 1: A mixture of 500 g. of acetylsalicylic acid and 100 g. of lactose were granulated with a 2% amylopectin solution. The granulate was sieved and dried, then mixed with 14 g. of Na CMC (1100/0.35 = polymerization degree/substitution degree) and 50 g. of talc, and the compressed into tablets of 700 mg. each. In the same manner tablets were prepared in which KCMC (1500/0.8), Na CMC (600/0.13) and Na CMC (1100/0.24) were incorporated as disintegrating agents in quantities of 8 g., 15 g. and 11 g., respectively.

Example 2: One gram of estriol was granulated with 24 g. of lactose and 2% amylopectin solution. This granulate was mixed with 0.5 g. of Na CMC (1250/0.28) and 2 g. of magnesium stearate, and then compressed into tablets of 250 mg. each. In the same manner tablets were prepared in which NH_4CMC (1500/0.43), KCMC (500/0.06), Na CMC (500/0.21) and Na CMC (1100/0.18) were incorporated as disintegrating agents in quantities of 0.6 g., 0.85 g., 0.7 g. and 0.6 g., respectively.

Example 3: A mixture of 50 g. of sodium bicarbonate and 50 g. of borax was granulated, sieved and dried, and then mixed with 2 g. of thymol and 2 g. of Na CMC (1400/0.38) and then tabletted. Further KCMC (1100/0.09) was used instead of Na CMC in a quantity of 2.5 g.

Granular Blends of Cellulose Derivative, Polymer and Fatty Acid Salt

Time release tablets are prepared by *A. Nakamoto, K. Ogwa and T. Ukigaya; U.S. Patent 3,629,393; December 21, 1971; assigned to Nikken Chemical Co., Ltd., Japan* including those where the active ingredient is penicillin, ethylphenylephrintheophylline, hydrocortisone, nicotinamide, butylbiguanide, and especially those compounds which are absorbed into the stomach and decomposed by gastric acids, such as penicillin G.

These are prepared by blending and compressing each of the following three types of granules: (A) granules comprising a medically active ingredient, a hydrophobic salt of a fatty acid, and a nontoxic polymer compound which is insoluble in the digestive fluids, (B) granules comprising a water-swellable, high molecular weight compound and a pharmaceutical carrier, and, (C) granules comprising a pharmaceutical carrier, and, if necessary, a medically active ingredient or a buffering agent.

The higher fatty acid salt used in granule (A) is preferably a salt of stearic acid, palmitic acid, oleic acid, or the like. Applicable metals for formation of the above salt include magnesium, calcium, aluminum. Suitable polymers which are insoluble in the digestive fluids include the vinyl polymers, such as polyvinyl acetate, polyvinylpyrrolidone; the methacrylic resins, such as polymethyl methacrylate; and the cellulose derivatives, such as cellulose acetate-phthalate.

The high molecular weight water-swellable compound used in granule (B) is preferably hydroxypropylcellulose, hydroxypropylmethylcellulose, sodium carboxymethylcellulose, gum arabic, sodium alginate, or the like. Any pharmaceutical carrier which is easily disintegratable may be used in granule (C) to provide release control or buffering. Suitable carriers include starch, lactose, calcium carbonate, calcium phosphate, sugar, glucose and the like.

Good results are obtainable when the ratio of granules (A), granules (B) and granules (C) is between 2 to (0.5 to 2) to (0.5 to 2). Where the proportions of granules (A) or granules (B) is increased, the speed of release becomes too slow. On the other hand, where the ratio of granules (C) is increased, the speed of release becomes too fast. The ratio of the three types of granules should be selected depending upon the required period of release time. The tablet of this process should be shaped by compression so as to have a hardness of 0.5 to 7 kg. In the following example, all parts are by weight, unless otherwise specified.

Example: 150 grams of potassium penicillin G were mixed with 120 grams of magnesium stearate and 100 grams of 30 weight percent solution of polyvinyl acetate in trichloroethane were added and the mixture was kneaded and passed through JIS 20 mesh sieves. After drying at 40° to 50°C., the mixture was granulated into particles having a size range of 18 to 24 meshes, (A).

Meanwhile 75 grams of calcium carbonate, 60 grams of starch, and 15 grams of hydroxypropylcellulose were mixed and kneaded after addition of trichloroethane and granulated with a JIS 20 mesh sieve in a manner similar to the above described procedure, (B).

The granules produced were mixed in a proportion of 30 grams of granule (A), 14.7 grams of granule (B), and 15 grams of granule (C), 0.3 gram of magnesium stearate was added as a lubricant. The mixture was compressed into tablets having a weight of 0.6 gram each.

Each tablet produced contains 150 mg. of penicillin G (potassium). The results of the time releasing tests conducted at 37.5°C. for the above tablets are shown in the table below. Artificial digestive fluids having a pH of 1.2 was employed for the initial first hour, whereas digestive fluids having a pH of 6.0 was employed for subsequent hours in the test.

Time Passed (hrs.)	Amount of Ingredient Released, %
1	26.0
2	47.6
4	69.8
6	85.5
8	94.6
10	100

Calcium Sulfate-Cellulose Derivative Matrix Blend

Most former sustained release tablets have been prepared by granulating the medicament, the water-insoluble retardant agent and the diluents with a solvent until granular aggregates form, screening the wet mass, drying it, and then tabletting. Tablets formed in this manner have been deficient in that they require a large amount of water retardant agent to maintain a tablet which will not disintegrate when exposed to gastric or intestinal fluids. This excess of retardant prevents the release of pharmaceutically desirable amounts of the drug in the early stages of medication. Reduction of the amount of water-retardant agent, however, has caused rapid disintegration of these tablets thus eliminating the sustained release function of this dosage form.

S.S. Kornblum; U.S. Patent 3,632,739; January 4, 1972; assigned to Sandoz-Wander, Inc. has disclosed a sustained release pharmaceutical tablet, prepared by dissolving the medicament and a retardant agent in a solvent, forming a slurry of the solution and a carrier, spray drying the slurry and tabletting the resultant free flowing powder.

The water-insoluble retardant agent is resistant to disintegration in the gastrointestinal tract and provides for a gradual release of the medicament in the tract. Among the water-insoluble pharmaceutically acceptable retardant agents which may be used either alone or in combination are ethylcellulose, methylcellulose, polyvinyl chloride, fatty acids, polyvinyl alcohols, hydroxypropylcellulose, fatty alcohols, shellac, vinyl acetate resins and the like. The amount of the water-insoluble retardant agent used is from 2.5 to 7.0% w./w. preferably 2.5 to 5.5% w./w. of the spray dried powder. This has been found to give a pharmaceutically acceptable sustained release of the drug for periods in excess of 5 hours, without appreciable disintegration of the tablet.

Water-insoluble carriers such as calcium sulfate and dicalcium phosphate may be used in the formulations but they must be nontoxic and inert to the other ingredients of the preparation. They provide a nucleus or center, upon which the drug and retardant agent may be carried, so as to form a tablet of acceptable size and weight. The solvent used must be a solvent for both the drug and the water retardant agent, so that upon evaporation during spray drying the carrier surface will be coated with the drug and water retardant agent.

By using this process, sustained release tablets can be prepared which have both a pharmaceutically acceptable first hour release rate of 40 to 45%, and a high resistance to disintegration (5 or more hours) in the gastrointestinal tract. This is achieved with a substantial and unobvious reduction in the amount of retardant agent necessary to achieve the sustained release action by former methods.

Example: Sustained release medicaments containing the following composition of ingredients (Formulation A) were prepared: isobutylallylbarbituric acid, 24.0%; ethylcellulose, low viscosity, 4.5%; methylcellulose 60 HG, 50 cp., 1.0%; calcium sulfate dihydrate, 65.6% and alginic acid 4.9%. Tablets were prepared from Formulation A containing per tablet: isobutylallylbarbituric acid spray dried powder, 250.0 mg. and magnesium stearate, 5.0 mg. The procedure for preparing Formulation A is as follows:

The isobutylallylbarbituric acid and ethylcellulose were placed in a stainless steel vessel containing 1,000 ml. of special denatured alcohol (90% ethanol; 10% methanol). A propeller-type mixer was used to stir until the solids were dissolved. Gentle heat may be employed. In another vessel, 200 ml. of purified water was heated to boiling and the methylcellulose 60 HG, 50 cp., slowly added to the vortex formed by the propeller mixer until the synthetic gum was completely dispersed. The hydrated methylcellulose was then slowly added to the alcoholic solution. Finally, the calcium sulfate dihydrate and alginic acid were added and mixed until a uniform smooth slurry was obtained.

A portable laboratory spray dryer having a centrifugal atomizing wheel functioning from air turbine drive with a velocity of about 40,000 rpm was used. The heated chamber of the dryer was kept at 150° to 160°C. and the outlet temperature at 90° to 100°C. The slurry was fed to the atomizing wheel using a pump which maintained the flow at the rate of 45 g./min. A cyclone collector was used to separate the spray dried powder from the solvent. The spray dried powder was blended with the magnesium stearate and compressed into tablets using a single-station machine (Stokes E Tablet Press) employing 8 mm. flat, bevel-edge punches.

Compounded Ethylcellulose Matrix

S.F. Jeffries; U.S. Patent 3,362,880; January 9, 1968; assigned to The Dow Chemical Co. has found that a highly desirable pharmaceutical preparation of the type containing a large proportion of an active ingredient can be made in the following manner:

(1) dry mix the active ingredient with an ethylcellulose: wet the dry mixture with alcohol; remove the alcohol from the mixture;

(2) make the foregoing mixture part of an aqueous granulation which may contain one or more additional therapeutic agents in addition to tragacanth, glyceryl monostearate and gum karaya; blend, dry, and sieve the aqueous granulation;

(3) coat the sieved material with an alcoholic solution of an ethylcellulose; dry the coated material;

(4) blend the coated material with running powders consisting of talc and magnesium stearate and compress the blend into tablets.

The foregoing composition in compressed tablet form provides a long-sustained therapeutic action of three and one-half to eight hours or more. Generally, this compressed tablet serves as a part of a composite tablet, either as a core which is further press-coated or as an initial layer which is compressed together with an additional composition to form a multilayer tablet in which at least an edge of each layer is exposed.

Suitable active major ingredients include aspirin; p-hydroxyacetanilide; binary mixtures of aspirin and p-hydroxyacetanilide; a mixture of aspirin, acetophenetidin and caffeine; a salicylate; a simple inorganic bromide; ascorbic acid; and physiologically compatible mixtures thereof. The acetylsalicylic acid and p-hydroxyacetanilide or other active major ingredients used in this process are customarily available in commercial quantities in particle sizes in the range passing a No. 20 to a No. 40 sieve, though finer powder grades may be used, if desired.

The ethylcellulose used is an organo-soluble, ethyl ether of cellulose. Any of the commercially available celluloses can be used which have an ethoxyl content of from 2.2 to 2.6 ethoxyl groups per anhydroglucose unit. This corresponds to an ethoxy range of about 45 to 49.5% weight. While both high and low viscosity types of ethylcellulose work, the medium viscosity types are to be preferred in making the preparation of the process.

In addition to the active ingredient employed in major proportions, the composition may include smaller proportions of therapeutic agents normally employed in lesser amounts. For example, it is often desirable to include decongestants and/or antihistamines with analgesics such as salicylate, aspirin, or p-hydroxyacetanilide. Examples of suitable decongestants are: phenylpropanolamine hydrochloride, pseudoepinephrine hydrochloride, cyclopentamine hydrochloride and phenylephrine hydrochloride. Examples of suitable antihistamines include pyrilamine, phenyltoloxamine citrate, prophenpyridamine maleate and chlorpheniramine maleate.

Example: As an example of the composition and process, 18 grams of acetylsalicylic acid in a granular form passing a No. 40 sieve, was dry mixed with an ethylcellulose having a viscosity of 23 cp. The dry, analgesic mixture was wetted with 9 ml. of denatured alcohol and mixed. The acetylsalicylic acid-ethylcellulose mixture was then dried with a stream of forced air at room temperature and sieved. Then 0.8333 gram of phenylephrine hydrochloride, USP, and 0.1333 gram of chlorpheniramine maleate, NF, were dissolved in about 7 ml. of water.

Two grams of tragacanth powder, USP, were admixed with the so-formed aqueous solution. Then 8 grams of glyceryl monostearate (Aldo 72) were mixed thoroughly into the aqueous mass, followed by 8 grams of karaya gum, NF. Upon completion of the addition of the karaya gum, the wet mass became a homogenous dough. The dough was added to the dried acetylsalicylic acid-ethyl cellulose mixture. The resulting mixture was thoroughly blended and allowed to dry overnight at room temperature. The dried mixture, granular in form, was then forced through a No. 16 sieve (U.S. Sieve Series) and dried for about an hour at 40°C. The dried granules were then coated with an alcoholic solution of ethylcellulose. The solution consisted of 0.5835 gram of an ethylcellulose, of a grade having a viscosity of 23 cp., dissolved in about 7 to 10 ml. of denatured alcohol.

The so-coated granules were dried with a stream of forced air at room temperature and then sieved through a No. 16 sieve before being blended with 0.395 gram of talc powder, USP, and 0.1 gram magnesium stearate powder, USP, and slugged at relatively high pressure in a conventional tabletting machine. The slugs were broken down by being passed through a No. 16 sieve. The screened material was blended with an additional 0.395 gram of talc powder, USP, and 0.1 gram of magnesium stearate powder, USP, and compressed into tablets on a standard tabletting machine to form 100 tablets, each weighing about 405 mg.

These tablets were tested according to a modified USP tablet disintegration test in which the test machine was regulated to oscillate 41 times per minute instead of 30 times per minute. In this test procedure, the tablets exhibited disintegration times of about 6 to 8 hours in either simulated gastric juice or artificial intestinal fluid. The composition of these sustained release tablets is as follows:

	Percent
Acetylsalicylic acid	44.4
Ethylcellulose	6.38
Phenylephrine HCl, USP	2.05
Chlorpheniramine maleate, NF	0.33
Tragacanth powder, USP	4.93
Glyceryl monostearate	19.73
Karaya gum, NF	19.73
Talc, USP	1.95
Magnesium stearate, USP	0.5

Cellulose Ether-Polymer Mixtures

Sustained release tablets for oral administration have been prepared by a process disclosed by *K. Eberhardt and H. Röthing; U.S. Patent 3,362,881; January 9, 1968; assigned to*

Boehringer Ingelheim GmbH, Germany. The active ingredient is first mixed with one or more gel-forming swelling agents and also with a water-insoluble polymer or film-forming agent in the presence of an organic solvent or organic solvent mixture in which the active ingredient is insoluble. The mixture is then pressed into tablet cores in the conventional manner. A particularly favorable embodiment of the process consists of first mixing the active ingredient and swelling agents, then granulating the mixture with a solution of the water-insoluble polymer or film former in the organic solvent or solvent mixture, and finally processing the granulate into pill cores in customary fashion.

The swelling agents which may be used are substances which swell and form a gel upon contact with water. Specific examples of such swelling agents are: cellulose ethers, such as carboxymethylcellulose (CMC), methylcellulose, hydroxyethylcellulose; polyacrylic acid (Carbopol 934); sodium alginate and pectin. Particularly preferred is the use of carboxymethylcellulose (sodium salt) and polyacrylic acid.

As water-insoluble polymers, polyvinyl acetate of medium viscosity is preferred. A suitable film-forming agent is cellulose acetate phthalate (CAP), which is used preferably in admixture with stearic acid. Other macromolecular substances with similar characteristics may also be used.

The amount of swelling agents in the sustained release composition may vary between 50 to 500% by weight, based on the weight of active ingredient, whereas the total weight of polymers and film-forming agents may vary between 10 and 50% by weight. By appropriate choice of the quantitative ratios of active ingredient, swelling agents and polymer or film-forming agent, the period of sustained release may be varied within wide limits. When a high initial release dose is desired, additional active ingredient may be applied or pressed, in the customary manner, onto the tablet cores obtained by the above process.

The selection of a suitable organic solvent or solvent mixture depends upon the particular active ingredient used which has to be insoluble, and further depends upon the nature of the water-insoluble polymer or film former, which has to be soluble in the solvent. Examples of suitable solvents are acetone, ethyl acetate and tetrahydrofuran. Also, a mixture of 90 parts of chloroform and 10 parts of isopropanol may be used to good advantage.

According to this process, sustained release tablets may be prepared even from those active therapeutic ingredients where all other methods have completely failed. For instance, no method has heretofore been found by which sustained release tablets could be obtained from which the antitussive, easily water-soluble 1-p-chlorophenyl-2,3-dimethyl-4-dimethylaminobutanol-(2) hydrochloride is sufficiently slowly released.

With this process, however, tablets may be prepared with these active ingredients from which the active ingredient is gradually and uniformly released over a period of 6 to 12 hours; the rate of release may be increased within wide limits by increasing the content of swelling agent, or it may be reduced by increasing the content of water-insoluble polymers or film formers.

Example: 100 g. of 1-p-chlorophenyl-2,3-dimethyl-4-dimethylaminobutanol-(2) hydrochloride were admixed with 140 g. of pulverized highly viscous carboxymethylcellulose and 30 g. of polyvinyl acetate of medium viscosity. The mixture was thoroughly kneaded in 80 ml. of acetone; the moist mass was dried at a temperature of 40°C. and the dry mixture was pulverized with the aid of a conventional pulverizer.

From the pulverized mass thus obtained, 1,000 pill cores were pressed, each having a weight of 270 mg. and a diameter of 9.5 mm. The pill cores, upon being tested for release rate of the active ingredient in distilled water at a temperature of 37°C., produced an initial release (measured after 1½ hours) of about 25% of the total amount of active ingredient. The remaining amount of the active ingredient was released at a uniform rate over a period of 7½ hours which is independent of the pressure with which the dried mixture is formed into pills, e.g., 7½ hours at either 11 or 5 kg. (Monsanto hardness test).

OTHER TABLET MATRIX MATERIALS

EFFERVESCENT MATRIX MATERIALS

Three-Step Granulation

In the customary manufacture of effervescent tablets, the effervescent mixture is prepared by mixing the alkaline bicarbonate in the dry state with the aliphatic polycarboxylic acid in the form of a powder and a variable amount of water is vaporized onto the mixture obtained in order to granulate it. The grains obtained are dried in a thin layer on sieves in an oven for a period of time varying from 2 to 3 hours according to the relative moisture content inside this oven.

The effervescent mixture is then added to the active mixture and again dried in a thin layer on sieves in an oven for 11 hours and finally made into tablets. It was found that in the granulation of the effervescent mixture by humidification, a chemical reaction takes place between the acid and the bicarbonate with the liberation of carbon dioxide gas leading to the swelling of the grains and with the formation of water which further accelerates the reaction. Due to this, it is absolutely necessary to stop this chemical reaction as soon as possible in order to limit the deterioration of the effervescent mixture.

The method developed by *G. Gergely; U.S. Patent 3,773,922; November 20, 1973; assigned to Societe Francaise de Developpement et de Recherche Sofrader, France* comprises the granulation of the effervescent mixture, possibly containing the medicine, in three main stages:

(1) the humidification of the effervescent mixture possibly containing the medicine, or of one of the constituents of the mixture by a quantity of water less than 1% by weight with respect to the alkaline bicarbonate, in order to initiate the chemical reaction between the alkaline bicarbonate and the citric acid in the presence of moisture with the liberation of carbon dioxide gas and the formation tion of water;

(2) the predrying of the humidified mixture, in a fluidized bed, by hot air, the temperature of which does not exceed 60°C. and the moisture content of which does not exceed 5 g./m.^{3} by a sequence of short drying operations each of 4 to 8 minutes by varying the speed of flow of the drying air in each operation from a maximum of approximately 6 to 8 m./sec. to 0 m./sec. at the end of the operation, and this is an order to stop the chemical reaction;

(3) the final drying of the granulated mixture, in a fluidized bed, by hot air, the temperature of which does not exceed 60°C. and the moisture content of which does not exceed 5 g./m.^{3} at the maximum speed of flow of the drying air until the residual content of water of the granules is less than 0.25% by weight, preferably comprised between 0.05 and 0.15%.

Generally, the overall duration of the predrying and of the final drying is from 25 to 30 minutes approximately (whereas, in the customary process, the duration of drying of the effervescent mixture is approximately 11 hours) such that the chemical reaction is quickly stopped. The effervescent mixture is then combined with the active mixture prepared separately and the final mixture is immediately made into tablets, without any necessity to dry it again. The tablet obtained dissolves in water very quickly (40 seconds to 1 minute). The process is illustrated by the following example.

Example: In this example, the manufacture of effervescent tablets of vitaminized aspirin having the following formula of an effervescent tablet weighing 3.50 grams is described.

	Grams
Acetylsalicylic acid	0.330
Ascorbic acid	0.200
Glycocoll	0.100
Sodium bicarbonate	1.743
Anhydrous citric acid	1.079
Sodium benzoate	0.048

The effervescent mixture is firstly prepared as follows, from the following ingredients:

	Kilograms
Glycocoll (binding agent)	7.500
Sodium bicarbonate	130.725
Anhydrous citric acid	80.925

These ingredients having been previously passed through a sieve having a mesh size of 2 mm. The sodium bicarbonate is introduced into a mixer of the Lodige FKM 600 D type equipped with antideposit blades and the apparatus is started for 1 minute then 1,125 ml. of demineralized water is sprayed in; then, the mixer is stopped and the citric acid and glycocoll are poured in, then the mixer is restarted for 3 minutes. The powdery mixture becomes compact. It is removed into a carrier and dried.

Solvent Treatment of Effervescent Tablets

Effervescent tablets having improved hardness and friability without reduction of solubility have been prepared by a process disclosed by *W.H. Schmitt; U.S. Patent 3,653,914; April 4, 1972; assigned to Alberto-Culver Company*. These tablets, formed by molding or compressing a matrix free of water insoluble polymers, are contacted with a volatile organic solvent in which one or more materials comprising the tablet are at least partially soluble. The volatile solvent is removed causing the organic solvent solubilized material to be redeposited in situ. This causes an increase in the hardness and a decrease in the friability characteristics of the tablet.

In practice, where compressed or molded tablets are contacted with volatile organic solvents, any of various techniques, including dipping, spraying, or the like, may be employed. Dipping of the tablets can conveniently be accomplished by placing a quantity of tablets on a screen and immersing them in a vessel containing the organic solvent for a time sufficient to permit the organic solvent to enter the tablet matrix. The screen, with the solvent containing tablets, can then be removed from the vessel, the excess organic solvent allowed to drain away, or, more desirably from a time-saving standpoint, the tablets can be subjected to an air stream to evaporate the excess organic solvent, and then heated to remove the organic solvent from the tablets and to dry them.

The length of time that the tablets are permitted to remain in contact with the organic solvent is variable. Generally speaking, it will not be necessary that the contact time exceed 1 or 2 minutes, generally less than 1 minute, commonly 5 to 10 seconds. In any event, the tablets should be permitted to remain in contact with the organic solvent for a time sufficient to allow the tablets to become saturated, or nearly so, with the organic solvent, but not for a time such that erosion or breakdown of the tablet structure occurs.

The volatile organic solvents used can be selected from a wide group. The uppermost considerations in the choice of such organic solvent, are that it be a solvent, or at least a partial solvent, for at least one of the ingredients comprising the tablets, that it be compatible with essentially all of the ingredients of the tablet, and that it be capable of reasonably ready removal, as by heating, from the tablets. Illustrative examples of organic solvents having utility in the practice of the method of this process are ethanol, 2-propanol, 1-butanol, propan-1,3-diol, amyl alcohol, ethyl ether, methylal, acetone, diacetone alcohol, and the like, as well as mixed solvents. The following example illustrates the preparation of improved tablets by this process.

Example:

Effervescent Molded Triturate Tablet

Ingredients	Parts
Citric acid powder	500
Sodium bicarbonate powder	655
Ethanol	25
Chloroform	150

The citric acid and sodium bicarbonate were triturated with the mixture of the ethanol and chloroform and the triturated mixture was molded on a Colton 720 power triturate machine to produce tablets 0.250 inch diameter, 0.140 inch thick, 125 mg. each, which were then dried at 80°C. A number of the tablets was placed on a wire mesh screen and dipped in 2-propanol/chloroform solution, 1:1 (V:V), for 5 seconds, drained and dried at 80°C. to remove the organic solvents.

Tablets	Strong-Cobb* Hardness, kg.	Friability,** % Loss	Dissolution in Still 2° to 4°C. Water, sec.
Untreated	0.5 - 1	19	7.5
Solvent treated	2 - 3	3.5	10

*This is a device which subjects the tablet to increasing pressure by pressing on the top of a tablet on an anvil, hardness being indicated by a measure of the pressure required to fracture the tablet.

**This is measured by a so-called Friabiliator in which a standard number of tablets is subjected to 25 six-inch falls per minute for a total of 4 minutes, friability being expressed as % loss of weight from the starting weight. The test measures the integrity of the tablet or resistance to dusting on shipping and handling.

The untreated tablets could not be satisfactorily handled or packaged. The solvent treated tablets were firm and resisted abrasion. The dissolution times were not markedly different.

PROTEIN AND GUM TABLETTING MATERIALS

Thiolated Gelatin

R.H. Johnson and E.L. Rowe; U.S. Patent 3,574,820; April 13, 1971; assigned to The Upjohn Company have described a dry solid medicinal dosage form comprising a medicinal agent, the reaction product of gelatin with N-acetylhomocysteine thiolactone having an average molecular weight of 10,000 to 500,000 and having an average of 3.5 to 30 –SH equivalents per 100,000 grams and accelerating agent and one or both of a nondigestible hydrophilic colloid and a water-soluble mineral acid salt. The dosage form containing the reaction product of gelatin with N-acetylhomocysteine thiolactone in the unpolymerized form, i.e., the product is not cross-linked and contains free sulfhydryl groups. The thiolated gelatin can be prepared by reacting a thiolactone, e.g., N-acetylhomocysteine thiolactone, with gelatin whereby free sulfhydryl groups (–SH) are attached through peptide bonds to the gelatin. The preparation can be accomplished in accordance with the method of Benesch and Benesch, *Proc. of Natl. Acad. Sci. U.S.*, 55 (9) 848 to 853, September 1958. The thiolated gelatin can comprise from 5 to 90% wt./wt. of the dry solid medicinal dosage forms.

Suitable accelerating agents are pharmacologically acceptable oxidizing agents, e.g., potassium iodate, cupric sulfate, ferric ammonium sulfate, dehydroascorbic acid, and iodosobenzoic acid; and bases, e.g., tribasic sodium phosphate and dibasic calcium phosphate. The accelerating agent can comprise both an oxidizing agent and a base and can be from 0.1 to 20% wt./wt. of the dosage form. The medicinal ingredient can be any therapeutic agent which is suitably administered orally or by pellet implant (parenterally) as well as agents usefully administered by suppository. Antibiotics, anticholinergics, tranquilizers, sedatives, steroids, antihistamines, vitamins, hematinics, anorexigenics and analgesics are advantageously administered by means of the dosage forms of the process.

The first ingredient, whose addition results in an improved tablet is a nondigestible hydrophilic colloid, for example, naturally occurring gums and polysaccharides such as sodium alginate, carrageenin, guar gum, pectin, pectic acid, and locust bean gum; clays; synthetic polymers such as styrene-maleic acid copolymer, polyvinylpyrrolidone, irradiated polyoxymethylene, polyvinyl methylether maleic anhydride and carboxypolymethylene; and cellulose and derivatives thereof. Mixtures of two or more colloids can be used, for example, sodium alginate and carboxypolymethylene are a preferred combination. The nondigestible hydrophilic colloid can be up to 90% wt./wt. of the dosage form with a preferred range of 5 to 70%.

The second ingredient whose addition results in an improved tablet is a pharmacologically acceptable water-soluble salt of a mineral acid having a cation selected from alkali metal and ammonium ions. Suitable salts are, for example, the chlorides, nitrates, iodides, sulfates, carbonates and bicarbonates of sodium, potassium and ammonia. Sodium chloride is preferred. The salt is present in 8 to 60% wt./wt. of the dosage form. It is also preferred that the salt pass a 20 to 200 mesh screen.

Example: 5,000 tablets are prepared from the following types and amounts of ingredients:

	Grams
Thiolated gelatin (12 to 13 –SH/10^5 gram)	500.0
Cupric sulfate	7.5
Sodium alginate	750.0
Carboxypolymethylene	325.0
Tetracycline hydrochloride	1,375.0
Sodium chloride	500.0
Magnesium stearate	40.0

The ingredients are mixed together and pressed into tablets. The tablets so prepared when swallowed orally, wet and swell rapidly in the stomach, remain in the stomach, and release tetracycline to the gastric fluids for a sustained period of time.

Collagen Fibril Matrix

J. Nichols; U.S. Patent 3,435,110; March 25, 1969; assigned to Ethicon, Incorporated has discovered that if collagen is present in a pharmaceutical tablettizing composition, it facilitates the break-up or disintegration of the tablet after administration and provides a matrix for the efficient release of the active pharmaceutical from the tablet. It is preferred to use collagen that has been processed to remove impurities that are associated with collagen in its native state. Collagen swells rapidly at the pH normally present in the stomach, thus rupturing the tablet and forming a gel-like network or matrix of interwining swollen collagen fibrils that occlude the active pharmaceutical. Thus, the active pharmaceutical that is close to the surface of the collagen matrix is almost immediately available and that portion of the active compound that is trapped deep within the collagen matrix will diffuse out slowly.

Tanning the collagen that is present in pharmaceutical compositions provides another means of controlling and prolonging the release of the active ingredients. Collagen that has been tanned with formaldehyde, or higher aldehydes such as acetaldehyde, glyoxol pyruvic aldehyde, glutaraldehyde, dialdehyde starch; or equivalent tanning agents, such as quinones, hydroquinones, dimethylol acetone, or divinyl sulfone, will not swell in acid solutions but is attacked by the enzymes that are present in the gastrointestinal tract at a rate that is dependent upon the tanning agent and the extent to which the collagen is tanned.

A long acting dosage formula can be conveniently prepared by compounding a pharmaceutical with untanned collagen and subsequently tanning various portions of the collagen-pharmaceutical mixture under different conditions to alter the rate at which collagen is absorbed in the gastrointestinal tract. The ultimate tablet is then formulated to contain the collagen-pharmaceutical composition in combination with controlled amounts of compositions containing the pharmaceutical and collagen that has been tanned to provide different digestive rates.

Yet another convenient and effective method of preparing a long acting dosage form is to coat a pharmaceutical tablet with a film of collagen in conventional pill-coating apparatus. The collagen coating may, if desired, be tanned to the extent that is calculated to produce the desired rate of release of the pharmaceutical, and the collagen coated tablet is subsequently coated with the pharmaceutical to provide a pharmaceutical layer overlaying the collagen coating. The product so obtained is then coated again with collagen and the outer layer of collagen may be tanned. In this manner successive alternate layers of the active pharmaceutical material and collagen may be built up to provide a dosage form that will release the pharmaceutical over a period of 10 to 12 hours. In the following examples all parts are expressed in parts by weight unless otherwise indicated.

Example 1: To 1,000 parts of a mass of swollen collagen fibrils prepared as described in Example 1 of U.S. Patent 3,123,482 is slowly added with stirring 8.8 parts of dextroamphetamine sulfate, the resulting mixture is thoroughly homogenized to obtain complete distribution of the pharmaceutical throughout the viscous mass of swollen collagen fibrils, the mixture is filtered through a 7 mil filter screen, and spray dried. The dried powder is screened and formed into 50 mg. tablets. Such tablets containing dextroamphetamine sulfate and collagen have utility as an appetite depressant; the collagen swelling several hundred times in volume under the acid condition present in the stomach to provide bulk and slow release of the dextroamphetamine sulfate.

Example 2: A first portion of the dried powder of Example 1 above, prior to tabletting, is entrained in a warm air stream containing 10 ppm formaldehyde. The temperature of the air stream is maintained at 50° to 60°C. and the dried powder is in contact with the formaldehyde vapor for 5 minutes.

A second portion of the dried powder of Example 1 above, prior to tabletting is entrained in a warm air stream containing 20 ppm formaldehyde. The temperature of the air stream is maintained at 50° to 60°C. and the dried powder is in contact with the formaldehyde vapor for 5 minutes.

To 15 parts of the powder described in this example that was tanned in an atmosphere containing 10 ppm formaldehyde and 15 parts of the powder of this example that was tanned in an atmosphere containing 20 ppm formaldehyde is added 15 parts of the powder described in Example 1 above. This mixture of three collagen-pharmaceutical polymers is mixed thoroughly in a conventional paddle mixer, screened, dried in a current of warm air and reduced in particle size to pass a 100 mesh screen. The resulting product is formed into 75 mg. tablets on conventional tablet-forming apparatus, these tablets provide a slow release of dextroamphetamine sulfate over a period of time and are useful as appetite depressants.

Guar Gum-Skim Milk Blend

Troches are prepared by *G.L. Christenson and H.E. Huber; U.S. Patent 3,590,117; June 29, 1971; assigned to Richardson-Merrell Incorporated* which provide a vehicle for various medicaments used in treating the oral cavity or for sublingual or transbuccal administration lasting for periods of one-half to eight hours or more, and preferably for at least one or two hours.

It was found that a troche containing dry skim milk powder and guar gum has a long-lasting dissolution time together with uniform dissolution without the objectionable features of the prior formulations. Experiments have shown that the addition of guar gum to various levels of dry skim milk powder resulted in a two to three-fold increase in total dissolution time.

Generally, the dissolution time is dependent on the percentage of dry skim milk powder incorporated in the troche, i.e., the dissolution time is longer when a larger percentage of dry skim milk powder is in the troche. It was further found, however, that a relatively small amount of guar gum synergistically increases the troche dissolution time by an amount greater than the sum of dissolution times for troches made with corresponding levels of the guar gum and no dry skim milk powder, or dry skim milk powder and no guar gum. The hardness of such troches is within a desirable level and in excess of 4 kg. as measured on a Pfizer hardness tester.

These troches contain from 3 to 6% of guar gum and from 15 to 85% of dry skim milk powder and preferably from 4 to 6% of guar gum and 30 to 75% of dry skim milk powder. The remainder of the troche can be a conventional water-soluble tablet diluent or base, preferably including minor quantities of a medicament and conventional pharmaceutical tabletting excipients such as lubricants, dyes and flavoring agents. The guar gum, dry skim milk powder, and the water-soluble tablet diluent are in finely divided powdery form, which is compressed into a troche.

The compressed troches can be made by either wet or dry granulation methods. Heat or moisture labile compounds can thus be included in the formulations and handled in a manner to maintain the compounds' integrity. The bland powders used as the troche matrix are readily flavored with a wide variety of fragrances to meet the varying products needs.

The medicaments used in the troche are preferably those which are useful in treating the oral cavity by sublingual or transbuccal administration. The medicament can be powdered or can be absorbed on the various powdered ingredients of the troche. Examples of drugs that may be used in these troches are: antiseptics such as thymol, phenol, cresols, hexachlorophene; quaternary ammonium compounds such as cetylpyridinium chloride; iodoforms and benzoic acid and its derivatives; antibiotics; corticosteroids; anesthetics; fluorides such as sodium fluoride; oxygenating agents such as potassium peroxymonosulfate and urea peroxide; antispasmodics and antinauseants such as dicyclomine; vitamins; anorexics such as diethylpropion; blood clearing and regulating agents such as heparin; and enzymes such as lipase. The quantity of medicament in the troche can vary from 0.05 to 15% of the troche and preferably 0.2 to 5%.

Example:

A

	500 Troches, g.
Guar gum (4%)	35.0
Dry skim milk powder (17%)	148.0

(continued)

	500 Troches, g.
Hydrocortisone	0.5
Cortisone	0.5
Cetylpyridinium chloride	2.5
Mannitol	614.8

B

Flavor	8.7
Talc	30.0
Carbowax 6000	30.0

Mix A powders in a suitable mixer and add sufficient deionized water to make a wet granulation. Dry the granulation in an oven at 120°F. to between 2 and 4% moisture. Pass the dried granulation through a No. 12 screen on an oscillator. Add B powders and mix well. Compress the mixture on a Stokes or suitable tabletting machine at approximately 4,000 psi into 1.74 gram troches with ¾ inch flat faced beveled punches.

Blended Gum Matrix

A sustained release tablet has been developed by *K.R. Klippel; U.S. Patent 3,558,768; January 26, 1971; assigned to Sterling Drug Incorporated* which is composed of a core comprising a medicament in a matrix of a compressed blend of a synthetic gum of the cellulose ether type, preferably methylcellulose, and corn protein, for example zein, and a shell comprising a medicament distributed in a matrix of a compressed blend of a synthetic gum of the cellulose ether type, preferably methylcellulose, and at least two natural hydrophilic gums, for instance, karaya, pectin, and sodium alginate, but preferably the latter two. The active ingredient: inert material ratio in each of the core and shell separately and in the core and shell together is between 1:1 to 1:20.

The preferred embodiment contemplates methylcellulose in conjunction with zein in the core of the tablet, and methylcellulose in conjunction with pectin and sodium alginate in the shell, particularly one in which the shell comprises a blend containing methylcellulose, pectin, and sodium alginate in a weight ratio of from 1:1:1 to 1:4:4. In this embodiment the synthetic gum-natural gum blend of the shell or the synthetic gum-corn protein blend of the core represents between 25 to 75% by weight of the shell or core weight granules, respectively, and the synthetic gum:natural gum weight ratio of the shell is preferably between 1:2 to 1:8, while the synthetic gum:corn protein weight ratio of the core is preferably between 1:1 to 1:2.

Optionally a portion of the essential ingredients of the core and shell, up to one-third of the matrix by weight, can be replaced by conventional inert diluents, for example lactose, talc, sucrose, starch, and by 1 to 3% by weight of a lubricant, for example, magnesium stearate, calcium stearate, or sodium lauryl sulfate, without adversely affecting the desired result.

It is believed that the sustained release characteristics of these tablets are due to a combined action of diffusion and erosion. Thus, the shell portion when exposed to the gastrointestinal fluids, hydrates to form a mucilagenous gel barrier through which the medicament is slowly released by diffusion with concomitant erosion of the outer layer. As the gastrointestinal fluids penetrate further into the shell, more gel layer is formed around the core with the core acting as a reservoir releasing the medicament into the gel layer of the shell to maintain the overall desired release pattern of the core-shell tablet combination.

Therapeutically-active ingredients suitable in these tablet formulations include a wide variety of medicaments for example, antispasmodics; barbiturates; antihistamines; analgesics; vasopressors; vasodilators; vitamins; hormones; antibiotics; and other antiinfective, sedative, hypnotic, hypotensive, etc. drugs. The dosage of the medicaments can be varied with the percentage of the medicament ranging from 5 to 50% by weight of the finished tablet weight.

The gum blend of either the core or shell can represent as little as 20% by weight or as much as 75% of the granule weight depending upon the dosage of active material required. The synthetic gums of the cellulose ether type include, for example, methylcellulose, hydroxyethylcellulose, carboxymethylcellulose, and hydroxypropylcellulose, while the natural gums contemplated can include, for example, acacia, pectin, guar gum, psyllium, locust bean gum, sodium alginate, karaya, etc. The following example will further illustrate the process.

Example: Compressed-coated tablets containing the following ingredients on a per tablet basis were prepared using conventional wet granulation procedures.

	Mg./Tablet
Core:	
Isoproterenol HCl	15.00
Sodium bisulfite	0.75
Methylcellulose	22.50
Zein	31.50
Talcum	3.75
Sodium lauryl sulfate	1.50
	75.00
Shell:	
Isoproterenol HCl	15.00
Sodium bisulfite	2.00
Methylcellulose	11.40
Sodium alginate	41.00
Pectin	41.00
Powdered sucrose	48.00
Sodium lauryl sulfate	1.60
Calcium stearate	2.00
	162.00

The completed granulation was compressed by press coating methods into tablets each weighing 237 mg. Release was determined in simulated body fluids by a standard method using 0.084 N hydrochloric acid and pH 7.5 phosphate buffer. At periodic intervals a sample was removed and the percent of medicament released determined with the following results:

Exposure Time (at end of)	Cumulative % Released
1st hour in gastric fluid	30.5
2nd hour in intestinal fluid	46.2
3rd hour in intestinal fluid	63.7
4th hour in intestinal fluid	76.4
5th hour in intestinal fluid	86.9
6th hour in intestinal fluid	93.8
7th hour in intestinal fluid	96.9

FAT AND WAX MATRIX MATERIALS

Lipid Silica Mixture

A process developed by *I. Lippmann; U.S. Patent 3,400,197; September 3, 1968; assigned to A.H. Robins Company, Incorporated* incorporates a pharmaceutically active agent such as a drug or other medicinal agent into a matrix comprising a gel of silica contained in a lipid material. The composition so formed is then compressed into tablets or provided in other dosage forms such as capsules, powder, liquid suspension, etc.

When so administered, the tablets or other dosage forms provide sustained release of the pharmaceutically active agent over a period which may be precisely controlled by varying the matrix composition. If it is desired to provide a means for the immediate release of a fraction of the pharmaceutically active agent, the tablets or other dosage forms so provided may be utilized as cores, and an additional amount of the active agent applied over the cores in the form of a concentrated coating. The resulting coated tablet, when internally administered, provides an immediate controlled dosage of the active agent, with the remainder thereof being released at a retarded rate over the sustained period determined by the composition of the core.

The lipid materials suitable for the preparation of the matrix may be selected from fatty alcohols having 16 to 44 carbon atoms, fatty acids having 12 to 28 carbon atoms, esters derived from alcohols having 2 to 44 carbon atoms and acids having 2 to 28 carbon atoms, esters of aliphatic polyhydroxy compounds having 3 to 6 carbon atoms with fatty acids having 10 to 28 carbon atoms, esters of aliphatic polyhydroxy compounds having 3 to 6 carbon atoms with fatty acids having 10 to 28 carbon atoms where at least some of the hydroxyl groups are esterified with fatty acids containing 2 to 4 carbon atoms, and waxes. The lipid should preferably have a melting point in the range of 50° to 90°C.

Of the suitable lipids listed above, the preferred members are stearyl alcohol, cetyl alcohol, stearic acid and palmitic acid, since these materials are readily available commercially, have reproducible specifications and provide reproducible results, and are relatively inexpensive. By far the best results are obtained by using colloidal silica having a maximum ultimate particle size of 20 mμ. The minimum ultimate particle size is not critical, and in fact, superior results may be obtained by utilizing silica having an ultimate size particle as small as is practically available.

Colloidal silica has a tendency to form weak agglomerates consisting of loose clusters of particles requiring only mild energy to effect their separation. As used here, the term "ultimate particle size" denotes the size of the individual particles within the agglomerates or clusters. Commercial products having an ultimate particle size of 2 to 20 mμ have been found to be highly satisfactory. In addition to particle size, a large surface area is highly desirable. Colloidal silicas having external surface areas of from 0.1 to 3,000 m.^{2}/g. may be utilized. The preferred range is from 100 to 400 m.^{2}/g.

Although the desired ratio by weight of lipid to silica depends somewhat on the nature of the materials themselves, as well as on the nature of the medicament, a preferred range of lipid to colloidal silica ratio by weight is 3:1 to 8:1. Because the method for providing sustained release dosage units and the compositions produced thereby are not limited by the physical or chemical properties of the drugs utilized, a large number of drugs of various physical and chemical properties may be embodied therein.

The matrix material is prepared by melting the lipid and then adding the colloidal silica to the melt. The colloidal silica disperses in the melt to form an optically clear gel, the viscosity of which may be increased by increasing the colloidal silica content. The desired pharmaceutically active agent, such as a drug, is pulverized to a fine powder, desirably less than 60 mesh, and mixed into the molten gel. The mass is then congealed, cut or broken into convenient granules, and compressed into tablets, or prepared in other dosage forms. In vitro testing of the rate of drug release of the composition demonstrates a uniform release rate over a prolonged period of time. Moreover, when the experiments are repeated utilizing the same compositions, consistently precise duplications of the original results are obtained.

Example: The preparation of phenobarbital-methamphetamine tablets is as follows. A composition for preparing tablets is provided by first measuring out the following ingredients in the stated amounts:

	G./10,000 Tablets
Methamphetamine hydrochloride	67
Phenobarbital	432
Sodium phosphate, tribasic, monohydrate	225

(continued)

	G./10,000 Tablets
Cabosil M-5 (silica)	230
Stearyl alcohol	1,046
Batch weight	2,000

The first three ingredients are mixed and comminuted to a fine powder. The stearyl alcohol is melted in a Hobart bowl. The Cabosil is added to the melt. Finally the powder mixture is added to the melt. The mass is congealed by cooling. Granules are prepared by use of an oscillating granulator with a 12 mesh screen. The granules are compressed on a rotary tablet machine, using $^{11}/_{32}$" deep concave punches. Tablets are finished by conventional pan coating, and methamphetamine hydrochloride and phenobarbital are applied to the coating so that the final tablet contains $^{1}/_{3}$ the amount of these ingredients in the coating.

Wax-Like Edible Matrix Materials

A. Cavalli and L. Drekter; U.S. Patent 3,584,114; June 8, 1971; assigned to Hoffmann-La Roche Incorporated have disclosed methods for producing free flowing, directly compressible compositions from poor flowing powders by mixing the poor flowing powders into melted waxy-like edible materials such as stearic acid, Carbowax, glyceryl monostearate and the like. These compositions can, if desired, be converted into tablets with excellent properties by direct compression.

This is accomplished by melting the waxy-like material, then adding the powder with stirring until the powder is completely incorporated into the melt. Subsequently, the melt is cooled with stirring, and the product is recovered as a finely divided granular powder. The product is comminuted, if necessary, to a particle size range of which 75% is larger than 40 mesh and smaller than 16 mesh. Mesh refers to a screen mesh of the U.S. Sieve series where 40 mesh is 38.02 meshes per linear inch and 16 mesh is 14.66 meshes per linear inch.

The poor flowing powders which are improved by this method are those generally used in vitamin compositions. This method, however, can be used in other applications, e.g., drug, food or feed additives, i.e., cornstarch. The characteristics of the powders treated by this method are that they have poor flow properties, are not amenable to direct compression into tablets or are not suitable for use in direct compression processes and have a particle size distribution where over 90% is finer than 80 mesh (85.47 meshes per linear inch).

Typical powders are cornstarch, multivitamin compositions containing cornstarch and/or ferrous sulfate, ascorbic acid, calcium pantothenate, vitamin A, niacin or mixtures thereof or similar pharmaceutically acceptable or edible poor flowing, difficult to compress powders. The amount of powder used in conjunction with the waxy-like material depends upon the particular powder treated and the final composition it is in. Generally, from 65 to 95% by weight of the powder is incorporated into the composition.

The waxy-like edible materials suitable for use in this process are those which are normally used as lubricants at a rate of 0.5 to 5% by weight in vitamin or other ingestible compositions. These materials, include, for example, stearic acid, glyceryl monostearate, Carbowax or the like. Preferably stearic acid is used. The amount of waxy-like material which is effective to improve the flow and compressibility of the treated powders is critical only insofar as a sufficient quantity is used. This quantity varies with the treated powder. Thus, for example, cornstarch requires 25 to 30% by weight of stearic acid, while ascorbic acid with 2% by weight of cornstarch requires 8% by weight of stearic acid. Multivitamin compositions require varying amounts of stearic acid, e.g., from 5 to 20% depending upon the particular formulation.

Example: In preparing B complex iron tablets stearic acid is first melted, and ferrous sulfate is then added with stirring until the mixture becomes uniform. Riboflavin, niacinamide, calcium pantothenate, Brewer's yeast and cornstarch are then added with stirring until the mixture is uniform. The remaining ingredients of the formulation given below are then added with mixing. The resulting granular powder, which has excellent flow, is compressed in a conventional tabletting machine to form hard tablets.

	Parts by Weight
Ferrous sulfate exsiccated	168.00
Thiamine mononitrate crystals	5.75
Riboflavin, fine powder	5.50
90% vitamin C, granular	96.00
Niacinamide, dense grade	31.50
Calcium pantothenate	3.00
Pyridoxine HCl	0.55
Vitamin B_{12} in gelatin (0.1%)	3.75
Inositol	20.00
Methionine	25.00
Choline bitartrate	25.00
Brewer's yeast, granular	50.00
Cornstarch	33.00
Lactose	33.00
Stearic acid	40.00

Using the same formulation but adding stearic acid as a powder results in a powder which has poor flow characteristics and is unsuitable for direct compression.

Low Melting Wax Matrix

Tablets were developed by *R.A. Cain and H.J. Federici; U.S. Patent 3,402,240; Sept. 17, 1968; assigned to Chas. Pfizer & Co., Incorporated* which comprises a matrix substantially insoluble in gastric and intestinal juices, a therapeutically bland or inert filler or extender and an active therapeutic agent or agents or drugs. The matrix is constituted of such materials as carnauba wax, candelilla wax, esparto wax, or ouricury wax, which have melting points between 65° and 90°C. Other materials which can be used are spermaceti, stearic acid and other edible hard and nontoxic waxes and materials mixed with one or more of the first mentioned group of waxes to provide a matrix having a melting point between approximately 65° and 90°C. These relatively low melting point materials can be satisfactorily mixed with carnauba wax or some other high melting point wax to provide a material for the matrix having the desired melting points. Synthetic waxes such as Durawax 1032 (MP 84° to 86°C.) can also be used as the matrix. For practical purposes carnauba wax is preferred.

The filler or extender may be any of the standard materials used in making medicinal tablets, such as calcium or sodium phosphate dibasic, magnesium stearate (serving also as a lubricant in tabletting), calcium phosphate tribasic, talc, calcium oxide, calcium stearate, sodium stearate and starch and mixtures thereof as used in the making of tablets and methylcellulose (serving also as a swelling agent in the gastrointestinal tract). The following is a detailed description of the materials used and the procedure followed in preparing the tablets using the specific active ingredients referred to in the example.

(1) The selected wax, preferably carnauba, in amount of 44 lbs. and 1 oz., in powdered form, is passed through a 30 mesh screen.

(2) Calcium phosphate tribasic, in amount of 61 lbs. and 11 oz., talc 8 lbs. and 13 oz., together with the carnauba wax of step (1), are mixed in a standard mixer for 15 minutes.

(3) Glucose in amount of 8 lbs. and 13 oz. and 18,000 cc of deionized water are stirred together with a paddle to facilitate dissolving the glucose and when nearly dissolved the mixture is stirred with an electric mixer until complete solution is obtained.

(4) The glucose solution is added to the mixed dry powders in the mixer in four equal amounts with 15 minutes of stirring between each addition. If necessary, to obtain satisfactory granulation, an additional amount of deionized water may be found necessary.

(5) Mixing is continued for one and one-half hours after the last addition of the glucose solution.
(6) The moist granulation is removed from the mixer and spread on trays and partially dried in an oven at 130°F.
(7) The partially dried granulation is passed through an oscillator fitted with #6 sieve, then spread on trays and again dried in an oven at 120°F. for 4 to 5 hours until perfectly dry.
(8) Magnesium stearate in amount of 10 lbs. and 12 oz., 1 lb. and 10 oz. of methylcellulose and 9 lbs. and 4 oz. of pure triethanolamine trinitrate biphosphate are mixed to a uniform powder mixture.
(9) The dry granulation of step (7) is passed through an oscillator fitted with a #30 sieve and the uniform powder mixture of step (8) is added thereto intermittently.
(10) The granulation of step (9) is then transferred to a mixer and mixed for one hour.
(11) It is preferred to take a small portion of the granulation and convert it into tablets and make an initial assay thereof.
(12) The granulation of step (10) is then converted into tablets by the use of a standard tabletting machine, such as a Stokes Rotary Tablet Machine.

The finished tablets will comprise the matrix consisting of an aggregate of the ground carnauba wax having interconnecting voids therein, in which are embedded an intimate mixture of the active ingredient and the filler.

Example: The vasodilator, comprising triethanolamine trinitrate biphosphate, for treating angina pectoris to prevent attacks or reduce their number and severity, is administered over prolonged periods. Each of such tablets, made as described above, has the following ingredients:

	Milligrams
Carnauba wax	50.00
Magnesium stearate	12.00
Triethanolamine trinitrate biphosphate	10.00
Calcium phosphate, tribasic and talc	80.00
Methylcellulose	2.00
Glucose (binder)	10.00

The filler in the finished tablet is comprised of magnesium stearate, calcium phosphate tribasic, talc and methylcellulose, each of the first and last mentioned agents also performing another function as indicated heretofore. Each finished tablet weighs 164 mg.; is 3.2 mm. thick; has a hardness of 4 to 6 kg. (determined by a Monsanto Hardness Tester) and a diameter of 5/16". When tested for 1 hour in simulated gastric juice and then for 7 hours in simulated intestinal juice, the weight of the wax is 47 mg.; the recovered filler removed from the matrix and found in juices, 63 mg.; the active ingredient has been substantially entirely leached out and the binder has been eliminated. About 6% of the matrix has been lost but structurally it remains intact.

Low Melting Wax Additives

Delayed release tablets are disclosed by *D.C. Hess and D.J. Allen; U.S. Patent 3,487,138; December 30, 1969; assigned to Merck & Company, Incorporated* where the drug is mixed with a suitable wax or wax-like substance which will melt at a temperature at which the drug will not decompose or be adversely affected. This wax or wax-like substance is called the wax additive and preferred ones are cetyl alcohol, castor wax, glycerol monostearate, stearyl alcohol, stearic acid, beeswax and solid polyethylene glycols. Lubricants and/or flow conditioners which are conventional in the tablet art may or may not be added with further intermixing. The mixture is then compressed to form tablets containing the desired weight of the drug. The tablets are coated with a suitable film-forming material, such as methylcellulose, which is not affected either by the molten wax or by the elevated temperature at which the wax melts. This coating material should not become tacky during the subsequent heating so as to prevent agglomeration of the tablets. The coated tablets are placed for a predetermined period in a drying oven set at a temperature higher than the melting point of the wax additive. This heating causes the wax additive to soften or melt and the coating serves to preserve the shape of the tablet and to prevent agglomeration of tablets. After cooling to room temperature the tablets exhibit the desired sustained release effect.

The wax-additives should have melting points above body temperature and should be slowly soluble or disintegratable by digestion in gastrointestinal fluids. Among them are those derived from both natural and synthetic sources, including such organic compounds as hardened fats and oils, for example, animal, mineral or vegetable fats or oils, such as animal fats and hardened vegetable oils, including hydrogenated fats and oils; higher fatty alcohols and acids such as octyl, decyl, lauryl, myristyl, cetyl or stearyl.

The coating which is applied directly to the wax-additive core, in addition to the methylcellulose mentioned above, may be ethylcellulose, cellulose acetate, cellulose acetate phthalate or a substituted alkylcellulose such as hydroxypropylmethylcellulose. Other conventional coatings may be used if it is known that it will not melt or become sticky during the heating step which melts the waxy core. Sufficient coating should be applied so that it will serve to retain the shape and also prevent agglomeration of the tablets during the time that the core is molten, and for this purpose the film should be from 0.03 to 0.1 mm. thick.

The heating temperature should be slightly above the predetermined melting temperature of the wax additive and it should be sustained for a period that will assure the melting of the entire wax additive. This will generally require a minimum of 30 minutes although the tablets may be heated for as long as an overnight period. The process is illustrated by the following example.

Example: Ingredients per core tablet are as follows:

	Milligrams
Potassium chloride (granular)	1,000
Cetyl alcohol	150

The ingredients are thoroughly intermixed and compressed to form tablets containing the desired weight (1,000 mg.) of potassium chloride. A coating solution of the following composition is prepared:

	Percent
Hydroxypropylmethylcellulose	2.0
Alcohol	50.0
Chloroform to	100.0

The film coating is applied to the tablets by a continuous spraying operation well-known to those in the industry. Thirty milligrams of coating are applied to each tablet. The tablets are then placed in an oven (110°C.) for 30 minutes. The finished product is obtained by cooling the tablets to room temperature. The dissolution time of the resulting tablet in water (75 ml.) was as follows:

Time, min.	% Dissolved
30	12
60	24
90	38
120	51
150	57
180	65
210	70
240	75

Compounded Wax Additives

I.C. Robinson; U.S. Patent 3,577,514; May 4, 1971; assigned to Pfizer Incorporated has disclosed a sustained release pharmaceutical tablet containing up to 70% by weight of a medicament, 15 to 50% by weight of a hydrophobic dissolution retardant, 0.1 to 5.0% by weight of an acid-insoluble release agent and 5 to 15% by weight of a water-soluble or dispersible binder.

Various types of medicaments can be used such as antihistamines, hypoglycemics, antidepressants, coronary vasodilators, bronchodilators, sedatives, decongestants, antispasmodics, vitamins, and the antibiotics. The hydrophobic dissolution retardants, by virtue of their water insolubility, function by retarding the dissolution and diffusion of the drug from the tablet or granulates into the gastrointestinal fluid. Among the hydrophobic dissolution retardants that have been found effective are the natural and synthetic waxes, resins and plastics. Of these are preferred carnauba wax, beeswax, spermaceti, and the commercial product Sterotex K-100, which is a hydrogenated cottonseed oil.

Enteric substances, insoluble in the acidic stomach juices, are the preferred acid-insoluble release agents. Of these are preferred cellulose acetate phthalate and the other acetate phthalates; the esters of the carbohydrate polymers; and the phthalic acid derivatives of polyacrylic acid. The effect of the water-soluble or dispersible binder is to insure a uniform release of the drug. Although the binders of choice are the polyvinylpyrrolidones, acacia and other water-soluble or dispersible binders may be used. Besides the above essential ingredients other conventional tabletting ingredients may also be included in the blend. Thus, antioxidants, e.g., ascorbic acid, sodium metabisulfite; lubricants, e.g., talc, magnesium stearate and sodium lauryl sulfate; fillers, e.g., calcium diphosphate; and colorants are generally added to further improve the product.

The tablets can be prepared from the blended ingredients in the usual manner, e.g., dry blending followed by compression into tablets, or dry slugging and granulating the blended ingredients prior to compressing them into tablets, etc. The tablets may also be prepared by first wet granulating the blend with a suitable solvent or binder solution or dispersion, such as alcohol or polyvinylpyrrolidone colloidal solution.

Example: The ingredients listed below are dry blended and directly compressed into tablets on a rotary or single punch tabletting machine.

	Grams/4,000 Tablets	Milligram/Tablet
Metamine and dicalcium phosphate*	146.80	36.70 (5.25%)
Dicalcium phosphate	383.08	95.77
Light brown dye	0.52	0.13
Cab-O-Sil	8.00	2.00
Magnesium stearate	12.00	3.00
Carnauba wax	197.60	49.40 (23.5%)
Polyvinylpyrrolidone Type C	84.00	21.00 (10%)
Cellulose acetate phthalate	8.00	2.00 (0.95%)
Total weight, ca	840.00	210.00

*Representing 30% active potency, 17.5% of total blend.

144 tablets are tested in the disintegration test described in *U.S.P. XVII.* For the first hour the tablets are contacted with gastric juice and for the remaining time with intestinal juice. At the end of each hour's testing, the apparatus containing the tablets is placed in a beaker containing fresh gastrointestinal fluid. The fluid containing the dissolved drug is filtered and an aliquot is taken and quantitatively assayed by a suitable method. The quantity of drug determined to have dissolved in the total amount of gastrointestinal fluid is converted to percent of total drug contained in the aggregate of tablets by dividing with the total amount of drug represented by the aggregate of tablets, and multiplying by 100%. The pertinent results are given in the following table.

Drug Dissolution Rate

Time, hr.	Total of Metamine Released, %	Total of Metamine Released/hr., %
1*	39.0	39.0
2	50.7	11.7
3	59.9	9.2
4	71.1	11.2
5	82.2	11.1
6	92.4	10.2
7	98.9	6.5

*First hour in gastric juice; thereafter intestinal fluid.

Wax-Fat-Carbopol Matrix Blends

A. Riva; U.S. Patent 3,459,850; August 5, 1969; assigned to Dr. A. Wander, SA, Switzerland has disclosed a sustained release tablet formed by integrally mixing a drug component with a digestible fat, an indigestible wax, and a solid polymer which swells when ingested and tabletting the resulting mixture. In the preferred embodiment the drug component is intimately mixed with the digestible fat and indigestible wax forming granules with the granules uniformly dispersed throughout the solid polymer which forms a sparingly water-soluble carrier for the granules. It has been found that, in the tablets prepared by this process, the release of active substance is governed by the following factors relating to the composition of the active substances and retarding agents present in the tablet:

(1) The ratio between the total amount of wax/fat and the active substance.
(2) The ratio between the total amount of wax/fat, the polymer and the active substance.
(3) The ratio between the indigestible wax and digestible fat.
(4) The total percentage component of the polymer.
(5) The combination of the preceding factors.

It is possible by varying these factors and their combination to make allowance for the properties of the active substance, with the result that a readily controllable protracted effect is obtained in vivo. The therapeutic activity level may be kept substantially constant, for example, over periods ranging from 8 to 12 hours, because the rate at which the active substance is released can be adapted to the excretion rate. This is illustrated in the following example.

Example: The composition of the coating of these sustained release tablets is the same for all the forms examined. It is prepared as follows:

	Grams
Ephedrine hydrochloride	50
Allobarbital	300
Theophylline	1,500
Caffeine	500
Emetine hydrochloride	4
Lactose	361
Maize starch	95
Polyvinylpyrrolidone	100
Stearic acid	80

These ingredients are mixed thoroughly together, the resulting mixture sifted through a No. 50 screen, mixed with 420 ml. of a solution consisting of 1 part of Eudragit E and 2 parts of ethyl alcohol, and then granulated through a No. 14 screen. After drying at 40°C., the resulting granulate is mixed with 118 grams of stearic acid, 179 grams of maize starch and 95 grams of talcum, and the resulting mixture pressed on to the cores. The composition of the cores is given in the following table.

Components of the Cores in Milligrams

	FC/1	FC/2	FC/3
Ephedrine hydrochloride	30	30	30
Hydrogenated castor oil	15	5	10
White wax	5	--	--
Carnauba wax	--	15	10
Calcium sulfate	25	25	25
Magnesium stearate	15	15	15
Colloidal silicic acid	10	10	10
Ethylcellulose	5	5	5
Carbopol 934	12	12	12
Magnesium stearate	4	4	4
Talcum	4	4	4
Totoal	125	125	125

The granulate is prepared as follows: the fat/wax mixture is melted on a steam bath. The finely ground ephedrine hydrochloride which has been sifted through a No. 70 screen is introduced into and then stirred with the melt until a homogeneous mixture is obtained. After cooling, the mixture is finely ground through a No. 60 screen. The ground mixture is then mixed with calcium sulfate, colloidal silicic acid and magnesium stearate, and granulated with a solution of the ethylcellulose in alcohol through a No. 16 screen. The granulate is mixed with Carbopol 934, magnesium stearate, talcum and then compressed. The coated tablet is prepared on a conventional machine: weight of core is 125 mg., weight of coating is 340 mg., total weight of the coated tablet is 465 mg. Compressive strength of the coated tablet is approximately 9.5 kg.

The results which were obtained from tests in vivo on human patients are given in the following table expressed as the total amount of ephedrine released in percent.

	Type of Tablet		
Excretion After	FC/1	FC/2	FC/3
2 hours	2.4	0.63	3.93
5 hours	14.5	9.0	14.08
8 hours	37.0	22.5	27.73
14 hours	62.5	39.3	53.33
23 hours	84.8	54.6	76.23
33 hours	97.0	61.6	94.48

These results show that the coated tablet FC/3 has the best protracted effect. It may be regarded as extremely good because its ephedrine excretion curve is practically the same as that obtained in the test using 3 normal tablets. Consequently, the conditions selected in this formulation FC/3 for producing the protracted effect may be regarded as the most suitable for the ephedrine hydrochloride.

MISCELLANEOUS MATRIX MATERIALS

Particle Size Control of Matrix Materials

A process has been developed by *J.R.A. Simoons; U.S. Patent 3,322,633; May 30, 1967; assigned to NV Koninklijke Pharmaceutische Fabrieken v/h Brocades-Stheeman & Pharmacia, Netherlands* for preparing controlled release drug forms. The method comprises forming an intimate mixture of the drug with the excipients and this is done by having the drug and excipient materials of about the same particle size. According to this process, the desired result is attained by bringing the drug for which a prolonged acting form is sought to the desired particle size, then intimately mixing it with an inert, insoluble substance having about the same particle size, while a hydrophobic substance and a binding agent, all having the same particle size, are added. The matrix is then formed with a granulating agent.

Substances selected from the group consisting of $CaSO_4 \cdot ½H_2O$, anhydrous calcium phosphate and Florite (a mineral mixture with aluminum oxide as main constituent) are preferred as inert insoluble matter. Suitable hydrophobic substances are the nonhydrophilic salts of the nontoxic alkaline earth metals, such as calcium or magnesium stearate or palmitate or the corresponding aluminum salts. Also hydrogenized and natural animal and vegetable fats and mineral waxes which are solid at body temperature may be used.

As a binding agent, water-swellable substances selected from methyl- and ethylcellulose, polyvinyl acetate, polyvinylpyrrolidone, cellulose acetate or prolamines, such as zein, kafirin, hordenine and gliadin, or a mixture of these substances may be used. As a granulating agent, such liquids as a solution of 3% colophonium in 77% alcohol, a solution of 2% colophonium and 1% polyvinylpyrrolidone in 80% alcohol, a solution of 1% colophonium with 1% polyethylene glycol in 80% alcohol or 70% alcohol may be used. The matrix formed from these materials is processed to granules by dry-granulating and then, if desired, the resulting granules are compressed to tablets in the customary manner.

Drying of the granulate should preferably be done at temperatures not exceeding 40°C.; the most feasible range has proved to be between 35° and 40°C. When preparing the granulate, care should be taken that the coarse granulated mass should not be subjected to drying until it has been hardened at room temperature. Compressing of the granulate will yield a strong tablet from which the drug can only be released by diffusion. As a result of this diffusion principle, influences from gastric and intestinal conditions are very nearly eliminated. Neither the acidity nor the possible presence of electrolytes affects the diffusion rate. The following examples will further illustrate the process.

Example 1: In making tablets the substances listed below are used in the proportionate amounts as indicated and the amounts referred to are for one tablet.

	Milligrams
Orphenadrine citrate	75
Ethylcellulose	30
Zein	80
Calcium stearate	20
$CaSO_4 \cdot ½H_2O$	145

The substances passed through the desired size of screen are thoroughly mixed. A granulate is prepared from this mixture by granulating with a sufficient amount of 3% colophonium in 77% alcohol. (For 20,000 tablets about 1,200 ml. is used.) The mass is divided into small fragments and pressed through a No. 10 screen, gauze width 2 mm. and left to harden for 12 to 24 hours at room temperature. The granulate is then dried in a drying cabinet at 35° to 40°C. The granules have a high degree of hardness and are passed through a dry granulator with a No. 20 screen, gauze width 0.8 mm. and are thoroughly mixed; no further additions are made. They are finally compressed to 350 mg. tablets with normal pressure using punches of 8 to 9 mm. diameter. If desired, the tablets may be coated in a conventional coating pan, colored and polished.

Example 2: Eleven-Hour Period – In preparing tablets the substances listed below are used in the proportionate amounts stated and the amounts refer to one tablet.

	Milligrams
Orphenadrine citrate	75
Ethylcellulose	30
Zein	80
Calcium stearate	20
Florite	45
$CaSO_4 \cdot ½H_2O$	100

Florite has a high water absorbing capacity. It is commercially available in the form of very fine granules, which, but for their mesh size, may be added to the other components without further processing. A solution of 3% colophonium in 77% alcohol is used for granulating (ca. 1,800 ml. is used for 20,000 tablets). Processing is completed as in Example 1. 350 mg. tablets are compressed with normal pressure with punches of 8 to 9 mm. diameter. They may be conventionally coated with a color-coating and polished.

Colloidal Magnesium Aluminum Silicate

M. Shepard; U.S. Patent 3,432,593; March 11, 1969; assigned to Key Pharmaceuticals, Incorporated has described a sustained release granule, capsule, or tablet with the active medicament adsorbed on a complex colloidal magnesium aluminum silicate. The individual granules may be further provided with one or more suitable retardant coatings, each of which provides a predetermined period of sustainment.

This complex magnesium aluminum silicate is a compound of variable composition, having a general formula $xMgO \cdot yAl_2O_3 \cdot zSiO_2 \cdot nH_2O$ in which x, y, z and n represents integers. It may be prepared by reacting stoichiometrical quantities of a soluble aluminum salt, a soluble magnesium salt, and an alkali metal silicate, whereupon the complex is precipitated, separated and dried.

Complex magnesium aluminum silicates of this type are known to be antacids. However, it was found, that they are also adsorbents for various medicaments. It was further found that granules of complex magnesium aluminum silicate having a medicament adsorbed thereon can be additionally treated to provide a sustained release type capsule or tablet. The colloidal magnesium aluminum silicate employed typically has an average chemical analysis as follows:

	Percent
Silicon dioxide	61.1
Magnesium oxide	13.7
Aluminum oxide	9.3
Titanium dioxide	0.1
Ferric oxide	0.9
Calcium oxide	2.7
Sodium oxide	2.9
Potassium oxide	0.3
Carbon dioxide	1.8
Water of combination	7.2

In the stomach, where an acid medium is present, the colloidal magnesium aluminum silicate having the adsorbed medicament forms a gel, which exerts a retardant action upon the release of the medicament, slowing the rate of absorption into the blood stream to as much as one-half the normal rate. A further retardant effect is provided by the acid neutralization capacity of the colloidal magnesium aluminum silicate.

The colloidal magnesium aluminum silicate is employed, in an amount ranging from 40 to 60% by weight of the amount of medicament to be adsorbed thereon, preferably 50% by weight. Any desired type of medicament may be adsorbed including herbs, botanicals, and various synthetic drugs, such as antihistamines, antibiotics, autonomics, cardiovascular agents, central nervous system depressants and stimulants, enzymes, gastrointestinal agents, hematological agents, immunological agents, hormones, renal acting and edema reducing agents, skeletal muscle relaxants, nutrients, and others.

It will be seen from the examples that, it is possible to mix uncoated granules of medicament adsorbed on magnesium aluminum silicate with enteric coated granules or with fat-wax coated granules, or with both, as desired. The process permits taking advantage of the fact that the magnesium aluminum silicate itself acts as a retardant in the stomach, and that when treated with the fat-wax coating, it acts as a retardant in the intestines. By treating the granules of magnesium aluminum silicate having medicament adsorbed thereon with retardant coatings, the liberation rate of the medicament is further controlled, thus providing control of release rate to a greater extent than was heretofore possible in preparations of this type.

Example: Vasodilator-Tranquilizer Combination, 10 Hour Release Rate – A vasodilator-tranquilized combination having a 10 hour release time was prepared in a batch size comprising 10,000 units. Each unit was designed to provide a dosage of 6.5 mg. nitroglycerine and 200 mg. lupulin NF. The starting materials were:

	Grams
Nitroglycerine (1 part nitroglycerine, 9 parts beta-lactose)	650
Lupulin NF VII	2,000
Magnesium aluminum silicate (flake)	1,325

These materials were thoroughly mixed and allowed to stand for 8 to 12 hours, followed by vacuum drying and screening into granules. The granules were divided into five equal portions. The first portion, 795 grams, was set aside. The second portion was sprayed with cellulose acetate-phthalate solution to coat it with 1% solids, yielding a total weight of 802.95 grams. The third portion of 795 grams was coated with a retardant solution having the composition:

	Grams
Glyceryl monostearate	225.10
Cetyl alcohol	2.38
Myristyl alcohol	2.38
Bleached white beeswax	7.14

This amount of beeswax was sufficient to add 5% of fat wax solids or 39.75 grams, and then a cellulose acetate-phthalate solution was added to give 1% by weight of solids, or 8.35 grams, making the total weight of the treated third portion 843.10 grams. The fourth portion of 795 grams of granules of adsorbate was treated with the retardant solution to add 10% fat wax solids or 79.50 grams, and then with cellulose acetate-phthalate to yield 1% solids or 8.74 grams, making a total weight of the treated fourth portion of 883.24 grams.

The fifth portion was similarly treated with retardant solution to add 15% fat wax solids or 118.75 grams, and an amount of cellulose acetate-phthalate solution to add 1% solids or 9.14 grams, making the total weight of this portion 922.89 grams. The third, fourth and fifth portions were then vacuum dried and screened into granules. All five portions were then blended, yielding a total weight of 4,247.18 grams. The mixture was tabletted by including conventional binder, filler and lubricant and compressing to provide a tablet containing a dosage of 6.5 mg. nitroglycerine and 200 mg. lupulin. A similar batch was made into capsules, each containing 0.4247 gram to yield the same individual dosage.

Enzyme-Substrate Matrix System

It has been found by *C.W. Hartman; U.S. Patent 3,493,652; February 3, 1970* that controlled release preparations of wide applicability and susceptible of close regulation can be prepared through the use of a combination of enzymes with selected substrates. Enzymes in combination with substrates can control, can increase or decrease, the release and absorption of a nonenzymatic medicament from solid, semisolid, or liquid dosage forms intended for either internal or external administration. By selectively choosing the substrate or substrates and the respective enzyme or enzymes for digestion of the substrate, as well as other components, and by varying the concentration of both the enzymes and the substrates, disintegration of and absorption from dosage forms can be regulated. These considerations are applicable to a variety of medicinal dosage forms, but are particularly adaptable to oral dosage forms.

The substrate can be any agent which is susceptible to the action of hydrolyzing or desmolyzing enzymes. The substrate is primarily the base or vehicle for the active medicament and, until it is separated from the medicament, prevents or retards its release. The base or substrate is therefore so chosen that it will retain the medicament under the various conditions it will encounter until the dosage form completes its function. That is, it may be chosen to resist moisture, acid, alkali, heat, body secretions or any combination of these. Various starches, fats, proteins and carbohydrates may be used, singly or in combination, as the substrate in these controlled release preparations. The enzymes used include hydrolases, desmolases or the other enzymes that add groups to double bonds. The hydrolases may be carbohydrases, esterases, glucosidases, proteases, amidases or coagulases.

The desmolases employed may be zymases, oxidases, dehydrogenases or reductases. In addition to the enzymes, enzyme precursors may also be used to alter the time of digestion of the dosage form, for example pepsinogen, chymotrypsin, etc. The enyzmes may be employed alone or in combination to effect a particular desired sequence of release for one or more medicaments. The pharmaceutical preparations may also contain other agents selected for particular effects in the various dosage forms according to conventional procedure. Thus, the compositions may contain stabilizing agents, surface active materials, coloring and flavoring materials and like ancillary agents where the particular function of that agent is necessary to or desirable in the preparation of the particular dosage form.

Example 1: The following ingredients are combined in the preparation of sustained release sulfanilamide tablets:

	Parts
Sulfanilamide	91.5
Takadiastase	3
Magnesium stearate	0.5
Starch (as starch paste)	5.0

A tablet granulation is prepared from these ingredients by mixing 30 parts of sulfanilamide with the three parts of takadiastase. The mixture is worked until it granulates and is then passed through a 24 mesh screen. The remaining 65 parts of the sulfanilamide is mixed with the starch paste and worked until granulation occurs. It is then passed through a 24 mesh screen, thoroughly admixed with the drug-enzyme granulation and the mixture is tray dried at 130°F. for 5 hours. The dry granulation is mixed with the previously sieved magnesium stearate and the resulting granulation is then compressed into tablets each containing 0.5 gram of sulfanilamide. This product disintegrates in less than 15 minutes in gastric fluid.

Example 2: Sulfanilamide tablets each containing 0.5 gram of the sulfonamide are prepared by granulating and compressing the following ingredients by the same procedure as described in Example 1:

	Parts
Sulfanilamide	70
Lipase (wheat germ)	5.0
Magnesium stearate	0.5
Starch (as starch paste) ca.	5
Hydrogenated cottonseed oil	20

This product disintegrates in the intestinal fluid within one hour.

Cation Exchange Resin

S. Borodkin and D.P. Sundberg; U.S. Patent 3,594,470; July 20, 1971; assigned to Abbott Laboratories have disclosed the process whereby pharmaceutical tablets containing basic-reacting drugs are made chewable and palatable by adsorbing the drug on a weak cation exchange resin and coating these particles before tabletting. The process consists essentially in absorbing the amino-group containing drug or a nontoxic, water-soluble acid addition salt thereof on a weakly acidic cation exchange resin with an exchange capacity of at least 6 meq./g. and consisting of discrete particles of 50 to 420 micron diameter to form a complex between the drug and the resin particles. The particles are coated wtih a film-forming, water-permeable polymer or polymer mixture, and compressed into a tablet, the coating polymer or polymer mixture being selected in such amount and manner that no more than 4% of the drug leaches out from the coated complex particles within two minutes after submerging the particles in artificial saliva.

Among the weakly acidic cation exchange resin, those with an exchange capacity of at least 10 meq./g. are preferred. Chemically, suitable ion exchange resins are those which have free carboxylic acid groups to which a basic reacting drug can be absorbed. The most common representatives of these resins are those based on polymers of acrylic acid, e.g., acrylic acid polymers and copolymers, methacrylic acid polymers and copolymers where the other monomer preferably is based on the same or similar matrices, e.g., styrene, methyl acrylate, methyl methacrylate, acrylonitrile, butadiene or other polymerizable vinyl compounds. Exchange resins with free sulfonic acid groups are not suited because the formed drug/resin complex is so strong that the drug is released too slowly or incompletely. Resins containing sulfonic acid groups have exchange capacities below 5 meq./g.

The above range of particle diameters is important in the process of making the chewable tablets. With particles of a diameter below 50 microns, processing is difficult due to dusting, poor flowability, slow flow-through rate, and other mechanical difficulties associated with small particles. Particles of a diameter above 420 microns result in tablets which, when chewed, create a peculiar and uncomfortable mouthfeel.

Example: (A) Five kilograms of Amberlite CG-50 (a weak cation exchange resin with a pK_a of 6.1) with a mesh size of 100 to 200 (particle diameters of 74 to 149 microns) is slurried in 50 liters of 1.0 N sodium hydroxide for 30 minutes. The slurry is placed in a 5 foot glass column of 12 inches diameter. Water is passed upwards through the resin bed for 2 hours to eliminate extremely fine particles with the flow rate adjusted to allow the resin bed to expand 2 to 3 times its settled volume.

Subsequently, 50 liters of 1.0 N sodium hydroxide solution is passed downwards through the column at a flow rate of 1 l./min. followed, in turn, by 25 liters of water to eliminate excess sodium hydroxide, 120 liters of a 5% acetic acid solution, and 25 liters of water. The resin is then removed from the column and tested for its extractable content. It is found to contain less than 0.2% volatile water-extractables. The resin is then placed in the column again and converted to its sodium form by passing 50 liters of 1.0 N sodium hydroxide through the column followed by 25 liters of water.

(B) A solution of 20 kg. of d-pseudoephedrine hydrochloride in water to make 200 liters of solution is passed through the column prepared above at a rate of 1 l./min., followed by 25 liters of water. The effluent is collected for recovery of unabsorbed pseudoephedrine. Vacuum is used to remove any excess solution. The pseudoephedrine/Amberlite complex formed is removed from the column and dried in trays at 50°C. under reduced pressure for 48 hours to yield 10.1 kg. of the dry complex. Assays show that the complex contains 54.9% pseudoephedrine which is equivalent to 670 mg. of pseudoephedrine hydrochloride per gram of complex.

(C) Three kilograms of the pseudoephedrine/Amberlite complex are charged into a 12 inches diameter air-suspension coating column and coated with 25 liters of a solution containing 40 grams of ethylcellulose (10 cp.), 10 grams of methylhydroxypropylcellulose (10 to 12 cp.), 0.03 gram of Yellow Dye, FD&C #6, and 500 ml. of methylene chloride per liter of solution, the remainder being ethanol. The fluidizing air is passed through the column at a rate of 144 scfm; the inlet temperature is maintained at 50° to 55°C. resulting in an outlet temperature of 40° to 45°C. After the coating solution is exhausted, fluidizing the bed is continued with air of sufficient temperature to maintain the outlet temperature at 45°C. Analysis of the coated complexed particles shows the following composition: 41.2% pseudoephedrine, 33.9% Amberlite, 19.9% ethylcellulose and 5.0% methylhydroxypropylcellulose.

(D) Chewable tablets are made from the above particles using the following:

	Grams
(A) Coated particles (equivalent to 60 grams pseudoephedrine HCl)	119.0
(B) Carbinoxamine maleate	2.5
(C) Mannitol	412.8
(D) Sorbitol, crystalline	70.0
(E) Yellow dye D&C Lake #6	0.167
(F) Sodium cyclamate	33.0
(G) Polyvinylpyrrolidone	28.0
(H) Carbowax 6,000, milled	14.0
(I) Magnesium stearate	5.5
(J) Flavor (tutti-frutti)	10.0
(K) Ethanol, 19 proof (enough for mashing)	--
Total	700

A mixture of (B), (E), (F) and (G) is milled in a Fitzmill grinder with a portion of (C). This blend is mixed with (D) and the remaining (C) and subsequently massed with (K), screened and dried in a warm-air oven. The dried granulation is passed through a 20 mesh screen, placed in a blender, blended with the remaining ingredients (A), (H), (I) and (J) and subsequently compressed into tablets using 17/32 bevel-edge punches with a bisect. Each tablet weighs 700 mg. and contains the equivalent of 60 mg. of pseudoephedrine hydrochloride. The tablets, when submitted to a trained taste panel for taste evaluation during and after chewing, are shown to have only very mild or almost unnoticeable bitterness.

CARBOHYDRATE COATING MATERIALS

SUGAR BASED COATING MATERIALS

Syrup Coating Without Subcoatings

It has been found by *S. Weinstein; U.S. Patent 3,361,631; January 2, 1968; assigned to Sandoz, Inc.* that hydraulically spraying a sugar syrup directly onto tablet cores at a nozzle pressure of 800 to 1,500 psi without using any subcoating or other preliminary preparation of the tablet cores produces excellent tablets which may have as little as 10% by weight of sugar coating based on the total tablet weight.

By so applying a sugar syrup under high hydraulic pressure, the drying of the coating is expedited and simplified due to the rapid evaporation of water from the fine mist spray delivered by the spray gun. By following this method the tablets can be coated more rapidly and with fewer coating steps as well as requiring less coating material. The method is also of such nature that the exposure of the tablets to aqueous sugar solutions for prolonged periods of time is eliminated. This is in direct contrast to finished sugar coated tablets made by conventional techniques where the coating amounts to approximately twice the weight of the core.

The hydraulic spray equipment used in carrying out this process is capable of spraying heated sugar syrups and sugar syrup suspensions at a nozzle pressure of 800 to 1,500 psi through a fine nozzle orifice. It is not absolutely essential to use this particular type of equipment, however, since any suitable or similar spray equipment can be employed. While it is not absolutely necessary to heat the sugar syrup, it is preferable to do so, in which case a temperature is used in the range of 80° to 170°F.

The sugar syrup or sugar syrup suspension may also contain any suitable approved coloring material. The spraying operation is carried out for a period of time ranging from 1 to 120 seconds following which drying is carried out for a period of time ranging from 1 to 15 minutes, depending on the number of tablets being coated in a given batch.

The spray coating and drying steps are repeated for a sufficient number of cycles to produce tablets of the required total weight, but, as pointed out above, it is possible to provide an adequate sugar coating which amounts to as little as 10% of the total tablet weight. The sugar syrup solutions and suspensions are made in accordance with accepted laboratory procedures and for heating they are circulated through a heater of any appropriate or known type. The following sugar solutions and suspensions are examples of those which have been successfully sprayed onto tablet cores without subcoating, rounding or other pretreatment.

Example 1:

	Grams
Sucrose powdered	91.00
Distilled water	54.75
FD&C color, q.s.	

Example 2:

FD&C Red #3	0.300
Dioctyl sodium sulfosuccinate	0.005
Titanium dioxide	50.000
Distilled water	125.000
Simple syrup, q.s.	250.000

In a particular coating operation, the coating solution or suspension is circulated through a heater until its temperature is raised to approximately 150°F., tablets are placed in a conventional coating pan and heated to 100°F. and the heated coating solution is then hydraulically sprayed onto the tablets at a nozzle pressure of 1,000 psi for 3 seconds following which the tablets are dried for 5 minutes and the spraying and drying cycle repeated for the necessary number of times to give a predetermined total tablet weight. The tablets were then polished in standard polishing pans in accordance with standard polishing procedure.

Lubricated Sugar Coatings

S. Lee; U.S. Patent 3,406,031; October 15, 1968; assigned to Geigy Chemical Corporation has developed coating compositions particularly adapted to producing smooth circumferential surfaces on pharmaceutical dosage unit forms in a minimum amount of time. These compositions are as follows.

	Percentages
Lubricating compound	0.1 - 10
Dispersing agent	0.0001 - 5
Colloidal material	0.01 - 10
Coating vehicle	50 - 99

In the above compositions the lubricating compound is part of the coating. The addition of this lubricating compound specifically enhances the passage of the dosage forms over each other in the rotating coating pan and superior circumferential surfaces are produced in less time. Another advantage of this coating procedure is a marked reduction in the breakage of tablets during coating and a reduction of seconds which must be discarded.

Among the lubricating compounds which are adapted for use in the coating compositions are water-insoluble nontoxic light metal salts of long chain fatty acids. Water-insoluble nontoxic lubricating compounds specifically adapted to the compositions are metal salts of long chain fatty acids, such as, magnesium stearates, oleates, laurates and myristates; aluminum stearates, oleates and myristates; calcium stearates, myristates and laurates; zinc stearates; iron stearates, etc.

Dispersing agents which negate the water repellent properties of the lubricating compound include nontoxic surfactants such as sodium 2-ethylhexane sulfonate, sodium di-(2-ethylhexyl)phosphate, sodium salt of sulfate ester of an alkyl phenoxy polyoxyethylene ethanol, oleic acid ester of sodium isethionate, sodium N-methyl-N-acyl taurate (commercially available mixture), and the like.

The coating is enhanced by the presence of an edible hydrophilic protective colloid. Among the useful water-soluble protective colloids are cellulose ethers; cellulose esters; natural carbohydrates such as water-soluble salts of alginic acid and acacia; and protein colloids such as casein and albumin. The coating vehicle comprises 50 to 90% solution or suspension of sucrose, glucose, dextrose, lactose, fructose, sorbitol or other innocuous materials and mixtures thereof in a volatile solvent such as water, alcohol, etc.

The coating composition may be prepared by dissolving the dispersing agent and lubricating compound in water. The colloidal matter may be added to this solution or to the coating syrup. Upon mixing the water solution and coating syrup an efficient coating composition is produced which can be used to simultaneously perform the functions of subcoating and coating. If a colored coating is desired an appropriate dye or pigment can be added to the coating composition so that upon subcoating and coating colored pharmaceutical dosage unit forms are produced. The following examples illustrate coating compositions and coating procedures used in this process.

Example 1:

Composition	Grams
Magnesium stearate	50.0
Sodium lauryl sulfate	10.0
Hydroxyethylcellulose	20.0
Water	120.0
Simple syrup USP	800.0
	1,000.0

The sodium lauryl sulfate is dissolved in the water and the magnesium stearate is then dispersed by light speed agitation until a translucent, smooth liquid is obtained. The cellulose compound is dissolved in the syrup by high speed agitation, avoiding the formation of lumps of undissolved colloid. Upon mixing these two colloidal solutions, an efficient coating vehicle is obtained. Within less than 1 hour, an entire batch of tablets is smoothly and roundly defined with a colorless, translucent coating.

Example 2:

Composition	Grams
Aluminum distearate	90
Dioctyl sodium sulfosuccinate	5
Methylcellulose (15 cp.)	15
Water	290
70% sorbitol solution	200
Sucrose	400
	1,000

The sulfosuccinate is dissolved in the water and the aluminum stearate then dispersed while mixing. With continued agitation, the methylcellulose is added and dissolved. The sorbitol solution is then added and the sucrose dissolved in this mixture. When applied to a batch of tablets rotating in a conventional coating pan this mixture will produce a smooth, circumferential coating on each tablet in less than ten steps.

Colored Sugar Coatings

A colored coating composition for tablets, pills or pellets has also been developed by *S. Lee; U.S. Patent 3,413,400; November 26, 1968; assigned to Geigy Chemical Corporation*. This process is advantageous over the prior procedures in that the number of steps required for coating is reduced by as much as 80%. Likewise by this method, colors can be consistently reproduced by semiskilled operators and the colors exhibit improved light stability.

The coloring medium comprises any water-soluble nontoxic dye, particularly any dye derived from coal tar which is certified as suitable for human consumption. A single concentration of each dye employed is used in the composition and method. Therefore, the color hues and shades are easily reproducible and the coating operation is not solely dependent on the skill of the operator. The following ingredients make up the composition.

	Percentages
FD&C or D&C dyes	0.0001 - 5
Pseudo laking agent	0.001 - 15
Coating vehicle	50 - 99
Colloidal material	0.01 - 10
Dispersing agent	0.0001 - 5

The FD&C or D&C dye is present within the above ranges in such quantities that the desired shade of color is produced. The pseudo laking agent is present in a stoichiometric relationship or greater. The pseudo lakes may be defined as a mixture of a water-soluble dye with a water-insoluble colorless material which does not form a physicochemical compound as in the case of a true lake. Nevertheless the pseudo lake acts as a lake through stabilization of the dye against ultraviolet degradation and migration.

Unlike a true lake, the dye remains water-soluble during the coating process and even after the coating is dried. Substances which serve as pseudo laking agents are nontoxic, water-insoluble salts wherein the cation has an atomic number of under 40, especially salts produced by the reaction of calcium, magnesium, strontium, aluminum, iron, zirconium and zinc; and as acid such as decanoic, dodecanoic, tetradecanoic, hexadecanoic, octadecanoic, octadecenoic, octadecadienoic, octadecatrienoic, carbonic, phosphoric, etc.

Premature pseudo laking is prevented by the presence of an edible, hydrophilic protective colloid which, upon drying, allows the pseudo laking to proceed. Among the colloids suitable for use are cellulose ethers; cellulose esters; natural carbohydrates such as water-soluble salts of alginic acid, acacia and amylo pectin; and protein colloids such as casein and albumin. The coating vehicle comprises a 50% or greater solution or suspension of sucrose, glucose, dextrose, lactose, fructose, sorbitol or other innocuous materials and their mixtures in a volatile solvent such as water, alcohol and the like.

The dispersing agent is a water-soluble, nontoxic FDA approved surfactant such as sodium 2-ethylhexane sulfonate, sodium di-(2-ethylhexyl)phosphate, sodium salt of sulfate ester of an alkyl phenoxy polyoxyethylene ethanol.

In preparing the coating composition the dye is dissolved in a portion of the water. The pseudo laking agent is then dispersed in the remainder of the water which also contains the dispersing agent and protective colloid. These are then mixed to form the lake precursor and the syrup then added.

Coating is accomplished by application of a coating composition containing one or more FD&C or D&C dyes and a pseudo laking agent. Alternately, the process can be carried out by the application of a coating composition containing the FD&C or D&C dyes and a separate coating composition containing a dispersed pseudo laking agent. During coating this composition is advantageous in that the buildup in the coating pan is at a minimum. The following example specifically illustrates coating compositions and coating procedures included in this process.

Example:

	Grams
FD&C yellow #6	16.0
FD&C red #2	1.1
FD&C blue #2	4.4
Aluminum octadecanoate	50.0
Calcium carbonate	180.0
Sodium lauryl sulfate	10.0
Hydroxyethylcellulose	10.0
Simple syrup, USP	600.0
Water	200.0

The dyes are dissolved in half of the water and the sodium lauryl sulfate in the other half.

The calcium carbonate and the aluminum octadecanoate are dispersed in the lauryl sulfate solution and the hydroxyethylcellulose dissolved therein by agitation. These solutions are mixed with part of the syrup to form the stock color base. This is further diluted with the remainder of the syrup to form the coating composition. One million 100 mg. oxyphenbutazone tablets may be coated to an attractive tan shade in 1 hour, with all the coating compound going on the tablets and only a negligible buildup of coating material on the inside of the coating pan being observed.

Textured Coatings

L. Carletti and A. Rigamonti; U.S. Patent 3,480,468; November 25, 1969; assigned to Società Farmaceutici Italia, Italy have developed the method for applying coatings to tablets which dry to give an outer wrinkled, orange peel-like appearance. The coated tablets produced in this manner have been given the name of farmoids.

The process comprises coating the tablets with a protective resinous material; heating the tablets at a temperature from 35° to 60°C. in a coating pan rotating at 5 to 30 rpm; and spraying, on the protected tablets, the solution or suspension for coating; the solution is maintained at a temperature of from 15° to 80°C. Farmoids have the advantages of coated tablets because of the protection from outside, sweet taste of the coat and agreeable outer aspect. Furthermore they show other advantages over coated tablets, some of which are listed below:

(1) average time necessary to prepare one lot of coated tablets is reduced from 30 hours to an average time of 2 hours for one lot of farmoids;

(2) less excipients are wasted because by spraying a perfectly continuous coat is obtained employing a relatively small quantity of coating mixture;

(3) less volume as direct consequence of (2); and

(4) lower production costs as a consequence of (1), (2) and (3), and because the coating process may be carried out by a nonhighly specialized staff.

In greater detail, the process may be carried out as follows. Into a coating pan are put from 2 to 80 kg. of tablets (according to the capacity of the pan itself), to which a film of protective resinous substance has been first applied. The coating pan is adjusted to a rotary speed, between 5 and 30 rpm. The heating is regulated so that the temperature of the tablets is between 35° and 60°C. The pan is also provided with an aspiration system to remove the excess of spray over that required for the coating.

As the heated tablets rotate, a coating mixture, at a temperature of 15° to 80°C. is sprayed over the tablets in the presence of sprayed air, at a temperature of 20° to 65°C. Farmoids so obtained may be optionally polished with a polishing solution, such as natural or synthetic gums and resins like benzoin, lac gum or carnauba wax dispersed or dissolved in suitable solvents. The equipment used for spraying the coating mixture comprises the following elements:

(a) a paint spray gun having external or internal mixer nozzles provided with a spray head to produce a rather large spray pattern. The pressure at which the liquid is sprayed is 0.5 to 2.5 atmospheres. For higher quantities of tablets, two or more spray guns may be used;

(b) a cup for paints under pressure from 0.1 to 1.5 atmospheres provided with a pressure regulator and a stirrer which is necessary, if the coating mixture contains substances insoluble in suspensions; and

(c) a heating system which may be embodied into the cup or inserted between the cup and spray gun. This system regulates the temperature of the coating mixture and of the air so that the required temperature is reached.

The spraying mixture consists essentially of a sugar solution having a density of between 1.15 and 1.37 at a temperature of 17.5°C. Sorbitol or saccharose may be employed as the sugar. The sugar solution may be suitably charged with an inert excipient, such as calcium carbonate, titanium dioxide, starch, talc, natural gum, etc. Among coloring substances, which may be used, are any of the nontoxic dyes, which have been certified for use, in particular indigo carmine (FD&C blue #2), sunset yellow (FD&C yellow #6), erythrosine extra yellowish (FD&C red #3), and the like.

Sometimes it is opportune also to add a plasticizing agent such as polyvinyl alcohol, polyethylene glycol or a surface active agent such as a polyoxyethylene ester of sorbitol, etc. Small quantities of water-miscible solvents, preferably ethyl alcohol and acetone, may be added. The coating liquid is sprayed onto the tablets by means of the spray gun in the form of a mist, in which the ratio of liquid:air is between 1:4 and 1:20.

Example: 25 kg. of tablets having an average weight of 500 mg. are placed into a copper pan with inside diameter of 84 cm. and provided with a suitable aspiration system. The tablets are rounded, rather hard and surrounded by a protective film of natural gums or artificial resins. The pan is rotated at a speed of 9 rpm, and at the same time heated by gas to a tablet temperature of about 50°C. Onto the heated tablet the following solution is sprayed:

	Grams
Saccharose	67
Distilled water to	100

To obtain a good vaporization, the coating solution is heated at 80°C., the air at 20°C. and the equipment is adjusted to provide a pressure of 2 atm. in the general circuit, and 0.6 atmosphere in the cup containing the solution itself. Spraying is continued without interruption until the desired coat is obtained. The average weight of the tablets, after such a treatment, is increased by about 30%. The time required for the whole process is about 1 hour and 30 minutes. Finally the farmoids may be polished by one of the systems used for the polishing of coated tablets, e.g., applying lac gum and carnauba wax.

Sugar-Glucoside Coating Compositions

Tablets are coated with a solution developed by *P. Sheth and L. Lachman; U.S. Patent 3,421,920; January 14, 1969; assigned to Ciba Corporation* which eliminates the need for prior subcoatings or smoothing coating operations. This enables one to form elegant and uniform thin film coated tablets in a total time ranging between 2 to 3 hours, depending upon the size and shape of the tablets to be coated. This has been accomplished through a physical-chemical approach to the factors governing the crystallization of the ingredients used in the coating formulation, the bonding of the coating to the tablets and the flow-out properties or the spreadability of the coating solution respectively.

Accordingly, this process concerns a sugar coating solution comprising in addition to the aqueous sugar solution used, an effective amount of at least: (a) a hexanehexol; (b) a water-soluble salt of a higher alkyl sulfosuccinate; and (c) a linear poly-1,3-β-glucoside containing on every third glucose moiety of the chain a 1,6-β-glucosido group. The sugar solution employed is that usually used for coated tablets. It may contain a mono- and/or disaccharide in the appropriate concentration, but preferably contains sucrose in an amount from 40 to 80%, especially 50 to 70%.

The hexanehexol used is preferably that obtained from natural hexoses by reduction, such as sorbitol, dulcitol or especially mannitol. The water-soluble salt of an alkyl sulfosuccinate is preferably an alkali metal or ammonium salt. The higher alkyl residue esterifying preferably both of the carboxyl groups contains advantageously 6 to 10 carbon atoms, such as 1-, 2- or 3-hexyl, 1-heptyl, 1-, 2- or especially 3-octyl, 1-nonyl or 4-decyl. The polyglucoside used, mainly has the formula shown on the following page. It is sold under the trademark Polytetran and the procedure for making it is found in Belgian Patent 639,361; April 30, 1964.

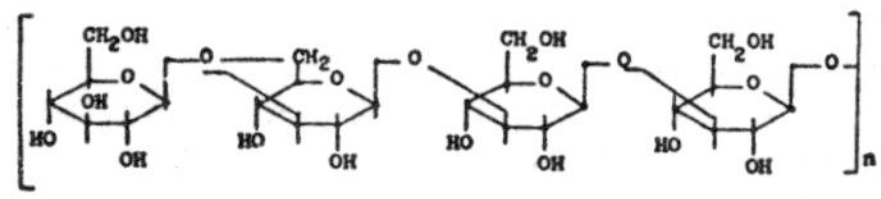

A preferred form is one which will give a final viscosity (after 5 hours) of about 2,400 to 3,000 cp., measured with a Brookfield viscosimeter using a No. 3 spindle and using a 1% aqueous solution at 24°C. in a pH range between 6.8 and 7.5. An especially valuable coating solution contains about 50 to 70% sucrose, about 4 to 6% mannitol, about 0.2 to 0.3% of di-3-octyl sodium succinate and about 0.02 to 0.05% of the polyglucoside.

The coating procedure is carried out according to known methods, preferably that described in U.S. Patent 3,141,792. The material is placed into the usual coating pan and is sprayed several times with the coating solution. Between the sprays, the coatings applied to the tablets are dried, preferably by directing heated air into the coating pan. The spraying and drying operations are repeated until the desired coating is obtained. Heat may not be applied to the last coat in order to obtain a smooth surface of the resulting coated tablets. If desired, they may be polished, preferably with the use of natural waxes, such as beeswax and carnauba wax, wax mixtures, or synthetic products, such as silicones.

Example: 8 kg. of a coating solution sufficient for 20 kg. of modified ball tablets each weighing 500 mg. are made up as follows.

	Grams
Sucrose	4,800.0
Mannitol	400.0
Di-3-octyl sodium sulfosuccinate	20.0
Polyglucoside	2.0
Titanium dioxide	40.0
FD&C lake yellow #5	4.0
Purified water	2,734.0

The di-3-octyl sodium sulfosuccinate, sucrose, mannitol and polysaccharide are dissolved in water in this order. The lake and titanium dioxide which have been previously milled are added and suspended well by adequate agitation. 20 kg. of the tablets are placed into a 30 inch coating pan and the above coating solution is sprayed onto the tablets with the following coating cycle.

Coating	Amount
1	100 ml.
2-8	Gradually increasing from 20 to 130 ml.
9-32	Each 130 ml.
33-45	Gradually decreasing from 130 to 110 ml.
Final	Each 110 ml.

Between the sprays the coatings applied are dried by a stream of air heated to 47°C. After the last spray no hot air is applied and the coated tablets are allowed to dry overnight in a drying cabinet. If desired, they can be polished using, for example, a suitable wax, such as carnauba wax, either as the powder or in solution, for example, in carbon tetrachloride, isopropanol or a hydrocarbon.

Sugar-Polymer Coating Mixtures

W. Daum, E. Nurnberg and H.J. Sippel; U.S. Patent 3,420,931; January 7, 1969; and U.S. Patent 3,554,767; January 12, 1971; both assigned to E. Merck AG, Germany have developed an improved method for producing dragées where the dragée coating solution comprises 35 to 60% by weight of sugar and 0.5 to 10% by weight of a vinyl polymer. This method permits automatic operation and markedly reduces the time conventionally used for producing dragées. By using this coating composition, it has been found that the entire coating process can be carried out with this composition alone since it can be applied manually or by suitable apparatus, with or without spraying, without any inconvenient sticking of the dragées. It has been found necessary to additionally introduce pulverulent substances such as talc, into the rotating vessel during the time of the coating process. With rationalized operation, the entire coating process can be carried out in one or two days. It was particularly unexpected that such a substantial improvement can be achieved by increasing the polymer from 0.325% of prior formulations to at least 0.5%, preferably to about 2%.

The preferred polymers include homopolymers of vinylpyrrolidone, vinyl acetate and vinyl alcohol and copolymers of vinylpyrrolidone, vinyl acetate, and vinyl alcohol. These polymers are characterized by their physiological compatibility. It has been particularly advantageous to apply commercial preparations of polyvinylpyrrolidone with a dry content of at least 94%, a maximal ash content of 0.02% and a maximal monomer content of 0.8%, molecular weights between 10,000 and 800,000, preferably about 20,000 to 30,000. Another polymer which is used advantageously is a commercial copolymer of 60% vinyl pyrrolidone and 40% vinyl acetate with the following characteristics: dry content at least 95%; maximal monomer content 0.8%; and nitrogen content about 7.6%.

As for the other essential ingredients of the coating, the percent by weight of sugar in the aqueous suspension is 1 to 60%, preferably 35 to 40%. Various types of sugars can be employed, such as sucrose, glucose, sorbitol, mannitol, etc.; it is preferable, however, to use sucrose.

The application of this coating dispersion can be adapted to different types of operation. It is possible to lay on the coating either manually, or semiautomatically or completely automatically. The suspension can be applied by spraying or it can be poured in liquid form directly onto the cores tumbling in an angularly oriented rotating kettle. The suspension is applied until the material to be coated is well moistened. The kettle is then allowed to rotate until the coated cores no longer adhere to one another but instead roll freely. Finally, the coated cores are dried under continuous rotation, preferably with the aid of a warm air stream, or an infrared lamp, or any other equivalent drying means.

These steps can be conducted continuously; and it is possible in this connection to shorten or even omit the rotating phase (second phase) during the first coating applications. It is also unnecessary to remove the dragées from the coating vessel during the course of the entire coating procedure in order to postdry them, perhaps under vacuum or in drying chambers. A further advantage of this method consists in that all of the process steps can be conducted at ambient temperature. In general each core is coated with 10 to 500, preferably 50 to 80 separate thin coats, each coat having a thickness of 0.5 to 200μ, preferably 5 to 20μ.

A particularly economical mode of conducting the process comprises passing a predetermined volume of the suspension through a relay controlled solenoid valve into the dragée coating vessel to cover the dragées rolling around therein. Suitably, a three-phase time relay is employed, such that in the first phase the suspension is passed through the solenoid valve; in the second phase the rotating operation is conducted, the duration of which can be varied; and in the third phase the heating device is actuated. The suspension can be applied onto cores whose surface is not pretreated. However, it is also possible to coat cores which have been previously provided with a sugarless coating, for instance, with a lacquer coating resistant to stomach acids. The following examples are those for the manufacture of the suspension to be employed in this process.

Example 1:

	Percent
Polyvinylpyrrolidone	4
Titanium dioxide	4.5
Calcium carbonate	4.5

(continued)

	Percent
Talc	14.5
Glycerine	2
Sucrose	38
Water	32.5

Polyvinylpyrrolidone is dissolved in water; then, the remaining components are added under constant stirring; thereafter, the mixture is passed through a fine sieve or a homogenizing device.

Example 2:

	Percent
Methylcellulose	0.5
Polyvinylpyrrolidone	2.0
Aerosil (particulate SiO_2)	4.0
Titanium dioxide	4.5
Calcium carbonate	4.5
Talc	14.5
Glycerine	2.0
Sucrose	38.0
Water	30.0

Sugar-Wax Coating Mixtures

Another process for coating dragées has been disclosed by *P. Rieckmann and H. Schalk; U.S. Patent 3,456,050; July 15, 1969; assigned to C.F. Boehringer & Soehne GmbH, Germany.* The coating comprises an aqueous sugar suspension containing in addition to 45 to 85% by weight of sugar and 5 to 20% by weight of solid fillers, 0.01 to 10% by weight of fat and/or wax.

By the incorporation of a small amount of wax and/or fat in the sugar-coating suspension, the tendency to stickiness at the start of the drying of the suspension is overcome, that is, the dragées do not stick to one another nor do they adhere to the kettle wall. There is, as a result, made possible a rapid, fully automatic dragée preparation suitable for the confectionery industry.

In preparing the dragées, the coating suspension is sprayed onto the pills or centers rotating in a coating kettle, the spraying interrupted and the sprayed dragée centers kept in rotation for a period of time and then dried with a current of warm air. These three steps in the sequence are repeated, if necessary, until the desired total amount of coating has been applied.

The aqueous sugar suspensions can be used cold so that they can be employed with the use of simple devices, without thermostatic control. In this way, there are obtained satisfactory sugar dragées in a substantially shorter period of time than with the old manual process (finishing time for one charge about one day), while saving the valuable manual work of skilled persons.

In addition to the fats and/or waxes, the dragée-making suspensions also contain 45 to 85% by weight sugar and 5 to 20% by weight of the conventional fillers, such as starch, chalk, gum arabic, kaolin, talc, alkaline earth metal phosphates and titanium dioxide and mixtures thereof. If desired, there can also be added any of the permitted emulsifiers, such as lecithin and the alginates, in order to ensure a fine dispersion of the fats and/or waxes in the suspension.

If an automatic dragée-making device is being employed, it is not necessary to use an emulsifier because the dragée-making suspension is, in this case, continuously circulated by a geared pump through a valve so that its homogeneity, especially during the period shortly before applications, is always ensured. The coating suspensions can be produced very simply without heat merely by stirring the components together and homogenizing the resultant suspension, for example, in a corundum disk mill or the like. The solid fats and/or waxes are advantageously added in a molten state. It is possible to add coloring material from the start of the process if desired, thus achieving a uniform coloration of the dragées. In the following table are illustrative examples of a number of dragée-making suspensions according to this process.

Composition of Dragée Suspensions in Percent

	1	2	3	4	5	6	7	8	9	10	11	12
Sucrose	60	60	52	54.5	52	53	50	46	50	50	50	54
Liquid glucose [1]			2.5			2.5	3	2.5	2.5	2.4	3	2.5
Starch		9.5			7.5	7.5				5		6.5
Chalk	9.5		10	9			8	10	8	7	8	
Titanium dioxide			2	1			2	2	2		2	
Palmitin	0.5	0.5	0.9	0.4								
Cocoa Butter											0.9	
Butter						1.0						
Cream								4				
Bees' wax									1			
Parting wax					0.4		1.8					0.9
Olive oil										0.5		
Lecithin						1.0	0.2	0.5	0.5			
Sodium Alginate			0.1	0.1	0.1					0.1	0.1	0.1
Coloring	Q.S.	Q.S.	Q.S.	Q.S.	Q.S.	Q.S.	Q.S.	Q.S.	Q.S.	Q.S.	Q.S.	Q.S.
Water ad	100	100	100	100	100	100	100	100	100	100	100	100

	13	14	15	16	17	18	19	20	21	22	23	24
Sucrose	46.5	49	52.4	55	55	55	56	56	57.5	60	60	65
Liquid glucose [1]	2.5	2.5	2.5	3.5	5	3.5	3.5	4.5	2.5	5	3	2.5
Starch					9	6	12	10				
Chalk	10	10	9						9		8	
Titanium dioxide	2	2	1			2						
Palmitin	3.4	1.4	5	0.5	1	0.3		0.5			2	
Margarine									1			
Olive oil										3		0.5
Peppermint oil						2						
Wax ("comprimatwachs")							0.5					
Milk powder				14		3						
Sodium alginate	0.1	0.1	0.1									

[1] The liquid glucose used is obtained by the hydrolysis of starch and contains glucose, maltose, and dextrines, together with about 20% water.
Q.S.—Quantum sufficit.

The following example illustrates a satisfactory procedure for the manufacture of dragées.

Example: 22 kg. of chewing gum cores (length 21.1 mm., breadth 11.1 mm., height 5.2 millimeters, weight 1,100 mg., number 20,000) were placed in a kettle having a diameter of 100 cm., which had been provided with a powerful exhaust system. The spray device was adjusted in such a manner that, per coating, about 170 ml. of the dragée-making suspension were sprayed onto the chewing gum cores within a period of 7 seconds. The cores were then allowed to circulate in the kettle for 1 minute without any external interference so that the suspension was uniformly distributed on the surfaces of the dragées.

Drying was subsequently carried out for 2 minutes using a current of air. These three steps (spraying, circulating, and drying) were repeated until 16 kg. of suspension had been applied. The pieces of chewing gum which have had smooth surfaces from the start of the process were now ready for waxing. The total production time amounted to 5.5 to 6 hr. During this time, no supervision of any kind was necessary. After the dragéeing had been completed, the individual pieces of chewing gum had a weight of 1,900 mg.

Sugar-Fatty Acid Ester Coatings

Coatings for hygroscopic medicaments have been developed by *R. Kawata, H. Kawada, T. Ohmura and S. Uematsu; U.S. Patent 3,639,564; February 1, 1972; assigned to Yamanouchi Pharmaceutical Co., Ltd., Japan.* The coating material comprises a sugar syrup containing at least one monoester, diester, or triester of sucrose and a higher fatty acid having 8 to 20 carbon atoms such as palmitic acid or stearic acid, the ester or ester mixture having a hydrophile-lipophile balance (HLB) of less than 11. This coating can be applied directly to tablet cores containing hygroscopic medicaments thereby avoiding such conventional pretreatment steps as waterproof-coating and subcoating.

The coating syrup may be prepared by dissolving or dispersing uniformly sugar and a sucrose higher fatty acid ester in an amount of less than 30% by weight, preferably less than 10% by weight to the sugar in warm water. The sucrose higher fatty acid ester has an HLB of less than 11 and preferably less than 7. In the preparation of the coating syrup, a coloring agent, a flavoring vehicle, a shielding agent and an extender which are usually used in a conventional sugar coating process may be added if necessary. This coating syrup may be applied to tablet cores by repeating the application and drying of the syrup using the ordinary sugar coating procedure.

In this case, a high degree of skill generally required in a subcoating procedure is unnecessary, i.e., dropping or spraying of the syrup on the tablet cores in the coating pan and drying. Also, the thickness of the sugar coating may be desirably determined on considering the size of the tablets, the properties of the medicaments contained in the tablet cores, etc.

The sugar coated tablets prepared by this process are resistant to the formation of cracks and the exuding, etc., under severe conditions of high temperature and high humidity, not only during the coating steps but also after the preparation of the coated tablet. Further, there is no change in the time required for disintegration of the tablets after swallowing even after such tablets are stored for an extended period of time as compared with conventional sugar coated tablets. The process can be illustrated by the following example.

Example:

Composition	Grams
Sugar	950
Sucrose distearate*	75
Water	450

*Nitto ester S-770

After heating 450 grams of water above 80°C., 950 grams of sugar and then 75 grams of sucrose distearate having an HLB of 7 were added slowly to the water, with stirring, to provide a homogenous coating composition. In a coating pan were placed 10,000 tablet cores each weighing 150 mg. and while rotating the coating pan, about 30 grams of the coating composition prepared above was applied onto the tablets. The coated tablet cores were then dried, in air at a temperature of about 50°C. By repeating the same procedure, sugar coated tablet cores each weighing 300 mg. were obtained.

Sugar-Starch-Glycol Coating Mixture

An inexpensive tablet coating composition which can be used on a wide variety of tablets and ingredients has been disclosed by *J.E. Small and S.F. Jeffries; U.S. Patent 3,751,277; August 7, 1973; assigned to The Dow Chemical Company.* The coating mixture contains a sugar, a cereal solids hydrolysate, starch, a solid polyethylene glycol and a liquid polyhydroxy compound. Several other ingredients may be added to the previously named ingredients in order to enhance the properties of the coating obtained from the composition. Among the more important of these additional materials are plasticizing agents of the humectant type, opaquing agents and coloring agents.

Preferred cereal solids hydrolysate ingredients have a dextrose equivalent of from 8 to 20, and have on a dry weight basis 0.5 to 2% dextrose, 4.5 to 8.5% disaccharides, 5 to 10% trisaccharides, 3.7 to 6% tetrasaccharides, and 3.7 to 5.5% pentasaccharides, the remainder of the hydrolysate being higher polysaccharides such as hexasaccharides, heptasaccharides, dextrins and the like.

A preferred hydrolyzed cereal solids ingredient is a low dextrose equivalent starch hydrolysate such as MOR-REX Code 1918, having a dextrose equivalent of about 9 to 13 and containing 0.5 to 1% dextrose, 4.5 to 5% disaccharides, 4.75 to 5.5% trisaccharides and 3.75 to 4.5% each of tetrasaccharides and pentasaccharides. For the sake of convenience, the cereal solids hydrolysate will be referred to as HCS (for hydrolyzed cereal solids). The pregelatinized starch used in the composition has high solubility in cold water, generally in excess of 90% on a solids basis; slightly acid pH; and fine particle size, about 90 to 95%

or more of the material passing a screen having 100 meshes to the inch. The liquid polyhydroxy compound can be glycerol or glycerin, propylene glycol or a lower polyethylene glycol having a pour point below about 85°F. The solid polyethylene glycol ingredient is a polyethylene glycol or mixture of polyethylene glycols having an average molecular weight of 5,500 to 8,000, preferably 6,000 to 7,500. Such polyethylene glycols are typically designated by the average molecular weight thereof. The liquid polyhydroxy compound can be glycerol or glycerin, propylene glycol or a lower polyethylene glycol having a pour point below 85°F. The following example is illustrative of the coating compositions and method of application.

Example: A tablet coating solution is made up according to the following formula.

Water	60 ml.
Sucrose USP	4 grams
HCS (MOR-REX Code 1918)*	8 grams
Pregelatinized starch	12 grams
Red coating shade (mixture of FD&C colors)	0.08 grams
Titanium dioxide USP	0.4 grams
Propylene glycol USP	1.6 ml.

*Approximate Composition	Percent
Dextrose	0.7
Disaccharide	4.6
Trisaccharide	5.2
Tetrasaccharide	4.2
Pentasaccharide	4.1
Higher saccharides	81.2
Dextrose equivalent between 10 and 13	

The above ingredients are mixed to dissolve the sucrose, HCS, starch, propylene glycol and color in the water. Four grams of solid polyethylene glycol (Carbowax 6000) are then added and mixed well. Water is added to make a final volume of 100 ml. and the mixture is stirred with a propeller-type stirrer to completely disperse the insoluble titanium dioxide.

About 200 ml. of the coating solution are used to coat 500 grams of tablets. The tablets are prepared from a starch, milk sugar and sucrose base, with gelatin and gum acacia binder and with talc and magnesium stearate as lubricants. The tablets are compressed in a ⅜ in. die and have an average weight of about 0.35 gram each.

The coating solution is applied to a moving bed of the tablets in a conventional rotating coating pan by spraying the solution onto the tablets using a conventional air pressure operated spray gun while a stream of warm dry air is directed onto the moving bed of tablets to facilitate evaporation of water therefrom. After about 2.5 hours, the tablets are removed from the coating pan and dried on a tray for an additional 4 hour period at a temperature of 40°C. to assure complete drying of the coating.

Visual inspection of the tablets removed from the coating pan during and after the final drying shows that the coating has a good gloss and is smoothly applied to all surfaces of the tablets without heavy build-up at the edges. The coating is not abraded or worn away at the tablet edges, nor does the coating crack or peel or become soft or tacky during drying. Tablets coated in this manner do not become tacky when stored for substantial periods at 55°C. or at 45°C., with a relative humidity of 80%. Disintegration tests carried out on the tablets show that the coating disintegrates in a short time in either water or artificial gastric fluid. Each tablet has about 25 mg. of coating which is somewhat similar in appearance to a thin film coating.

Sugar-Calcium Sulfate Dihydrate Mixtures

Coatings having good elastic and mechanical strength have been developed by *W.E. Becker;*

U.S. Patent 3,753,767; August 21, 1973; assigned to Colgate-Palmolive Company. The coatings are an aqueous sugar syrup comprising 45 to 65% by weight of sugar and 5 to 30% by weight of calcium sulfate dihydrate or, as it is also known, terra alba. In the preferred practice, the tablet cores to be coated are placed in a side vented coating pan and the coating solution is hydraulically sprayed directly upon the tablet cores, preferably at a nozzle pressure of 800 to 1,500 psi.

When a predetermined amount of syrup has been sprayed on the cores, the tablet cores are rolled for 2 to 5 minutes to uniformly distribute the coating on all surfaces of the tablet cores. The coated cores are then dried under air pressure with heating. If desired, minor amounts of coloring materials and waxes may be added to the coated tablets.

The method lends itself to automation because it eliminates much of the operator handling which was necessary with traditional sugar-coating methods. For example, in the past it was often necessary after each addition of insoluble powders for the operator to hand roll the tablets in order to get an even distribution of a coating material. This process is further illustrated by the following example.

Example: An Accela Cota No. 24 side vented tablet-coating pan is loaded with 5.25 kg., or approximately 50,000, of $\frac{9}{32}$ inch lactose tablet cores. The reservoir of a Grayco tablet coater hydraulic spray system is charged with a syrup containing 17.84% by weight of calcium sulfate dihydrate, 54.08% by weight of sucrose and 28.88% by weight of water. The nozzle of the spray gun is equipped with a 0.021 inch spray tip and is positioned 8 to 10 inches from the tablets. The spray system is connected to an air pressure source providing a theoretical fluid pressure at the nozzle orifice of about 1,120 psi.

A Dayton 500°F. maximum heat gun is positioned 12 inches from the side of the pan. The pan is then rotated at 30 rpm, the pan vent opened and the exhaust system turned on. The hydraulic spray system is activated for 9 seconds with the pan rotating. In 9 seconds approximately 90 ml. of coating syrup is applied to the tablets. The tablets are then rolled with the pan blower turned off but the central exhaust system turned on for 2 minutes 25.5 seconds. The heat gun is then turned on at maximum temperature and the blower turned on for 2 minutes 25.5 seconds.

The pan is permitted to revolve at 30 rpm during the entire spraying, rolling and drying cycles. The complete coating cycle, which consists of the spraying, rolling and drying cycles, is repeated 55 times. At that time a colored subcoating syrup containing 10 parts of the original subcoating syrup and 1 part of Opalux AS 3162 Green by volume is substituted for the original sugar-coating syrup. The spraying, rolling and drying cycles are repeated five more times using the new colored subcoating syrup. The tablet cores are then removed from the pan and found to be uniformly smooth and of desired shape.

The total lapsed time for the described coating operation was about 5 hours. The tablets were weighed and found to have increased in weight by 90% as compared to the tablet cores. The subcoated tablets were then color coated and polished in the conventional manner. The finished tablets were then tested for elastic and mechanical strength and found to be equivalent to tablets which have been prepared by conventional coating techniques which had required 3 to 4 working days for completion. Tablets coated by this practice have been found to possess all of the desirable characteristics of tablets prepared by known methods which employ adhesives and lubricants.

CELLULOSE BASED COATING MATERIALS

Hydroxypropylmethylcellulose (HPMC) Coatings

N.F. Brindamour; U.S. Patent 3,383,236; May 14, 1968; assigned to Merck & Co., Inc. has developed a spray coating method for coating scored, engraved, or embossed tablets so that these markings and the tablet are uniformly covered without obliterating the desired markings. This is a one cycle continuous process requiring no drying or polishing cycles or steps. It has been found that a continuous nontoxic film coating may be produced on shaped cores containing pharmaceutical ingredients by the deposition of a continuous film of a compound selected from methylcellulose and hydroxypropylmethylcellulose (HPMC).

The film forming composition is applied to the shape cores containing pharmaceutical ingredients by the steps of (1) establishing a rolling bed of shaped dosage units of a pharmaceutical ingredient; (2) continuously spraying the dosage units with a solution of methylcellulose or hydroxypropylmethylcellulose in substantially equal amounts of ethanol and chloroform in an atomized state; (3) continuously evaporating the ethanol and chloroform from the sprayed dosage units at a rate such that the dosage units maintain a substantially dry appearance and where there is materially no transfer of film per se or of film forming solution from tablet to tablet; and (4) continuing the simultaneous rolling, spraying and evaporating, and controlling the relative spray rate and evaporation in such a manner as to prevent transfer from tablet to tablet until a continuous film of the desired thickness and quality has been established on the dosage unit.

The most important factors contributing to the process are the particle size of the suspended particles and spray droplet and the impact velocity. These are controlled by regulating the orifice sizes of both the air and fluid nozzles, the pressure on the atomized material which flows through the fluid orifice, and the pressure of the atomizing air if such is used. They are also controlled by regulating the viscosity and solids content of the coating composition, the number of nozzles, the spray distance, the size and shape of the spray pattern, the direction of the spray in relation to the travel of the tablets, and the spray angle. The number of nozzles does not vary directly as the weight of the pan load.

An equally important factor is the ratio of spray rate to drying rate. This is readily controlled by the use of flow meters and the control of bed temperatures which is a function of solvent evaporation rate. The temperature of the bed is monitored and kept within specified limits. At no time in the coating process are the tablets allowed to become wet. The tablets feel quite dry at the end of the spraying cycle. The following example will describe the process more fully.

Example: 60.75 liters of anhydrous ethanol (SD3A) were placed into a stainless steel container equipped with a high speed air driven agitator. While stirring, 2.673 kg. of hydroxypropylmethylcellulose (HPMC), NF, 50 cp. were added slowly to avoid clumping. Then there was added in order, 0.668 kg. of diethyl phthalate and 60.75 liters of chloroform USP, the contents then being mixed until the HPMC was dissolved.

After the solution had been effected, and while stirring, 3.645 kg. of titanium dioxide USP, 1.215 kg. of talc, USP, and 0.365 kg. of tartrazine FD&C Yellow No. 5, aluminum lake were added, and the stirring continued until a uniform suspension was obtained. This suspension was then passed through a Manton-Gaulin SMD homogenizer at 5,000 psi at a rate of 73 gph, 25 psi suction.

The coating procedure is as follows. 40.5 kg. of compressed cores containing 0.25 gram 1-α-methyldopa each were placed in a 42 inch stainless steel coating pan equipped with an air blower and exhaust system. The exhaust was turned on and drying air was directed toward the bottom of the tablet bed and adjusted to a temperature of approximately 190°F. The pan was then rotated at approximately 19 rpm, which caused the cores to take on a uniformly tumbling motion.

A manifold of 4 No. 2050 fluid nozzles (Spray Systems) equipped with a No. 120 air nozzle and cleanout assembly was arranged to continuously coat the full area of the pan occupied by the cores. The previously prepared suspension was contained in a reservoir located 10 inches above the manifold and fed by siphon to the nozzles. 40.5 liters of the suspension were sprayed from the nozzles using an atomizing air pressure of 46 psi pressure. The spray was directed at an angle to the face of the pan impinging to the left and in the opposite direction to the tablet flow. The average distance between the spray nozzles and the pan load was in the range of 7 to 8 inches. The suspension flow rate was in the range of 0.225 to 0.250 kg./minute, and the pan load was maintained at a temperature of 28° to 33°C. with the exhaust damper completely open. After completing the spraying the film coated tablets were transferred by plastic scoops to lined drying trays and dried in a forced air cabinet for approximately 18 hours at approximately 135°F. The resulting tablets had a clear colored continuous film coating formed thereon, which coating took a high polish when tumbled in carnauba wax.

HPMC-Polymer Coatings

A moistureproof, thermally stable film for coating tablets, pills and granules has been developed by *Y. Tuji; U.S. Patent 3,477,864; November 11, 1969; assigned to Sumitomo Chemical Co., Ltd., Japan.* The coating also contains hydroxypropylmethylcellulose dissolved in a mixture of at least one low boiling aliphatic halide and at least one other solvent, which may be an alcohol, mixtures of alcohol and a ketone or mixtures of water and an alcohol, and a sealing agent which may be a copolymer of butyl methacrylate and dimethylaminoethyl methacrylate, shellac or a prolamin.

The hydroxypropylmethylcellulose used in the coating is a cellulose derivative which contains about 7 to 12 weight percent of hydroxypropyl groups and about 28 to 30 weight percent of methoxy groups and the viscosity in 2% aqueous solution is below 10 cp. at 20°C. Thus, even when used at a high concentration, it does not hinder the coating operation so that the time for processing is shortened, the solvent saved, the procedure for coating much simplified and a uniform and smooth film formed easily. The dimethylaminoacrylate resin is a copolymer of butyl methacrylate and dimethylaminoethyl methacrylate. It dissolves below pH 2 and considerably swells at pH 3 to 6 to let water permeate through the same.

When employed alone, the former of the two polymers shows poor moistureproof property and, on coating by spraying, forms a less glossy surface. The latter has a peculiar color tone and causes difficulty in the coating operation. The combined use of these two polymers, however, can provide an ideal film. The use of shellac or a prolamin, i.e., zein, in place of the dimethylaminoacrylate resin may also furnish an improved moistureproof property and an excellent glossy surface to tablets without affecting their disintegration time in artificial gastric juice.

Example 1: 20 grams of 12.5 weight percent solution of dimethylaminoacrylate resin in a mixture of acetone and isopropanol and 20 grams of hydroxypropylmethylcellulose are dissolved in a mixture of 220 grams of ethanol and 80 grams of trichloroethylene. To the resultant mixture, there are added 1 gram of castor oil, 6 grams of diethyl phthalate and a hot solution of 2 grams of carnauba wax and 1 gram of hardened castor oil in 60 grams of trichloroethylene.

In the resulting mixture, there are suspended 2 grams of magnesium stearate, 3 grams of titanium dioxide and 15 grams of talc by the aid of a homogenizer or the like. An appropriate amount of the thus obtained coating solution is sprayed with an air spray gun on 3,000 convex surface tablets consisting of 22 parts of sodium chloride, 22 parts of sucrose, 33 parts of lactose, 22 parts of cornstarch and 1 part of magnesium stearate and rolling in a sugar coating pan, each tablet being 9 mm. in diameter and 280 mg. in weight. Instantly after the spraying is completed, hot air is blown into the pan to dry the tablets. This procedure is repeated to form a film weighing 15 to 20 mg. per tablet. The coated tablets thus prepared have a white, glossy and graceful appearance. Their moisture barrier, thermostability and facility of disintegration are satisfactory.

Example 2: 20 grams of 12.5 weight percent solution of dimethylaminoacrylate resin in a mixture of isopropanol and acetone and 20 grams of hydroxypropylmethylcellulose are dissolved in 80 grams of ethanol and 80 grams of trichloroethylene. Separately, there is prepared a homogeneous suspension of 2 grams of magnesium stearate, 3 grams of titanium dioxide, 15 grams of talc, 0.1 gram of saccharin sodium, 0.9 gram of sodium cyclamate and 1 to 2 grams of a color lake in 40 grams of ethanol. The suspension thus obtained is mixed with the above prepared solution. To the resulting mixture there is added a hot solution of 3 grams of isopropyl myristate, 3 grams of polyoxyethylene stearate, 1 gram of castor oil, 1.5 gram of carnauba wax and 1 gram of hardened castor oil in 60 grams of trichloroethylene. The tablets employed in Example 1 are coated with the resultant coating solution in the similar manner to produce the coated tablets having a glossy and graceful appearance. Their moisture barrier, thermostability and facility of disintegration are satisfactory.

HPMC-Erythrosine Coatings

E. Prillig; U.S. Patent 3,639,565; February 1, 1972; assigned to Abbott Laboratories has disclosed a composition consisting essentially of hydroxypropylmethylcellulose (HPMC) and erythrosine which is substantially insoluble in gastric juices but readily soluble in intestinal juices. It provides an excellent coating composition for tablets, granules and powders intended for dissolution in the intestines and for tablets, granules and powders containing a drug sensitive to the acidic environment of the stomach.

The coating is prepared from HPMC and erythrosine (sodium tetraiodofluorescein, more commonly known as FD&C Red No. 3) and a low-boiling solvent or solvent mixture, with the erythrosine being present in an amount between 0.5 and 50% of the HPMC. The amount of solvent or solvent mixture can vary but preferably, the coating solution contains between 1 and 10% of the above solids. Suitable low boiling solvents include methanol, ethanol, propanol, methylene chloride, chloroform, water and the like or their mixtures.

A particularly useful solvent system consists of 40 to 60% methylene chloride and 60 to 40% of ethyl alcohol. This mixture may contain other inert materials to a minor extent, e.g., other dyes, lakes or pigments, flavoring agents, and the like. All reference to erythrosine also includes the dye in form of its lake.

The above mixture can be provided in the form of a concentrate to which an additional solvent or solvents are added to give a suitable viscosity for the particular coating process used or it can be initially prepared in a viscosity range suitable for use in the available coating equipment. The mixture can be applied to tablets in the standard fashion, e.g., dip coating, pan coating or by suspension coating, the latter also being applicable to granules and powders.

Materials coated in this manner are resistant to gastric juices and are essentially impervious to liquids of a pH below 5.5. However, the films applied to tablets, powders and granules with the above coating composition readily dissolve at a pH above 7 and therefore offer no resistance to the juices in the intestines. This composition thus provides an excellent means for enteric coating of medicaments sensitive to gastric juices and can be used for proper release timing of orally administered drugs by providing the proper thickness of the coating. For ordinary protection toward the acidic passage of the alimentary channel, a coating thickness of between 0.05 and 0.1 mm. is sufficient.

Example: HPMC of 50 cp. viscosity and FD&C Red No. 3 were mixed in various ratios and dissolved in a mixture of 55% by volume of methylene chloride and 45% by volume of ethanol. Free films were prepared by casting the solution on glass plates with a Gardne Applicator. After drying, the films were removed from the glass plates and cut into discs with a 21 mm. diameter cork borer. The thickness of each disc was measured with a micrometer prior to testing; the average thickness was 0.06 mm.

The film pieces were individually placed in beakers containing artificial gastric juices, artificial intestinal juices, or deionized water. All film compositions were made from a mixture of 2% by weight of HPMC, dissolved in a mixture of 45% by volume of ethanol and 55% by volume of methylene chloride but contained different amounts of erythrosine. The following dissolution rates were observed.

Erythrosine	Gastric juice	Intestinal juice	Water
10 g./l.	Insoluble	Dissolved in 10 min.	Dissolved in 5 min.
5 g./l.	do.	Dissolved in 14 min.	Do.
2 g./l.	do.	do.	Do.

Methylcellulose Dicarboxylate Coatings

It has been discovered by *C.J. Malm, J.W. Mench and J. Emerson; U.S. Patent 3,504,082; March 31, 1970; assigned to Eastman Kodak Company* that dicarboxylic acid esters of methylcellulose are valuable as enteric coatings for medicaments, where the coated medicament is insoluble in stomach secretions but is soluble in alkaline intestinal fluids.

The dicarboxylic acid esters of methylcellulose are prepared by reacting methylcellulose with a mixture of glacial acetic acid, dicarboxylic acid anhydride particularly phthalic anhydride and an alkaline catalyst such as sodium acetate, potassium acetate or the like added or formed in situ. The methylcellulose used as a starting material may be that which is obtainable commercially such as having a methoxy content of 25 to 35%. It is desirable that the starting material have sufficient esterifiable hydroxyl groups that a substantial dicarboxylic acid radical content is added.

Although the phthalates are of particular importance, anhydrides of other dicarboxylic acids such as succinic anhydride, hexahydrophthalic anhydride, tetrahydrophthalic anhydride, maleic anhydride and the like may be used. The following example illustrates the preparation of this coating material.

Example: One part of methylcellulose having a methoxy content of approximately 28% and a viscosity of approximately 15 cp. was dissolved in a mixture of 4 parts of glacial acetic acid and 1.8 parts of phthalic anhydride with continuous stirring on a steam bath. Upon completion of the solution 0.9 part of anhydrous sodium acetate was added and the heating and stirring was continued.

After 2 hours reaction time the product was separated from the bath by diluting with acetic acid and precipitating into acidified water. The product was washed and dried and was found to have a combined phthalyl content of 38.7%, and an intrinsic viscosity in acetone of 0.82. The dibasic acid ester of methylcellulose thus obtained was readily soluble in organic solvents for instance acetone, and was easily soluble in aqueous 1.5% sodium bicarbonate solution and in aqueous 1% ammonia.

The medicaments to be coated in pill form can be pan coated with a solution of the esters or it may first be coated with or enclosed in gelatin or the like and then pan coated or otherwise coated with the solution of the cellulose derivative. The thickness of the coating can be controlled by varying the concentration of ester in the solvent. A plurality of immersions to form a layer of several coatings can also be used.

If desired, the ester may be formed into capsules composed of separate telescoping units into which the medicament can be placed and sealed with solution applied at the edge of the telescoping segments. The medicament may be enclosed in gelatin capsules which may then be pan coated or otherwise coated with a solution of the cellulose derivative.

Methylcellulose phthalate was compared as to effectiveness with cellulose acetate phthalate. In the case of each 400 salt tablets were coated with 100 ml. of a 15% solution of the esters in acetone. Twenty-five tablets were removed after 25, 50 and 75 ml. of the coating solution had been applied. The remaining 325 of the original tablets were given the 100 ml. level of coating. Thus a total of 400 tablets coated with methylcellulose phthalate and another 400 coated with cellulose acetate phthalate were obtained. After coating, the tablets were oven cured overnight at 50°C. to completely remove solvent. The test consisted of two parts: (1) treating with 0.25% concentrated hydrochloric acid solution (gastric juice) at 100°F. followed by (2) removability of the coating with aqueous 1.5% sodium bicarbonate (simulating intestinal conditions).

Methylcellulose-Polyalkylene Glycol Mixtures

R.H. Johnson; U.S. Patent 3,539,380; November 10, 1970; assigned to The Upjohn Co. has found that coating compositions consisting essentially of a solution of methylcellulose and a polyalkylene glycol having an average molecular weight of 200 to 9,000 can be applied to solid medicinal dosage forms to form a coating having superior properties. In addition, the coating compositions can contain minor amounts of adjuvants such as coloring agents, flavoring agents and sweetening agents. Active drugs can be dissolved or suspended in the coating fluid and added to the coat. Such coating compositions also have use in nonpharmaceutical applications, for example, the food and agricultural chemical fields.

These coating compositions have all of the advantages common to former film coatings, namely protection from chipping and breaking, masking of disagreeable taste and odor and providing a colored and attractive surface. These compositions also unexpectedly provide additional advantages. For example, the film coating is extremely thin, e.g., less than 10 mils and yet capable of adequate protection. Such a thin coating requires less labor and material in its application and does not appreciably increase the size of the tablet and does not obliterate embossing, scoring, or imprinting.

In spite of its thinness the film coating does not disintegrate prematurely, stick together or mottle in the presence of hot and/or humid atmosphere. Additionally the film coating process in eliminating the need for a sealing coat (e.g., shellac coat), or final polishing coat and, being soluble in volatile anhydrous solvents, is advantageous for coating water-sensitive dosage forms. Further, the film coating is uniformly deposited over the surface of the tablet and remains pliable and capable of withstanding shock or ageing. In addition, ageing does not discolor or unduly alter its rapid disintegration.

The coating compositions are prepared by dissolving the methylcellulose and polyethylene glycol in a suitable volatile solvent, or preferably in a system of two or more miscible cosolvents. In the preferred solvent system, a solution of chloroform, methanol and water is used in a ratio by weight of 55 parts chloroform, 35 parts methanol and 10 parts of water. The water can be omitted from the solvent system when water-sensitive tablets are to be coated. Additional suitable volatile solvents which can be used include methylene chloride, ethylene dichloride, ethanol, isopropanol, butanol and formamide.

The coating solutions are particularly advantageous for use in the air suspension coating machines, such as illustrated by Wurster in U.S. Patent 2,799,241 and in the *J.A. Ph. A.*, Scientific Edition, August 1959, at page 451. By use of the air suspension machine, tablets or other solid substances (e.g., small particles and granules) are suspended and tumbled in a current of air with the coating composition being blown into the system. The compositions have a particular advantage for use in this system in that the rotating substances do not stick together during the coating process.

The coatings can also be applied using conventional coating apparatus and procedure. For example, tablets can be placed in a standard rotating coating pan and the coating composition can be sprayed onto the tablets or poured over the tumbling tablets from a ladle. Applications of the coating composition can be made from time to time. Removal of the volatile solvents can be facilitated by means of a current of warm air being blown into the pan. The following example is illustrate of the process.

Example: 88 grams of methylcellulose USP, 10 cp. is wetted with 845 grams of absolute methanol. Sufficient chloroform is added to make 2,200 grams and stirred until the methylcellulose dissolves. 22 grams of polyethylene glycol 1000 is added together with about ½ gram each of FD&C Yellow No. 5 and No. 6. The solution is filtered through cheesecloth. A coating solution so prepared was applied to 2,000 grams of tablets. The tablets were 7/16 inch oval weighing 0.605 gram each. The tablets were placed in an air suspension machine and coated with about 2,150 grams of the filtrate obtained above. The following results were obtained.

Coating per tablet	30.4 mg.
Thickness:	
Edge	3.15 mils
Side	3.60 mils
Disintegration time: *U.S.P. XV*	
Coated tablets	10 min.
Uncoated tablets	4 min.
Difference due to film	6 min.

Nitrogen-Containing Cellulose Coatings

P.M. Grant, B. Fulkerson and J.W. Mench; U.S. Patent 3,562,806; February 9, 1971; and U.S. Patent 3,697,640; October 10, 1972; both assigned to Eastman Kodak Company have discovered that materials intended to be administered orally to ruminants can be protected from the rumen environment if the materials are first coated with a cellulosic material that resists not only the extremely corrosive microorganism environment of the rumen, but also the solubilizing action of the in vivo rumen fluid (which has a pH of 5.5 to 6.5 or more).

The cellulosic materials that have been found particularly useful in this respect are reaction products of organic nitrogen-containing bases (where there is at least one replaceable hydrogen connected directly to a nitrogen atom) with unsaturated cellulose ethers, unsaturated cellulose ester and unsaturated mixed ethers and esters of cellulose.

For example, the unsaturated esters may be aliphatic or unsaturated mononuclear aryl and aralkyl esters of cellulose such as cellulose crotonate, cellulose oleate, cellulose cinnamate, cellulose tiglate, cellulose linoleate, or cellulose ricinoleate. The useful, unsaturated cellulose ethers can be the simple unsaturated aliphatic ethers such as allylcellulose, vinylcellulose, or crotonylcellulose or of the cylcic series, as for example, styrylcellulose. Not all the substituent groups on the cellulose molecule need be unsaturated.

The organic bases can be aliphatic, alkyl, aromatic, or alicyclic and preferably should contain from 1 to 20 carbon atoms. They can be either primary or secondary amines, with secondary amines being preferred. Still further preferred are the cyclic secondary amines such as, for example, piperidine, morpholine and the like.

Some of the most valuable medicament or nutrient compositions are those coated with cellulose propionate 3-morpholinobutyrate having certain ratios of its various substituents on the cellulose backbone. Particularly preferred cellulose propionate 3-morpholinobutyrates are those containing 13 to 30% of propionyl, 0 to 4 weight percent of hydroxyl, and 22 to 50 weight percent of morpholinobutyryl. In the following examples all parts are by weight unless otherwise specified.

Examples 1 through 10: Into a stainless steel sigma blade mill are introduced 75,000 parts of (82% active) chlorotetracycline (CTC), 25,000 parts of a blend of (1) cellulose propionate 3-morpholinobutyrate containing 2% hydroxyl, 19% propionyl, 43% 3-morpholinobutyryl, and having an average molecular weight of 45,000, with (2) 125 parts of butylated hydroxyphenol (an antioxidant), and 125,000 parts of methylene chloride. The resulting mixture is blended for 20 minutes, air dried to remove the methylene chloride, and then ground to pass through a U.S. standard 16 mesh screen.

The product is then blended with a complete lamb feed at the level of 20 grams of CTC per ton of feed. After 10 weeks, the average weight gain of 10 lambs fed with this feed composition has increased more than 5.5 lbs./lamb (15.8%) as compared with the weight gained by a control group of 10 lambs that had been fed the same type of treated feed, except that the CTC was not blended with any of the nitrogen-containing cellulosic materials. It is particularly noteworthy that not every cellulosic material that is resistant to the action of the in vivo rumen environment is useful in this process. For usefulness however, the coating or protecting material must be resistant to the in vivo rumen environment, but must also readily dissolve in the more acidic abomasal fluid. Data set out in the table below illustrates these points. To obtain the data a piece of thin film of the test material is fastened inside a nylon fabric bag, which in turn is suspended for 24 hours inside the rumen of a living sheep.

The weight of the film before and after such treatment indicates the resistance of the film to the in vivo rumen environment. An acceptable material must be practically completely resistant to degradation under this test. An acceptable material must also dissolve in a strong aqueous acid environment; the solubility of the tested materials after 10 minutes exposure in in vitro abomasal fluid (pH is 2.5) is shown in the table.

Evaluation of Polymers for Rumen Stable Compositions

Example No.	Polymers	In Vivo Rumen Stability*	Solubility in Abomasal Fluid
2	Cellulose propionate 3-morpholinobutyrate	97	yes
3	Cellulose acetate	100	no
4	Cellulose acetate butyrate	97	no
5	Ethylcellulose	100	no
6	Copolymer**	2	partly
7	Copolymer***	97	no
8	Poly(1-methylamido-4-dimethylaminobenzene)	90	no
9	Cellulose acetate N,N-dimethylaminoacetate	78	yes
10	Deacetylated chitin	100	no

*Figures show percent of original weight recovered after exposure.
**25% dimethylaminoethyl methacrylate, 67% methyl methacrylate, 8% ethyl acrylate.
***15% dimethylaminoethyl methacrylate, 67% methyl methacrylate, 18% ethyl acrylate.

Cellulose Acetate Films

In a process described by *G.P. Polli, C.E. Shoop and W.M. Grim; U.S. Patent 3,538,214; November 3, 1970; assigned to Merck & Co., Inc.*, a tablet containing the drug is coated with a composition which will form a membranous film through which the drug will be leached out slowly. This slow leaching action will occur because gastrointestinal fluids can but slowly pass through the coating film to reach the drug in the tablet core and the drug which then becomes dissolved in the gastrointestinal fluids can but slowly pass out through the coating film and into the stomach and/or intestines. As the film remains substantially intact throughout the time that all the drug is being leached out the escape of the drug is prolonged and the rate of drug administration remains about uniform.

The coating composition is made up of a plastic having a low water vapor permeability such as cellulose acetate, a film modifying agent, a solvent such as acetone and, if desired, a plasticizer and/or a coloring material. The plastic should be insoluble in gastrointestinal fluids. Suitable plastics in addition to cellulose acetate are ethylcellulose, cellulose nitrate, low water-soluble polyvinyl alcohols and the other plastic pharmaceutical coatings.

The film modifying agent should be chosen so that it will be selectively but readily soluble or digestible in either the stomach fluids or in the intestinal fluids so that when it is partially or fully removed from the coating film the plastic which remains is of a membranous or dialytic nature. For removal in the stomach, suitable film modifying agents are calcium carbonate, calcium phosphates (mono-, di-, tri-), magnesium citrate, magnesium oxide, sodium bicarbonate, potassium bicarbonate, tetraethanolamine, lactose, polyvinylpyrrolidone and solid polyethylene glycols. Satisfactory results have been obtained when from 0.1 to 30 parts by weight of the plastic substance has been combined with 1 part by weight of modifying agent. Most satisfactory results have been obtained when from 1 to 3 parts by weight of the plastic substances have been combined with 1 part of the modifying agent. For removal in the intestines, suitable film modifying agents are benzoic acid, propionic acid, sorbic acid, salicylic acid and cellulose acetate phthalate. These agents are used in the same relative amounts set forth above for the other film modifying agents.

The film-forming composition is applied as a coating to the tablet cores, the amount and thickness being dependent upon the desired rate of release of the medicinal agent. In practice, it has been found that satisfactory results may be obtained when an average pharmaceutical tablet is coated with 5 to 100 mg. of the coating composition, although the amounts of the composition may be varied in accordance with the medicament and the amount of control of release desired.

To apply this coating, conventional tablet coating practices are used. This may use a tumbling barrel into which the coating composition is sprayed or it may use the fluidized column technique in which the coating composition is sprayed upwardly through the bed.

Example:

Ingredients for the Tablet Core	Mg./Tablet
Potassium chloride (granular)	572
Glyoxalated gelatin	572
Stearic acid	6

The potassium chloride and glyoxalated gelatin are intimately mixed. A portion is removed and mixed with the stearic acid. This is then passed through a number 12 sieve and added to the remaining potassium chloride glyoxalated gelatin mixture. The resultant mixture is then slugged, and the slugs are crushed and fed through a Fitzmill fitted with a 2A screen, and the resulting granules are compressed to form tablets having the desired weight of potassium chloride.

Ingredients for the Membranous Coating	Percent
Nitrocellulose	3.0
Calcium carbonate	1.0
Castor oil	1.0
Propylene glycol	1.0
Acetone to 100.0%	

The nitrocellulose is first wetted with a small amount of acetone, and agitated until all of the nitrocellulose is dispersed. The calcium carbonate is dispersed in some of the acetone, and the castor oil and propylene glycol in the remaining acetone. To the nitrocellulose dispersion the calcium carbonate, castor oil and propylene glycol dispersion is added with stirring. By passing the product through an homogenizer or mill, the incidence of nozzle clogging in the subsequent spraying operation is reduced significantly. 8 mg. of dry coating are applied to each matrix tablet by a continuous spraying operation. The tablets prepared in the example were tested in simulated gastric fluid and simulated intestinal baths and the results are tabulated in the table below.

	Test fluid[1]	Percent drug released time, hrs.			
		1	2	3	5½
Wt. of coating, mg.:					
8	A	75.0			
8	B	100.0			
12	A	5.0			
12	B			60.0	100.0

[1] A=Simulated gastric fluid; B=Simulated intestinal fluid.

Sodium Ethylcellulose Sulfate

A coated medicament has been developed by *R.R. Crawford, P.M. Grant, M.E. Rowley and W.D. Slowig; U.S. Patent 3,574,860; April 13, 1971* wherein the coating is glossy, smooth and hard; less bulky than sugar; dissolves in volatile organic solvents for rapid application and drying, yet disintegrates rapidly in gastric fluids; and can also be tailored to control the rate of disintegration in gastric fluids.

This coating consists essentially of sodium ethylcellulose sulfate which is applied to the medicament, either alone or in combination with a water-insoluble cellulose derivative and/or a plasticizer. The different cellulose derivative makes it possible to vary the solubility of the coating by varying the ratio of sodium ethylcellulose sulfate to the water-insoluble cellulose derivative in the mixture. A suitable plasticizer acts to lessen any tendency of the tablets to stick together in the coating pan, and also adds desirable flexibility to preformed capsules and other coatings to reduce brittleness.

Sodium ethylcellulose sulfate, the principal ingredient of this coating composition is a cellulose derivative described and claimed along with its method of manufacture in U.S. Patent 3,075,962. When this compound alone is to be applied as a coating on a medicament, it is dissolved in a suitable, easily evaporated organic solvent, such as methyl alcohol, or a mixture of acetone or methylene chloride with methyl alcohol, and then is repeatedly applied to the medicament with evaporation of the solvent taking place between repetitions until a protective coating or layer is built up.

When the coating contains not only the sodium ethylcellulose sulfate but also a different cellulose derivative and/or a plasticizer, it is applied in a similar manner, taking care that the solvent or appropriate mixture of solvents is one which will dissolve all ingredients of the composition. Among the operable cellulose derivatives are ethylcellulose and such cellulose esters of mono- and dicarboxylic acids as cellulose acetate phthalate, cellulose acetate and ethylcellulose phthalate. In general, a 2 component cellulose derivative coating should consist essentially of between 10 and 90% by weight of sodium ethylcellulose sulfate, the balance being the different cellulose derivative, the proportions depending upon the rate of solution of the coating desired when subjected to the action of gastric fluids.

The plasticizers can be any of the well-known compounds used for this purpose as long as they are compatible with the animal system to which they are to be introduced with the medicament. In a 3 component coating, plasticizer advantageously can comprise an effective amount up to 45% by weight, advantageously between 10 and 45% while the sodium ethylcellulose sulfate is between 10 and 80% and the different cellulose derivative is between 10 and 75%. Among suitable plasticizers are the polyethylene glycols, the propane diols and diethyl phthalate. The tablets can be coated by standard methods as shown in the following examples.

Example 1: A solution was prepared containing 10 grams sodium ethylcellulose sulfate and 5 grams cellulose acetate phthalate dissolved in a mixture of 75 ml. acetone and 25 ml. methanol. Small portions of the solution were added to about 100 tablets (deep concave 11/32 inch core, tricalcium phosphate-starch granulation) contained in a 1 liter beaker, continuously swirled. After each portion of the solution was added, the tablets were dried with a cold air stream. After 10 coats of the solution had been applied, the tablets were air dried for 25 hours. The tablets disintegrated in simulated gastric fluid in 35 seconds.

Example 2: A solution was prepared containing 6 grams sodium ethylcellulose sulfate and 9 grams ethylcellulose dissolved in 100 ml. methanol. Fifteen coats were applied. The tablets disintegrated in simulated gastric fluid in 15 seconds.

OTHER COATING MATERIALS

POLYETHYLENE GLYCOL BASED COATINGS

Quick Dissolving Coatings

Coatings which rapidly disintegrate in aqueous and gastric media but which can be applied in organic solvent solutions has been developed by *J.A. Sjogren and R.G.H. Persson; U.S. Patent 3,371,015; February 27, 1968; assigned to Aktiebolaget Hässle, Apotekare Paul Nordströms Fabriker, Sweden*. The coating comprises an inner layer 0.005 to 1.0 mm., preferably 0.05 to 0.03 mm., thick of a nontoxic-plastic substance soluble in water and organic solvents, preferably polyethylene glycol, and an outer layer of a nontoxic water-insoluble, film-forming thermoplastic substance soluble in a volatile organic solvent. The expression volatile here refers to substances or mixtures having a boiling point of 50° to 100°C.

Suitable organic solvents of this type are acetone, methyl ethyl ketone, methanol, ethanol, propanol, t-butanol, chloroform, ethyl propyl ether, dipropyl ether, diisopropyl ether, butyl methyl ether, carbon tetrachloride, trichloroethylene, ethyl acetate, isopropyl acetate, benzene, cyclohexene and dioxane. Suitable mixtures of organic solvents are, for instance, ethylene glycol monomethyl ether/acetone, methanol/acetone, ethanol/acetone, dioxane/methanol and chloroform/acetone.

Compositions having a coating in accordance with the process are satisfactorily covered as regards both taste and appearance, and at the same time the coating has a satisfactory tenacity and a suitable speed of disintegration in water and gastric juice, i.e., the coating disintegrates in from 10 seconds to 10 minutes. Another important advantage of this coating is that the application of the coating does not demand the same manual skill as older methods.

Although the course of the disintegration of the coating in water or gastric juice is not fully elucidated, it is probable that its superior properties may be ascribed to the combination of the inner, relatively thick coating of a plastic substance soluble in water and organic solvents which has good covering ability and adheres well to the core and at the same time is rapidly dissolved by water and gastric juice, and the very thin outer layer of water-insoluble, film-forming plastic which makes the objects as durable to handling as lacquered objects and effectively prevents the taste of the core being detectable in the mouth. The application of the coatings may be performed in known coating apparatus. Solutions of the substances constituting the two layers are separately poured or sprayed on the cores, which are at the same time kept in continuous movement, for instance, in a rotating pan. At each application of solution the cores should be evenly moistened, after which drying is performed by blowing on air at a suitable temperature, so that a thin layer of the plastic remains on the cores. The procedure is repeated until a coating of the desired thickness is obtained. The process is illustrated by the following example. The tablets used weigh 550 mg. each and have the following composition:

	Milligrams
Ascorbic acid	220
Succinic acid	150
Ferrosulfate, sicc.	100
Starch	31
Talcum	22.5
Magnesium stearate	2.5
Polyvinylpyrrolidone	24

These tablets had a disintegration time according to *British Pharmacopeia,* 1958, page 964, of 12.5 minutes.

Example: A solution was made of the following composition:

	Parts by Weight
Polyethylene glycol, molecular weight 6,000	50
Chloroform	35
Acetone	15

The solution obtained was poured on to the tablets tumbling in a coating pan so that the tablets became evenly moistened on the surface. The tablets were dried by blowing on air. The procedure was repeated 20 times after which the tablets showed an even, thin coating of polyethylene glycol suitable, if desired, for engraving. A solution of the following composition was prepared:

	Parts by Weight
Cellulose acetate phthalate	6
Methyl ethyl ketone	45
Acetone	49

The solution obtained was poured over the rotating mass of tablets so that the tablets became evenly moistened on the surface after which the tablets were dried by blowing on air. Six applications of this kind were made, after which the coated tablets were carefully dried. They showed a glazed, hard surface which did not turn smeary on handling. The coating obtained showed the following thicknesses of the layers: inner polyethylene glycol layer 0.100 mm. and outer cellulose acetate phthalate layer 0.015 mm.

Polyethylene Glycol-Carboxyvinyl Polymer Mixtures

N.E. Brindamour; U.S. Patent 3,379,554; April 23, 1968; assigned to Merck & Company, Incorporated has disclosed an improved series of coating compositions based on the combined use of known film-forming materials. One ingredient is chosen from high molecular weight polyethylene glycols and their esters and the other ingredient is chosen from a group of high molecular weight carboxyvinyl polymers. The resulting coating has the following particular advantages:

(1) The vinyl polymer imparts water solubility to the coating.
(2) The vinyl polymer is used in smaller amounts than if it were used alone.

This coating formulation gives a continuous, nontoxic, glossy film having the required solubility characteristics on shaped cores containing pharmaceutical ingredients by the deposition of a solution of 5 to 10 parts by weight of (1) the polyethylene glycol and 1 part by weight of (2) the water-soluble carboxyvinyl polymer. Minor amounts of gelling, suspending, opacifying, plasticizing, solubilizing, coloring, glossing, tack reducing, and alkalizing agents of the kinds commonly used in pharmaceutical manufacture may or may not be used.

Solvents suitable for the process may be water, methanol, ethanol, isopropanol, propanol, acetone, methyl ethyl ketone, chloroform, methylene chloride, carbon tetrachloride, Chlorothene, dimethylacetamide, methyl acetate, ethyl acetate, ethyl lactate, dioxane, benzene, toluene, Freons (the groups of low boiling alcohols), aldehydes and ketones, and mixtures or blends of the above. These ingredients may be used in the following ranges in making up the liquid composition to be applied to the tablet to form a film coating:

	Percent
Carboxyvinyl polymer	0.01 - 3
Polyethylene glycol 4,000 to 20,000	0.05 - 30
Gelling, tack reducing, suspending agent	0 - 5
Opacifying agent	0 - 10
Tack reducing, glossing agent	0 - 20
Organic or inorganic alkalizing agent	0 - 10
Plasticizing agent	0 - 5
Surfactant	0 - 0.5
Coloring agent	0 - 5
Solvent, q.s.	

In using this composition it is possible to use a conventional pear shaped rotating coating pan and to spray it on the tumbling tablets. However, best results are obtained if one uses a rotating coating pan and its associated equipment.

Example: Coating Solution – Two grams of Carbopol 934 and 20 grams of Carbowax 6000 were dissolved in enough methanol to make 100 ml.

Coating Procedure – Five hundred grams of $^{10}/_{32}$" standard curvature placebo tablets each weighing 270 mg. were placed in the coating pan equipped with a blower to direct dry air on the tumbling tablets and with an exhaust system to suck air from the interior of the pan. A paint container and spray nozzle operated at 30 pounds air pressure and having a 10" fluid head pressure was placed to continuously coat the plane of the tablet flow surface. The solution was sprayed in such a direction that the plane of the tablet flow surface formed a right angle with the line of spray, the spray distance to the tablets being three inches.

The drying air input and exhaust were adjusted to prevent the tablet load from becoming wet as the film was deposited on the individual tablets. The temperature of the tablet bed was kept within 20° and 30°C. The solution sprayed at the rate of 5 ml./min. until 100 ml. had been consumed. The tablets were allowed to roll for 15 minutes after the final application of the solution. The resulting tablets were glossy, smooth, and homogeneously coated. The disintegration time of both the coated and uncoated tablet was the same. A gas chromatogram of the coated tablet showed no residual solvent. The coating is not softened when exposed to either 50°C. or to a 75% relative humidity atmosphere for a period of two weeks.

Solventless Spray Coating Solutions

A process for spray coating tablets with a coating which contains no organic solvent has been developed by *P.A. Tuerck; U.S. Patent 3,383,237; May 14, 1968; assigned to Richardson-Merrell Incorporated*. The superior film coatings provided by the process are tough and pharmaceutically elegant. They are economical in that no volatile solvents are employed and the hazards during manufacture of toxicity and explosion are obviated. The coatings are water-soluble, may be colored with dyes, lakes, or pigments, and may be applied continuously without interruption for drying during the application. These coatings comprise essentially polyethylene glycols having an average molecular weight of 1,000 to 9,000 modified with 10 to 40% by weight of natural or synthetic gum or resin such as shellac or sucrose benzoate, or mixtures thereof. The process is practiced by warming the tablets, capsules, or granules to 30° to 45°C. in a conventional tablet coating pan. The tablets may be warmed by heating the pan itself, by means of steam or hot water jacketing, or by the application of an open flame. Alternatively, the tablets may be preheated in an oven before introduction into the pan.

The coating compositions are melted and maintained in liquid state in a container or reservoir heated above the melting point of the coating composition. The melted coating composition is fed by gravity or suction through a heated pipe to a steam jacketed spraying head. A preferred form is a pneumatic spraying head which depends upon air pressure to break the melted liquid into a fine spray. Spraying heads designed for airless spraying are also suitable if means are provided for preventing congealing of the coating composition in the spraying head.

The hot melted spray is directed onto the warmed tablets while they are tumbling in a rotating coating pan. The temperature of the melted composition and the pressure applied to the spray nozzle are regulated so that the melted material congeals soon after striking the tablets. When the melting point of the coating composition is too high, the sprayed material congeals before it strikes the tablets and satisfactory coatings cannot be achieved. If the temperature of the melted coating composition is too high, the coating remains liquid long enough to cause clumping of the tablets.

Example: Placebo tablets were prepared using a mixture of 85% lactose, 10% cornstarch, and 5% soluble starch. This mixture was blended, granulated with water, dried, placed through a No. 12 mesh screen, lubricated with 1% magnesium stearate and compressed into 7⁄16" diameter tablets weighing 415 mg./tablet. Three hundred grams (722 uncoated tablets) were placed in a stainless steel coating pan of 6½" in diameter and warmed to between 35° to 45°C. by applying heat to the rotating pan. At this point the heating was discontinued and the tablets were sprayed with a molten coating solution maintained between 110° and 140°C. The coating had the following composition:

	Percent wt./wt.
Sucrose benzoate	10
Dry shellac	10
Cetyl alcohol	5
Polyethylene glycol 4000	74.5
D&C Yellow #11	0.5

It was prepared by placing the dry shellac in a container and heating to 120°C. followed by the addition of the sucrose benzoate, cetyl alcohol, polyethylene glycol, and dye, with stirring, until all of the materials were in solution. The solution was sprayed upon the tablets with the pan rotating at 43 rpm through a steam jacketed pneumatic spray head ¼ JBCJ, employing a No. 2850 fluid nozzle and No. 70 air nozzle.

Low pressure steam is introduced into the steam jacketed spray head to keep the spray head hot during the spraying operation. Air at 12 psi is introduced into the air intake orifice of the spray head. The molten coating material is continuously sprayed on the tablets until an increase in weight of 73.8 mg./tablet is obtained. This spraying operation requires approximately 20 minutes. The sprayed tablets are allowed to tumble in the rotating pan for approximately 5 minutes after the spraying operation in order to cool them. The finished tablets had a pharmaceutically elegant appearance. The coating disintegrated in water within 6 minutes when tested by standard procedures.

Semipermeable Film Coatings

A continuous process for applying coatings to pharmaceutical tablets at low temperatures has been disclosed by *G. Pitel; U.S. Patent 3,476,588; November 4, 1969; assigned to Societe d'Etudes Scientifiques et Industrielles de l'Ile-de-France, France*. The composition employed for coating tablets by this process comprises a mixture, in suitable organic solvents, of:

(a) a substance that is insoluble in water but has the property of forming plastic films by evaporating a solution in an organic solvent; e.g., ethylcellulose; and
(b) a solid that is soluble both in water and in the selected organic solvent or solvents, e.g., a polyglycol having a molecular weight of at least 6,000. Polyglycol has the property of converting the water-insoluble film formed by the ethylcellulose into a film semipermeable to water and enables the tablet to disintegrate.

The solvents in which the coating composition is dissolved comprise a mixture of two solvents which solubilize both polyglycol and ethylcellulose and which are volatile under specific conditions, so that they enable the coating solution to be continuously applied without the tablets sticking together and, on the other hand, without there being any sliding in the centrifuge where the coating is carried out. The most favorable solvent is a mixture of equal quantities of an alcohol, e.g., methyl alcohol, ethyl alcohol, or isopropyl alcohol, and a chlorinated organic solvent, e.g., chloroform, methylene chloride, or 1,1,1-trichloroethane. Instead of one alcohol and one chlorinated organic solvent, a plurality of alcohols and chlorinated solvents may be used.

Being noninflammable and nonexplosive, chlorinated solvents enable the coating operations to be carried out in complete safety. The use of 1,1,1-trichloroethane is of particular advantage because of its low price and the fact that it is less toxic than methylene chloride or chloroform. Fillers may be added either to obtain an opaque or colored covering. For example, talc or titanium oxide, colors approved as complying with the requirements of the U.S. Food, Drug and Cosmetic Act, water-insoluble pigments, such as aluminum lacquers or nontoxic metallic oxides, such as iron oxide, may be used for this purpose.

The physical properties of the film obtained on the tablets may be modified by varying the proportions of ethylcellulose and polyglycol or by modifying the viscosity of the ethylcellulose used. Thus, increasing the percentage of ethylcellulose reduces the perviousness of the film formed to water, and conversely increasing the percentage of polyglycol makes the film more pervious. Moreover, ethylcellulose of low viscosity (10 cp.) forms films which are more flexible and more pervious to water, and conversely ethylcellulose of higher viscosity (100 cp.) produces coverings which are harder and less pervious.

Alternatively, substances designed to produce special effects may be added to the coating solvents. Resistance to water, for example, is increased by adding paraffin or a hard fat. Addition of wax gives a brighter coating. The addition of a fatty acid such as stearic, palmitic or lauric acid leads to a film which has a certain resistance to dissolution in the stomach. The apparatus conveniently used for applying the coating solution comprises a coating centrifuge equipped with a hot air blowing and vapor suction system, and equipment, including a spray gun, for atomizing the coating solution.

The process comprises placing the tablets in a centrifuge, rotating them, blowing in hot air in a quantity sufficient to bring the tablets to a temperature of 35° to 40°C., then atomizing the coating while regulating the discharge so as to obtain instantaneous drying. Application of the coating solution is continued until a film of the desired thickness is obtained on the tablets. In the majority of cases, it has been found satisfactory to apply 750 ml. of solution per kilogram of tablets. The application time is not generally longer than 4 hours for 35 kilograms of tablets.

A more comprehensive understanding of this process is obtained by reference to the following examples in which a mixture of the ingredients indicated in each example, forms a solution with or without solid filler, e.g., titanium oxide substantially uniformly dispensed therein, and such solution is applied to the tablets as above described.

Example 1:

Ethylcellulose (50 cp.)	3.50 g.
Polyglycol 6,000	7 g.
Ethyl alcohol	50 ml.
Chloroform	50 ml.

Example 2:

Ethylcellulose (50 cp.)	3.50 g.
Polyglycol 20,000	7 g.
Titanium oxide	3 g.
Talc	1 g.
Ethyl alcohol	50 ml.
1,1,1-trichloroethane	50 ml.

POLYMERIC COATING MATERIALS

Compressed Coatings of Polyvinyl Acetate

The technical problems inherent in developing compressed enteric coatings are quite different from those of the pan coating method. In the latter, one is mainly concerned in the development of solutions of coating substances capable of forming smooth and uniform films on the tablet surface. A major objective in the compression coating method is the development of coating granulations that will uniformly fill the die cavities and yield upon compression, tablets with centrally positioned cores and a coating of strongly coherent granules with a minimum of void space or interstices throughout the coating.

E.A. Hotko and L. Lachman; U.S. Patent 3,325,365; June 13, 1967; assigned to Ciba Corporation have found that tablets can be compressed coated by using an enteric coating granulate composition containing a polyvinyl acetate copolymer as the film-forming copolymer and a substrate. This process is carried out according to known methods, preferably by using a machine capable of compressing a coating around a preformed core tablet. The latter contains the physiologically active components, which is intended to pass unaltered through the acidic medium of the stomach and to be absorbed in the alkaline medium of the lower intestine.

The granulate composition is prepared by known methods. For practical reasons, a homogenous mixture of the bulking material and the lubricant agent, both screened through suitable screens, is first formed in one of the mixers used to prepare the substrate. The latter is then granulated by adding a solution of the polyvinyl acetate copolymer and of any plasticizer while agitating.

The solution is prepared by dissolving the polyvinyl acetate polymer and any plasticizer in a suitable organic solvent, particularly ethyl acetate, or in a mixture of solvents containing preferably ethyl acetate and another miscible organic solvent, e.g., methanol, ethanol, isopropanol, acetone and the like; a preferred solvent is a 1:1-mixture of ethyl acetate and ethanol. The resulting wet granulation mass is screened and dried, usually while passing air over it, and, if necessary, at an elevated temperature. The dried granules are then passed through a mill and screened to yield granulate particles of a certain maximum size.

Example 1: An enteric coating granulate composition suitable for a tablet compression coating procedure and containing 15.7% of a polyvinyl acetate copolymer consisting of vinyl acetate and crotonic acid as the comonomers, is prepared as follows:

Ingredients	Grams
Calcium lactate	630.0
Hydrogenated castor oil	70.0

(continued)

Ingredients	Grams
Polyvinyl acetate copolymer	151.0
Triethyl citrate	105.7

The calcium lactate and the hydrogenated castor oil are sifted through a 30 mesh screen and mixed in a suitable mixer for 30 minutes. A solution of the polyvinyl acetate copolymer and the triethyl citrate plasticizer in a sufficient quantity of the 1:1-mixture of ethyl acetate and anhydrous ethanol is prepared, and added to the mixer to form the granulate. The wet mass is passed through a No. 8 sieve, dried at room temperature and ground through a mill using a screen with 0.063 inch (about 1.6 mm.) openings.

In the above example, the particular polyvinyl acetate copolymer may be replaced by another polyvinyl acetate copolymer using as comonomers vinyl acetate and acrylic acid, vinyl acetate and acrylic acid amide, vinyl acetate and maleic acid, vinyl acetate and itaconic acid, vinyl acetate and methyl acrylate, vinyl acetate and vinyl chloride, and the like. The triethyl citrate plasticizer may be replaced by another suitable plasticizer, e.g., diethyl phthalate, benzyl benzoate and the like.

Example 2: Enteric tablets containing 0.3 gram of acetylsalicylic acid as the physiologically active component and having a compressed enteric coating are prepared as follows (for 20,000 tablets):

Ingredients	Grams
Acetylsalicylic acid	6,000.0
Cornstarch	340.0
Colloidal silica	80.0
Stearic acid	80.0

The acetylsalicylic acid, cornstarch, colloidal silica and stearic acid powders are sifted through a 16 mesh screen and mixed for 30 minutes. The powder mass is made compact by slugging, and the slugs are broken through a 16 mesh screen. The resulting material is compressed into cores weighing 0.325 gram each, using $^{12}/_{32}$ inch punches. An enteric coating is compressed around the resulting cores using the enteric coating granulate composition described in Example 1 and $^{15}/_{32}$ inch punches; the resulting enteric tablets weigh 0.65 gram each and have an average Strong Cobb Hardness of 20 units.

Polyvinyl Acetal Copolymer Coatings

Tablet coating compositions which are water insoluble but readily soluble in weak acid solutions of the hypoacidic or anacidic patients have been developed by *H. Negoro, E. Awada, Y. Ikegami, S. Akagi and K. Matsui; U.S. Patent 3,477,995; November 11, 1969; assigned to Sankyo Company, Limited, Japan*. They found that (1) synthetic resins obtained by esterifying polyvinyl alcohol, partially butyralized polyvinyl alcohol or hydrolyzate of copolymer of vinyl acetate and crotonic acid with monochloroacetic acid, acetalizing the esterified product with an aliphatic aldehyde containing 2 to 4 carbon atoms and aminating the resulting acetal with a di(lower alkyl)amine containing 1 to 4 carbon atoms on each alkyl moiety and (2) synthetic resins obtained by esterifying polyvinyl alcohol with monochloroacetic acid, etherifying the esterified product with dihydropyrane and aminating the resulting ether with a di(lower alkyl)amine containing 1 to 4 carbon atoms on each alkyl moiety can be with advantage used for coating oral preparations which are to be dissolved in the stomach.

Coating of pharmaceutical preparations with these coating compositions may be carried out in any convenient manner, and is applicable to the coating of pharmaceutical preparations adapted for oral administration, such as tablets and pills. The coatings are thus conveniently applied from solutions in suitable solvents such as ethanol and isopropanol, for example, by spraying, dipping, or tumbling by using conventional techniques. In the example below, the disintegration test is carried out by making measurements according to U.S.P. XVI method at 37°C. without disk.

Example: To a solution of 156 grams of polyvinyl alcohol having a degree of polymerization of 500, trade name Gohsenol NL-05, in 468 grams of water are added 475 grams of monochloroacetic acid. The mixture is heated at 100° to 110°C. for 4 hours. After chilling to 40°C., 220 grams of paraldehyde are added to the reaction mixture, followed by stirring.

To the resulting mixture are added 75 ml. of 50 vol./vol. percent sulfuric acid, followed by stirring at 40°C. for 2 hours. Solid matter thus formed is separated from the aqueous layer, washed and dissolved in 1,560 ml. of acetone. The acetone solution is added dropwise to 15 liters of water with stirring by an agitator to precipitate a white fibrous substance. The intermediary product is separated by filtration, washed with water and dried; weight 198 grams. This product, softening point 90° to 95°C. and decomposing point 140° to 145°C., is readily soluble in acetone, ethyl acetate and chloroform, but is insoluble in methanol and ethanol.

To a solution of 150 grams of the intermediate in 1.5 liters of acetone are added 55 grams of diethyl amine and the mixture is heated on a steam bath under reflux for 2 hours. After cooling, the acetone reaction solution is added dropwise to 15 liters of water with stirring by an agitator to precipitate white fibrous substance, which is separated by filtration, washed with water and dried in blowing air at 40° to 50°C. Polyvinyl acetoacetal diethylamino acetate weighing 117 grams is obtained; yield 99% on the basis of weight of starting material. This product, softening point 85° to 95°C. and decomposing point 100° to 110°C., is readily soluble in methanol, ethanol, ethyl acetate, chloroform and acetone. It is also rapidly dissolved in synthetic gastric juice.

Tablet preparations may be coated with the material thus produced. For example, to a powdered mixture of 1,300 grams of lactose and 200 grams of dextrine are added 500 grams of 5% starch paste. The resulting mixture is well mixed, subsequently passed through a No. 14 mesh screen and dried. The resulting matter is granulated through a No. 12 mesh screen. The granules are mixed with 2% of talcum and 1% of magnesium stearate for lubrication and then tabletted to tablets each weighing 310 mg. and having a diameter of ⅜" and a radius of curvature of $^{17}/_{64}$".

The coating material obtained as above, weighing 50 grams, is dissolved in 225 grams of acetone and 225 grams of methanol. Three thousand uncoated tablets placed in a coating pan of a diameter of 8 inches are subjected to consecutive coatings with 5 portions of 100 grams of the aforementioned solution to obtain tablets each weighing 320 mg. The coated tablets remain unchanged after immersion in distilled water for 4 hours, but are disintegrated in synthetic gastric juice in 16 minutes. This disintegration in gastric juice is the same as that of uncoated tablets.

Styrene-Maleimide Copolymers for Rumen Resistant Coatings

Rumen resistant coatings have been developed by *T. Kralt and J.A.C. Kroesen; U.S. Patent 3,488,417; January 6, 1970; assigned to U.S. Philips Corporation* which are styrene-maleic anhydride copolymers imidified with an alkylenediamine. Examples of suitable diamines include: N,N-diethylethylenediamine, N,N-dimethylpropylenediamine, N,N-dimethylethylenediamine, N,N-dipropylethylenediamine, N,N-dibutylethylenediamine, N,N-diethylpropylenediamine, N,N-dipropylpropylenediamine, and N,N-dimethylbutylenediamine. N,N-diethylethylenediamine, however, is preferred.

Suitable nutrients or medicines for mixing with the preparations are, for example, hormones, carbohydrates, such as dextrines and glucose, antibiotics such as penicillin, tetracycline, zinc bacitracine, vitamins, for example A and E, amino acids and proteins, such as lysine, methionine, cysteine and blood proteins, furthermore liver fluke and lung worm preparations and other medicines. The preparations may be produced in methods known per se. Cores of active substance may be pressed, mixed if desired with excipients, the cores being enveloped in the coating, for example, by applying the coating dissolved in a volatile solvent to the cores in the form of a dust. It is possible to mix the rumen resistant material as a powder or a granulate with the substance to be protected. The mixture may then be extruded under elevated temperature and pressure. Thereupon the product may be cut down to a desired size. A rumen resistant preparation may be prepared from the following ingredients: 4.4 grams of copolymer of styrene and maleic acid anhydride amidified to imide with N,N-diethylethylenediamine having an intrinsic viscosity in dioxane at 20°C. of 0.1 to 0.05 l./g.; 30 ml. acetone; 600 mg. vitamin A-acetate; and 50 to 100 mg. of a mixture consisting of equal parts butylated hydroxy anisole (BHA) and butylated hydroxy toluene (BHT). Such a composition containing vitamin A marked C^{14} was tested as follows with regard to effectiveness.

Two comparable groups of bucks were treated. One group received 0.5 standard units of vitamin A per buck, incorporated in small lumps of calf fodder; the other group received an equal quantity of vitamin A coated according to this process, also incorporated in small lumps. (A hole was made in the lumps and the preparation was brought therein after which the hole was further filled with powder obtained in boring the hole.) Fifteen days after the administration the animals were killed and the quantity of vitamin A stored in the liver was assessed. The animals which had received a coated composition had stored twice the quantity of vitamin A as compared with the animals of the control-group.

Methyl Vinyl Ether-Maleic Anhydride Copolymers

A coating composition is described by *J.T. Carstensen and J.J. Vance; U.S. Patent 3,407,157; October 22, 1968; assigned to Hoffmann-La Roche Incorporated* which contains, as essential ingredients, (a) a water-soluble interpolymer of methyl vinyl ether and maleic anhydride, (b) glyceryl monostearate, polyoxyethylene sorbitan monooleate, dioctyl sodium sulfosuccinate or a mixture thereof and (c) acetone, ethyl acetate or a mixture thereof as an inert organic solvent for the interpolymer.

Additionally, the coating can contain, as optional ingredients, many of the adjuvants which are normally found in the coatings, for example, plasticizers, pigments, lake dyes, FD&C dyes, D&C dyes, dusting agents, etc. The high molecular weight polymer which is used in formulating the composition is a linear polymeric anhydride which, chemically, is the interpolymer of methyl vinyl ether and maleic anhydride having an average molecular weight of 250,000. A polymer of this type, which has a structure corresponding to a one to one molar ratio of vinyl ether to anhydride, is available commercially under the trade name Gantrez AN-119. The coating process is disclosed in more detail in the following examples.

Example 1: In this example 20.0 grams of Gantrez AN-119 was added to, and dissolved in, 450 cc of acetone at room temperature. To this solution, there was added 8.0 cc of castor oil, 4.0 mg. of Aerosol OT (dioctyl sodium sulfosuccinate) and 100.0 mg. of D&C Yellow #11. Thereafter, 20.0 grams of titanium dioxide, containing 1% by weight of Cab-O-Sil (colloidal silica), 4.0 grams of talc and 4.0 grams of FD&C Yellow #5 Lake Dye was added to the solution. The suspension, thus obtained, was homogenized. The above suspension, was applied to tablets containing 7-chloro-2-methylamino-5-phenyl-3H-1,4-benzodiazepine-4-oxide as the active ingredient. The tablets were prepared by mixing the following in the portions indicated:

Ingredient	Mg./Tablet
7-Chloro-2-methylamino-5-phenyl-3H-1,4-benzodiazepine-4-oxide	10.25
Microcrystalline cellulose	18.00
Cornstarch	12.00
Dicalcium phosphate	79.15
Calcium stearate	0.60

The microcrystalline cellulose which was used was the product marketed under the trade name Avicel. The mixture was passed through a screen and it was compressed into tablets weighing 120.0 mg. using a standard concave punch. In the coating operation, the medicament-containing tablets were placed in a conventional, standard coating pan and a sufficient quantity of the coating composition, was run into the pan to wet the tablets completely. The coating pan was rotated continuously until all of the liquid coating composition was taken up by the tablets. The coated tablets were then dried by cool air for a period of 15 minutes. A second, third, fourth and fifth coat was applied in the same manner as the first coat, care being taken in each coating operation not to over-wet the tablets with the coating composition. After the fifth coat had been applied, the pan was permitted to continue its rotation until the tablets had lost their tackiness and had begun to take on a glossy appearance. At this point, the tablets were removed from the coating pan and then they were placed in a rotating polishing pan where they were dusted to a high gloss with powdered carnauba wax. There was thus obtained, tablets having an attractive appearance and completely satisfactory hardness, friability and disintegration characteristics.

Example 2: In this example, 4.5 grams of Gantrez AN-119 was dissolved in 100 cc of acetone at room temperature. To the solution thus obtained there was added the following named ingredients in the quantities herein indicated: 2.0 cc of diethyl phthalate, 2.0 mg. of Aerosol OT and 50.0 mg. of D&C Yellow Dye #11. Thereafter, 10.0 grams of titanium dioxide, containing 1.0% by weight of Cab-O-Sil, and 2.0 grams of FD&C Yellow #5 Lake Dye was added to the solution with agitation. The suspension, which was thus produced, was homogenized.

The suspension described above was evaluated as a tablet coating composition in the manner described in Example 1. In this instance, however, the suspension was applied in ten separate applications. The tablet which was coated was produced as described in Example 1, such tablet containing 7-chloro-1-methyl-5-phenyl-3H-1,4-benzodiazepin-2(1H)-one as the active ingredient thereof. Tablets having an attractive appearance and completely satisfactory hardness, friability and disintegration characteristics were obtained.

Aminopolyamide Coatings

G.J. Marco, E.J. Prill and E.G. Jaworski; U.S. Patent 3,492,398; January 27, 1970; assigned to Monsanto Company have developed additives for ruminant feeds where the biologically active material is enclosed in an aminopolyamide resin containing from 1 to 4.2 weight percent of amino nitrogen, from 83 to 87.5 weight percent of hydrocarbon and 8.3 to 16 weight percent of amide, the resin being nondispersible in the gastric and rumen fluids while being substantially dispersible in the intestinal fluids.

The expression aminopolyamide resin identifies a polyamide resin which contains a substantial quantity of unreacted amino groups. These are prepared by condensing polyamines, polycarboxylic acids, monocarboxylic acid, monoamines and amino acids selected and proportioned so that the resins consist substantially entirely of amide groups, amino nitrogen atoms and hydrocarbon groups.

These polyamide resins containing free amino radicals are condensation polymers prepared by the interreaction of polyamines and polycarboxylic acids, which may include as reactants monofunctional amine and carboxylic acid to provide chain end groups whereby the molecular weight and other properties can be controlled. Useful monofunctional amines include octadecyl amine, dodecyl ethyl amine, lauryl amine, benzyl amine, isooctyl amine, n-butyl amine and other alkyl amines of up to 22 carbon atoms, or mixtures thereof. Useful monocarboxylic acids include oleic acid, benzoic acid, abietic acid, pimaric acid, palmitic acid, hypogeic acid, caproic acid, butyric acid, behenic acid and other saturated or unsaturated acids of up to 22 carbon atoms or mixtures thereof. Since the preparation often involves heating at temperatures above the boiling points of some of the lower molecular weight monoamines and monocarboxylic acids, those of higher weights are usually more practicable. A partial list of amine-containing polyamide resins is shown in the table below.

Resin No.	Reactants	Equivalents
1	Dimer acid*	2.020
	Diethylene triamine	3.135
	Oleic acid	0.150

(continued)

Resin No.	Reactants	Equivalents
2	Dimer acid**	1.220
	Diethylene triamine	2.085
	Oleic acid	0.230
3	Dimer acid**	1.000
	Diethylene triamine	1.500
4	Dimer acid**	1.000
	Diethylene triamine	1.290
	Ethylenediamine	0.290
	Oleic acid	0.150
5	Dimer acid**	1.000
	Diethylene triamine	0.435
	Ethylenediamine	0.860
	Oleic acid	0.150
6	Dimer acid*	1.000
	Diethylene triamine	1.500
	Oleic acid	0.003
7	Isophthalic acid	0.500
	Dimer tetraamine***	2.000
	Oleic acid	0.050
8	Dimer acid**	0.550
	Diethylene triamine	0.750
	Stearyl amine	0.100
9	Dimer acid**	0.155
	Methylimino bispropylamine	0.255
	Oleic acid	0.022
10	Azelaic acid	0.200
	Dimer tetraamine***	0.480
	Oleic acid	0.040

*Commercial polymerized unsaturated fatty acids consisting primarily of linoleic acid and containing 95% dimers, 4% trimers and 1% monomers; average neutral equivalent of 292.

**Commercial polymerized unsaturated fatty acids consisting primarily of linoleic acid and containing 75% dimers, 22% trimers and 3% monomers; average neutral equivalent of 295.

***The tetraamine prepared by the hydrogenation of the biscyanoethylated dimer diamine; equivalent weight of 180.

Preparation of the biologically active composition is shown in the following examples.

Example 1: Eighty grams of Resin No. 3, described above, was blended with 320 grams of procaine penicillin G on a two roll mill at 140°F. The resulting product was sheeted off at a thickness of ¼" and cut into strips of ½" wide. The strips were fed into an extrusion mill with a circular die. The product was drawn down to a diameter of 1.5 to 2 mm. After cooling, it was cut into pieces 1.5 to 2 mm. long using a rotary chopper.

Example 2: A 40 gram sample of the calcium salt of the hydroxy analogue of methionine (with hydroxyl radical replacing the amino group) was blended with 10 grams of Resin No. 6. The resin was converted into particles of 1.5 to 2.0 mm. in diameter by 1.5 to 2.0 mm. in length for use as an animal feed supplement.

Aminoalkyl Acrylate Copolymers

Coatings for tablets, dragees, granules, and the like are being prepared in increasing numbers from synthetic polymers because these materials, in contrast to the natural substances, permit the solubility properties of the coating to be chosen at a desired value. For example, acrylic resins having basic groups in the polymeric resin dissolve in the stomach juices and there liberate the enclosed effective ingredient, whereas acidic groups make the coating resistant to stomach juices and first permit solution in the alkaline environment of the intestinal juices.

K. Lehmann, G. Markert and G.W.E. Rothgang; U.S. Patent 3,520,970; July 21, 1970; assigned to Rohm & Haas GmbH, Germany have developed materials which permit the preparation of coatings which have a solubility, or permeability for the material coated, which are variable within wide limits. These coating solutions contain, in an organic solvent, soluble copolymers comprising: (1) at least one ethylenically unsaturated monomer forming a water-insoluble homopolymer and (2) at least one polymerizable quaternary ammonium compound. The monomers (1) and (2) are present in the copolymers in a weight ratio between 5:95 and 95:5.

As the polymerizable quaternary ammonium compounds, quaternized aminoalkyl esters and aminoalkyl amides of acrylic acid and methacrylic acid are of principal importance, for example β-methacryloxyethyltrimethylammonium methosulfate, β-acryloxypropyltrimethylammonium chloride, and trimethylaminomethylmethacrylamide methosulfate. The quaternary ammonium atom can also be part of a heterocycle, as in methacryloxyethylmethylmorpholinium chloride or the corresponding piperidinium salt, or it can be joined to an acrylic acid group or a methacrylic acid group by way of a group containing hetero atoms, such as a polyglycol ether group. Further suitable polymerizable quaternary ammonium compounds include quaternized vinyl-substituted nitrogen heterocycles such as methylvinylpyridinium salts, vinyl esters of quaternized aminocarboxylic acids, styryltrialkylammonium salts, and the like.

From a practical viewpoint, it is not necessary to have a special copolymer at hand for each coating having a desired solution rate. Rather, it is suitable to have a small number of polymers having different proportions of quaternary amine. The tolerance of these polymers for each other is assured because of their similar structures, so that any desired value of solubility rate or swellability can be obtained by the mixing of two or more polymers.

The polymers are easily soluble in organic solvents such as alcohols, ketones, esters, halohydrocarbons, or mixtures thereof. Copolymers comprising a large fraction of quaternary ammonium compounds are water-soluble. For tablet coating, 10 to 20% solutions are preferably used. Of the solvents, isopropyl alcohol, ethyl alcohol, and methylene chloride or their mixtures are preferred. The amount of solution used depends on the surface to be coated and on the polymer content of the solution. Ten milligrams of a coating solution of the concentration mentioned above per square centimeter of tablet surface area generally give a film of sufficient strength and thickness.

Example 1: Glucose tablets were coated in a coating kettle with a 15% solution of a copolymer comprising 24% by weight of trimethylmethacryloxyethylammonium chloride, 56% by weight of methyl methacrylate, and 20% by weight of ethyl acrylate in a mixture of isopropyl alcohol and methylene chloride. About 10 mg. of solution were used per square centimeter of tablet surface area. A coherent film 10 microns thick was produced. The tablets dissolved in water at 37°C. in 3 to 5 minutes. In synthetic digestive juices having a pH of 2 (stomach juices), and pH's of 5 to 8 (intestinal juices), the same decomposition time was measured.

Example 2: A copolymer comprising 10% by weight of trimethylmethyacryloxyethylammonium chloride, 60% by weight of methyl methacrylate, and 30% by weight of ethyl acrylate was used to coat glucose tablets as in Example 1 from a 15% solution in isopropyl alcohol/methylene chloride. In water at 37°C., the tablet coating swelled, but did not dissolve. The amount of glucose released from the tablet interior by diffusion increased steadily and amounted to 80% of the amount originally within the tablet core after 120 minutes.

Coatings Containing Dispersed Plastic Particles

Coatings which have uniform color, do not fade, have high impact resistance, and good resistance to atmospheric conditions have been developed by *R. Kawata, H. Kawada, T. Ohmura, S. Uematsu and T. Kohinata; U.S. Patent 3,692,562; September 19, 1972.* This coating comprises a coating material or base and 0.1 to 30% based on the coating material of fine particles of a plastic material, such as nylon, polytetrafluoroethylene, polyethylene and polypropylene. The use of fine particles of a solid plastic material in coating composition for tablets was not known. Also it had not been expected that advantageous results would be obtained by the incorporation of fine plastic particles in the coating composition. There are many kinds of solid plastics which can be used. For example, any material which can be finely pulverized and is insoluble in a solvent for the coating material, such as water, alcohols, acetone and ethyl acetate may be used. Typical examples are nylon, polytetrafluoroethylene, polyethylene, polypropylene, organosilicone oxide polymer, polyvinyl chloride, polymethylmethacrylate and the like. The diameters of the fine plastic materials are generally less than 50 microns, preferably 1 to 10 microns. As a suitable coating material or base, there can be used sucrose, gelatin, shellac, polyethylene glycol, cellulose acetate phthalate, etc., for film coating.

The coating composition is prepared by dispersing in a solvent the coating material and the fine particles of the solid plastic in a proportion of 0.1 to 30%, preferably 0.1 to 10% of the coating material. As the solvent for the coating composition, water or an organic solvent such as an alcohol, acetone, and ethyl acetate may be used according to the nature of the coating material to be employed. In addition, if the medicaments contained in the tablets are unstable to water, solvents other than water are preferably used.

One can add to the coating composition a coloring agent, a taste improving agent, a flavoring agent, a lubricant, a filler, a shielding agent, etc. However, the fine particles of plastic material act sufficiently as a shielding agent and thus even in the case where the use of an additional shielding agent is required, as in a conventional case, the purpose can be attained by using this coating composition without using an additional shielding agent. Moreover, if it is required to use such a conventional shielding agent such as titanium dioxide, together with the coating composition, the use of a surface active agent is unnecessary since this coating composition is characterized by good dispersibility. Also, where a coloring agent is used, it is preferable to use the fine particles of, e.g., nylon initially dyed by an acid dye and thus the coated tablets have a distinct color and a high fading resistance, which are not accompanied by uneven coloring and oozing of colors.

In order to coat tablets with this coating composition, the tablets may be immersed in the coating composition and withdrawn followed by drying or may be coated with the coating composition by a conventional manner using a coating pan. The process will be further described by the following examples.

Example 1:

	Grams
Cellulose acetate phthalate	100
Fine particles of nylon	10
Acetone	430
Isopropyl alcohol	430

In a mixture of acetone and isopropyl alcohol was dissolved cellulose acetate phthalate and then the fine particles of nylon (SP powder, made by Poyo Rayon Co.) were uniformly dispersed in the solution thus obtained to provide the coating composition. In a coating pan were placed 10,000 tablets each being 150 mg. in weight and while rotating the coating pan, 10 grams of the coating composition prepared above was uniformly sprayed over the surfaces of the tablets. The tablets were, thereafter, dried by a warm blast of air of 50°C. By repeating the same procedure, the coated tablets each being 160 mg. in weight were prepared.

Example 2:

	Grams
Hydroxypropylmethylcellulose	50
Fine particles of colored nylon	5
Methylene chloride	400
Methanol	400
2-Ethoxy ethanol	100

After dissolving hydroxypropylmethylcellulose in a mixed solvent of methylene chloride, methanol and 2-ethoxy ethanol, the fine particles of nylon dyed by a food red dye #3 were uniformly dispersed in the resultant solution to provide the coating composition. In the same manner as Example 1, the coated tablets each being 160 mg. in weight were obtained.

SHELLAC COATING FORMULATIONS

Plasticized Shellac Coatings

J.A. Butler and W. Valentine; U.S. Patent 3,297,535; January 10, 1967; assigned to Hoffmann-La Roche Incorporated have found that compositions which comprise a mixture of (1) a wetting agent, (2) an opacifying agent, (3) a plasticizer uniformly distributed throughout, and (4) an organic solvent solution of a food grade shellac are well suited for use as protective and decorative coatings for tablets. Such compositions form continuous, opaque films on the surface of articles to provide a coating which is both useful and attractive.

One may use any conventional wetting agent which may be anionic, nonionic or cationic in character. The wetting agent which is preferred is dioctyl sodium sulfosuccinate. However, wetting agents such as polyoxyethylene glycol sorbitan esters of higher molecular weight fatty acids, for example, polyoxyethylene sorbitan monolaurate, polyoxyethylene sorbitan monostearate, polyoxyethylene sorbitan monooleate, etc., can also be used. Any conventional opacifying agent can be used in preparing the coating compositions, however, titanium dioxide is preferred. In lieu of titanium dioxide, iron oxide pigments, carbon black, etc., can be used as the opacifier in the compositions.

Plasticizing agents which have been found to be particularly well suited for use include, among others, castor oil, diethyl phthalate, ethyl lactate, acetyltriethyl citrate, glyceryl triacetate, etc. Additionally, certain acetylated monoglycerides, as well as certain alkylaryl phosphates, are useful as the plasticizing agents of the compositions. If desired, mixtures of suitable plasticizing agents can be employed. Castor oil is, however, the plasticizer which is used in the formulation of the preferred products. In addition to the essential ingredients, the compositions may contain also certain optional components. For example, it has been found that a form of colloidal silica is advantageously incorporated, particularly where titanium dioxide is employed as the opacifier.

Example: In this example, 170.0 grams of shellac were dissolved in 619.95 grams of ethyl alcohol. Then, 0.05 gram of dioctyl sodium sulfosuccinate, 200.0 grams of titanium dioxide and 10.0 grams of castor oil were incorporated into the solution, with agitation. The mixture, was homogenized by passage through a roller mill.

The above liquid composition, was used to coat pharmaceutical tablets as follows. The medicament-containing tablets were placed in a standard coating pan and a sufficient quantity of the coating composition was run into the pan to wet the tablets completely. The pan was rotated continuously until all of the liquid coating composition was taken up by the tablets. The film-coated tablets were then dried by cool air for 25 minutes.

The second, third and fourth coats were applied in the same manner as the first, with care taken in each coating operation not to over-wet the tablets with the coating composition. After the fourth coat was applied, the pan was allowed to continue rotating until the tablets had lost all of their tackiness and the tablets had begun to take on a glossy appearance. At this point, the tablets were removed from the pan and placed in a rotating-polishing pan where they were dusted with powdered carnauba wax. Rubbing was continued until tablets of high gloss were obtained.

Coatings Using Water-Soluble Shellac

Shellac which has been made water-soluble is incorporated into tablet coating compositions by *A.B. Rednick and M. Secora; U.S. Patent 3,390,049; June 25, 1968; assigned to Smith Kline & French Laboratories*. When this coating composition is applied to pharmaceutical forms it is possible to obtain a fast drying, thin, transparent film coat. Sugar coating with all of its build up steps is completely eliminated. The time required to coat the tablets is reduced from days to minutes because of the relatively few coats that are necessary. The thin, transparent film allows for the monogramming and scoring of the compressed tablet. Furthermore, the constituents of the film are all materials readily used for human consumption. The tremendous reduction of the number of coats also results in the production of a much smaller finished tablet. This feature allows for a more pharmaceutically elegant tablet which is much easier for the patient to swallow.

The coating composition is prepared from wax-free shellac which is rendered water-soluble by dissolving the shellac in water and ammonia until a solution results. Other ingredients such as plasticizing agents, opaquing agents and coloring materials may be added to the coating solution to enhance the properties of the coating. Preferably the shellac will be present in an amount of from 0.1 to 5% by weight, advantageously from 1 to 3% by weight of the total coating composition. Preferably twice as much water and 28% ammonia solution (USP) used in a ratio of 10:1 to 30:1 is used to dissolve the shellac. If desired an organic solvent may be added to the above shellac concentrate to hasten the evaporation of the coating.

Most advantageously solid polyethylene glycol and polyvinylpyrrolidone are used either alone or preferably a mixture of both as plasticizers and results in a coating composition which is more flexible and smoother. Further, solid polyethylene glycol also acts as an antitacking agent and prevents the sticking of the tablets to one another as they are rotated in the coating pan. Finally, the use of a solid polyethylene glycol, such as for example, polyethylene glycol 6000, adds gloss to the tablet coat and eliminates the necessity of a final separate polish coating. Other ingredients such as coloring materials, opaque fillers and the like may also be added to the coatings.

Example: Shellac Concentrate –

Solution A

Ingredients	Percent wt./vol.
Wax-free shellac	15.34
Polyvinylpyrrolidone	15.34
Carbowax 6000	14.32
Strong ammonia solution 28% (USP)	1.53
Water, q.s., 100.00 ml.	

The shellac, polyvinylpyrrolidone and Carbowax are dissolved in the strong ammonia solution and water with the aid of heat to form a shellac concentrate.

Solution B

Ingredients	Amount
Shellac concentrate	300 ml.
Isopropyl alcohol	4,500 ml.
Chloroform	600 ml.
Titanium dioxide	180 g.
FD&C Yellow #5 Lake	18 g.

The shellac concentrate, isopropyl alcohol and chloroform are mixed and the titanium dioxide and FD&C yellow No. 5 lake are suspended in the mixture with continued agitation to form the coating composition. Tablet cores of $\frac{12}{32}$" diameter containing trifluoperazine and filler are placed in a rotating 12 inch coating pan and are thoroughly and evenly wetted by spraying on the above coating composition. The tablets are dried while being rotated and passing air over them. This procedure is followed until approximately 15 coats have been applied having a hard thin film coat on the tablets.

Opaque or Colored Shellac Sealing Coatings

J.R. Zingerman; U.S. Patent 3,427,182; February 11, 1969; assigned to American Cyanamid Company has developed an opaque or colored sealing coating for tablets which reduces the number of outer sugar coatings required to produce tablets having good appearance. This coating is formed from a water-insoluble resin, such as shellac, dissolved in a suitable solvent such as a lower alcohol.

With ordinary sealing coats, which are of course at least translucent, a relatively large number of coats of the colored film coating composition are often required in order to hide imperfections in the tablet itself. This is undesirable as the amount of dye used builds up, and although when using certified dyes, the toxicity of which is fairly low, dangerous concentrations may not occur if the color is relatively light. The toxicity of the soluble dyes is not zero and there has been considerable concern in recent years on the part of the Food and Drug Administration because in certain instances very large amounts of certified dyes have produced undesirable effects. Accordingly, rather stringent limitations on the amount of dye permitted have been set and, of course, even if a colored tablet falls within the limitations, it is never desirable to have more dye than is necessary. The process is described in greater detail in the following examples.

Example 1: About 35,000 ⅜" standard concave tablets of tetracycline hydrochloride were placed in an 18" coating pan. A sealing composition was prepared by blending 30 grams of titanium dioxide into 500 ml. 4 lb. cut confectionary glaze (shellac solution), with the aid of a Waring Blendor. The tablets were maintained at 60°C. at all times and after each shot were dried by blowing warm air over them. The sealing coat was applied in three shots, the first using 100 ml., the second 60 ml., and the last 50 ml., with ten minutes drying time between each shot. Also, after each shot kaolin was added to reduce stickiness. A film coating formula was then prepared having the following composition:

10 centipoise methylcellulose	150 g.
Alcohol	2,000 ml.
Chloroform	1,500 ml.
600 molecular weight polyethylene glycol	30 g.
Distilled H_2O	150 g.
D&C Yellow #11	3 g.

The above film coating formula was applied to the tablets by spraying in 30 applications of 15 ml. each at the rate of 1 ml./sec. Drying was effected between each coating. The final tablet, after polishing, had a deep yellow color, there was excellent coverage, and no evidence of spotted cores through the film.

Example 2: About 20,000 ⅜" tetracycline hydrochloride tablets were placed in an 18" coating pan. The tablet cores had a uniform yellow color. 800 mg. of D&C yellow dye No. 11 were dissolved in 400 ml. of confectionary glaze, as in Example 1, and a sealing coat was produced with two shots of 50 ml. each, with a ten minute drying time between shots and application of kaolin dust to prevent stickiness. The seal-coated tablets were then colored with the film coating composition of Example 1 but with the D&C yellow dye omitted. Twenty-five applications were made as described in Example 1, and after polishing the tablets showed a uniform color coating with no spots showing on the tablet surface.

Alternate Shellac and Sugar Coatings

A process has been disclosed by *C.A. Signorino and T.E. Jamison; U.S. Patents 3,524,756; August 18, 1970; and 3,576,663; April 27, 1971; both assigned to Colorcon Incorporated* whereby compressed tablet cores are coated with alternate layers of a tacky material, e.g., shellac, zein or gum arabic, and layers of a nontacky sugar composition. This process seals the cores against moisture and also gives a smooth even film with good color.

In accordance with this process, compressed tablet cores are screened to remove dust, and are deposited in a rotatable coating pan. A sufficient quantity of a shellac color suspension is applied to thoroughly wet the tumbling tablet cores. After the suspension is uniformly distributed about the cores for 1 minute, warm air is applied until the tablet cores start to break loose from each other and become less tacky. The warm air is applied to the rolling tablets for 4 minutes. Then the pan is stopped and is intermittently jogged every minute for 10 minutes. The jogging comprises rotating the coating pan for one-half revolution so as not to let the coated cores sit in the pan and adhere to each other.

After 10 minutes of jogging, the first coating is sufficiently dry to take a second coating. This second coating may be another coating, one-half the volume, of the shellac suspension if a double sealing layer of shellac is desired. The second shellac layer is more tacky than the first shellac layer, but this tackiness is not a serious problem. Instead of applying a second coating of shellac immediately, it is preferred to apply sugar syrup as the second coating. The sugar coating may be applied by ladling plain sugar syrup into the coating pan onto the tablet cores and rolling the sugar layer dry in 5 minutes.

Instead of plain sugar syrup, a sugar suspension of 10 to 25 lb. cut, preferably a 16 to 22 lb. cut, of sucrose syrup is formed into a sugar suspension by adding 1 to 5% by weight of a shellac suspension. By 10 to 25 lb. cut sucrose syrup is meant 10 to 25 lbs. of sugar dissolved in one gallon of water. This sugar suspension containing the small amount of shellac suspension has the advantage of etching or softening the previous shellac layer slightly to form a better or more secure bond of the sugar coating to the shellac coating. Since the shellac suspension is colored, its addition to the sugar suspension gives color to the sugar suspension and therefore the sugar coating aids in adding color instead of just forming a colorless base for the next color application.

The sugar suspension aids in developing the color of the tablet more rapidly. The sugar layer adheres well to the first layer of shellac and provides a flat, nontacky surface for a third coating layer which may be of shellac. After the sugar is dried in the second coating layer, a layer of shellac is applied to form the third coating layer. This third layer is applied by ladling a sufficient amount of shellac suspension onto the tablet cores to wet them completely, then rolling the tablet cores until they break free from each other, then jogging the coating pan every minute for 10 minutes to dry the tablet cores.

This procedure of applying alternate coating layers of shellac and sugar may be continued until the desired full color of the tablet is achieved. Advantageously, the anhydrous suspension may comprise a shellac coating suspension including, by weight, 30 parts of 4 lb. cut shellac (4 lbs. of shellac dissolved in a gallon of alcohol), 3 parts of slip and levelling agents, 25 parts of pigment solids, and ethyl alcohol, denatured. Also, the shellac suspension may include 2 parts of polyvinylpyrrolidone. The slip and levelling agents may be in the range of 0 to 6 parts, the pigment solids 10 to 30 parts, and the polyvinylpyrrolidone 0 to 5 parts.

The slip agents are included in the shellac suspension in order to chemically reduce the tacking of the shellac so that the tablet cores slip by instead of picking. The slip agents may include cetyl alcohol, glycol monostearate, and talc. The levelling agents are included in order to help spread the shellac suspension evenly over the tablet cores. The levelling agents may include sorbitan monooleate, and sorbitan monostearate. Acetylated monoglyceride may be included in the shellac coating suspension as both a levelling and a slip agent.

The polyvinylpyrrolidone is included in the shellac suspension to reduce the tendency of the shellac to polymerize and to modify the shellac film to help stabilize it. The pigment solids may include all the FD&C and D&C lakes, soluble and insoluble dyes, opacifiers, titanium dioxide, calcium carbonate, silica, iron oxides and channel black formulated to desired color. The following example of specific shellac suspension will show the preparation of the coating.

Example:

Ingredients	Amounts
4 lb. cut bleached shellac	11 lbs., 14 oz.
Cetyl alcohol	3.5 oz.
Isopropyl alcohol	4 lbs., 2.5 oz.
Sorbitan monooleate	5 oz.
Sorbitan trioleate	5 oz.
FD&C Yellow #5 Lake	2 lbs., 13 oz.
FD&C Blue #1 Lake	15.75 oz.
Titanium dioxide	9 lbs., 9 oz.
Talc	2 lbs., 8.5 oz.
Polyvinylpyrrolidone	3 oz.

The tablets are coated by alternately applying a layer of a shellac suspension and a layer of sugar suspension to the tablet cores, drying one layer before applying the next layer. The suspensions are applied by ladling them onto the tablet cores being rotated in a coating pan, and this procedure is repeated as often as necessary to obtain the desired coloring and depth of film coating.

Polyvinylpyrrolidone Modified Shellac

Shellac coating materials that do not harden on storage are disclosed by *C.A. Signorino; U.S. Patents 3,738,952; June 12, 1973; and 3,741,795; June 26, 1973; both assigned to Colorcon Incorporated*. The shellac is mixed with polymeric materials that contain basic groups. Such materials include polyvinylpyrrolidone (PVP), polyvinylpyridine, and polyamide resins containing free amino groups. Such polymers block the carboxyl group of the shellac from cross-linking by providing an acid-base reaction between the shellac and the polymer. The basic group of the polyvinylpyrrolidone complexes with the carboxyl group of the shellac to block esterification.

Adding any quantity of a basic polymer ties up some of the carboxyl groups and reduces the amount of carboxyl groups available for cross-linking, thus retarding the unwanted cross-linking in the shellac. Adding too much basic polymer, more than is needed to retard the unwanted cross-linking, produces a film having the characteristics of the polyvinylpyrrolidone and this is undesirable because polyvinylpyrrolidone does not seal against the penetration of moisture. The sealing characteristics of the shellac film are desirable in tablet coating, and the coating must be formulated to insure stability of the shellac without markedly modifying its desirable properties. This formulating requires a knowledge of the stoichiometry of shellac and the basic polymer used.

Shellacs vary as to composition, depending on the source and treatment of the shellac including the amount of rain, the health of the trees, whether the shellac has been dewaxed, how the shellac was decolorized, etc. Because of these variations, one mol of free carboxyl groups may be found in 600 grams of shellac solids, or may be found in 900 grams of shellac solids, or may be found anywhere between those weights of shellac solids. On the other hand, the polyvinylpyrrolidone is a synthetic material and may be made to a desired specification. One mol of basic groups may be found in 111 grams of polyvinylpyrrolidone.

The preferred stoichiometric ratio by mol of shellac-free carboxyl groups to polyvinylpyrrolidone-free basic groups is 1 to 1. However, because of the variation in the acid value of the shellac, the ratio by weight of the shellac to polyvinylpyrrolidone may be in the range of 600 to 900 grams shellac to 111 grams of polyvinylpyrrolidone. The ratio by weight of other basic polymers to the shellac, to give the 1 to 1 mol ratio, may be worked out in the same manner as the shellac-polyvinylpyrrolidone weight ratio, with a knowledge of the stoichiometry of the basic polymer.

The method of making a sealing film for coating tablets and the like comprises the steps of taking a desired quantity of shellac, titrating a specimen of the shellac to ascertain the number of mols of acid in the shellac, adding a quantity of polyvinylpyrrolidone having the same number of mols of base, and mixing the shellac and polyvinylpyrrolidone together in a solvent. The method may also include the steps of mixing a detackifier into the stabilized shellac to prevent picking in the tablet coating operation, mixing a plasticizer into the film to increase flexibility of the film, and mixing a colorant into the film to color the tablet. The method may further include the steps of applying successive layers of the film to tablet cores as they are being tumbled in a coating pan. The stabilized shellac sealing film provides a sealant against moisture for cores containing water-sensitive material, such as cores made of various medicaments.

Example 1:

Ingredients	Amounts, oz.
6 lb. cut refined shellac in ethyl alcohol	160
Polyvinylpyrrolidone	10
SDA 3-A alcohol	102

The polyvinylpyrrolidone is dissolved in the alcohol and then the shellac is stirred into the mixture. The 6 lb. cut refined shellac in ethyl alcohol contains 45% shellac solids so that of the 160 oz. of this ingredient there is present 72 oz. of shellac solids and 88 oz. of ethyl alcohol.

Example 2:

Ingredients	Amounts, oz.
6 lb. cut refined shellac in ethyl alcohol	160
Polyvinylpyrrolidone	10
Acetylated monoglyceride	10
SDA 3-A alcohol	136

The polyvinylpyrrolidone and the acetylated monoglyceride are dissolved in the alcohol and then the shellac is stirred into the solution. The 6 lb. cut of refined shellac in ethyl alcohol is 45% shellac solids so that of the 160 oz. of this ingredient, there are 72 oz. of shellac solids and 88 oz. of ethyl alcohol. The acetylated monoglyceride is a plasticizer that reduces brittleness and increases the flexibility of the stabilized shellac film.

The solutions of Examples 1 and 2 are stable in storage, and the films they form on tablets and the like are quite stable after deposition. The solutions of Examples 1 and 2 may be used to produce a sealing coating on tablets, candies, nuts, or any sort of solid piece. These solutions may also be used effectively to produce a film on sugar coated pieces that provides a print base or prewaxed base or seal against gases and moisture penetration.

WAX BASED COATINGS

Paraffin-Fatty Acid-Talc Coating Mixtures

Protracted release pharmaceutical preparations are prepared by a process disclosed by *G. Renwanz, K. Credner and E. Glantz; U.S. Patent 3,437,728; April 8, 1969; assigned to Diwag Chemische Fabriken GmbH, Germany*. The process is characterized in that the active ingredient is embedded in paraffin in a known manner and compressed with conventional adjuvants to form tablet cores, or tablet cores containing the active ingredient but free from paraffin are impregnated with molten paraffin, and the crude cores thus obtained are coated with a protective diaphragm of talc or other acid- and alkali-proof mineral materials and a mixture of paraffin and stearic acid or other higher fatty acids or with acetylcellulose or mixtures of these materials.

Paraffin as the embedding agent has been used only as a minor additive to stearic acid and its mixtures with other fatty acids which have been preferred, obviously due to their solubility in the alkaline intestine secretions. In contrast, pure paraffin in the tablet core is unattackable and serves as a skeleton substance permitting protraction of the release from the core of water-soluble active ingredients and tablet adjuvants. The achievable delay of the release of the active ingredient is unsatisfactory even when using paraffin. It is possible either by an increase in the amount of paraffin and/or in the compression pressure used in preparing the tablets to protract the release of the active ingredient sufficiently during the first hours, but at the expense of the final release during the last hours which is delayed beyond the degree desired (first type cores), or the amount of paraffin and/or the compression pressure are reduced to give cores which release the active ingredient within a much shorter period of time, e.g., within four hours rather than within eight hours (second type cores). For example, cores of this type release as much as 58% of the active ingredient as early as after one hour, 83% after two hours and 94% of the amount of active ingredient after four hours.

Uniform release of the active ingredient from the core can be obtained in a simple and economic manner by coating second type cores with a skeleton layer which consists of talc in a similar acid- and alkali-resistant mineral material and a mixture of paraffin and stearic acid and/or other higher fatty acids as bonding agent. For example, release of the active ingredient at a rate of 15% per hour is achieved if second type cores having a weight of 160 mg. are moistened with a few coatings each consisting of 3 mg. of a 1:1 mixture of paraffin and stearic acid dissolved in methylene chloride or another suitable solvent and each core is dusted immediately thereafter with 18 mg. of talc. The release of the active ingredient can be controlled conveniently by reducing or increasing the amount of talc.

The use of talc as an additive to enteric coating compositions for tablets is already known. However, in all these cases, talc serves only the improvement of the mechanical properties of the protective coating proper, uniform distribution of this filter being very essential. In contrast, the talc applied in this process is an essential ingredient of the protective coating and does not constitute a continuous film but forms a relatively irregularly built diaphragm about the core. If an acid- and alkali-resistant acetylcellulose coating is used in the physiological area, this coating assumes part of the function of the paraffin-stearin-talc diaphragm and, in addition, improves the mechanical strength of the dragée core.

Example 1: An active ingredient (1 kg.) which is soluble in water and insoluble in paraffin is added, to the same amount of molten paraffin, kneaded with ten times the amount of lactose, granulated in conventional manner and tabletted after addition of 1 kg. of talc. The resulting crude cores are provided, in a coating drum, with a protective coating of talc which is dusted in portions to the cores which are previously wetted with a solution of a 1:1 mixture of paraffin and stearic acid in methylene chloride. A total of 1.4 kg. of talc is applied to the surface of the tablet cores by means of 260 grams of paraffin-stearic acid mixture.

Example 2: If, on a dragée core of 160 mg. coated in accordance with Example 1 with a diaphragm of 1:1 paraffin-stearic acid mixture and 18 mg. of talc, one-third of the amounts given above of paraffin, stearic acid and talc is replaced by 1.to 1.5 mg. of acetylcellulose, the mean error of the individual measurement is reduced to one-half. While 7.2 ± 1.0 mg. of the total amount of active ingredient of 15.0 mg. contained in the core are, for example, released to the gastric juice within the first three hours when using no acetylcellulose, rates of 6.9 ± 0.5 mg. are found when using acetylcellulose. Reliable reduction in the spread requires uniform application of acetylcellulose from a sufficiently diluted solution (maximum, 5%). Examples of suitable solvents include methylene chloride and tetrachloroethane.

High Luster Wax Coatings

A.H. Cheiken and J.F. Bavitz; U.S. Patent 3,576,665; April 27, 1971; assigned to Merck & Company, Incorporated describe a method of imparting a high luster coating to ingestible tablets by coating with a liquid composition which is 30 to 40% powdered carnauba wax, 10 to 20% wax white and 40 to 60% methylchloroform or petroleum benzin.

In the past the luster of film coated tablets has been achieved by a so-called dry polishing operation in which the tablets, in a dry condition, are dusted with a dry, ground wax mixture and then continually rubbed against each other in a conventional tumbling barrel. This constant frictional contact serves to achieve a generalized polishing effect but the resulting tablets failed to attain a high degree of luster. Sugar coated tablets, on the other hand, require a very critical so-called set-up step during the process just prior to the application of the dry waxes in order to finally achieve a high luster. The use of the liquid wax mixture induces a high luster onto film coated tablets and eliminates the set-up in the sugar coating process. The composition which is applied to the tablets has the following relative proportions on a weight basis: 30 to 40% of carnauba wax powdered, 10 to 20% of wax white USP, and 40 to 60% of solvent.

The solvent may be either Chlorothene (methylchloroform) or petroleum benzin or a combination of them in any relative proportions. The general characteristic of the methylchloroform is that it boils between 73° and 75°C. Petroleum benzin boils between 35° and 80°C. The solution is applied at room temperature to the tablets in a tumbling barrel by pouring it onto them. It is applied either continuously or discontinuously and at such a rate that 1 to 2 mg./kg. of tablets is applied in 10 minutes. The amount applied per tablet will average less than 1 mg. for a ⅜" diameter tablet and a smaller or larger tablet will require a corresponding amount based on its surface area. Usually, the total application time will be 35 to 45 minutes, at the rate stated above, and thereafter a final drying period may be expedited by a blast of warmed drying air as in conventional practice. Representative examples are the following.

Example 1: Ten kilos of pharmaceutical tablets having a conventional sugar coating and which were ⅜" in diameter and 3/16" thick were placed in a tumbling barrel and rotated at 25 rpm. 15 ml. of a previously prepared solution by weight of 35% powdered carnauba wax, 15% wax white USP and 50% methylchloroform was poured onto the sloping surface of the tablets. The tablets continued to tumble for 10 minutes at which time a second application of 15 ml. was applied. After ten additional minutes of tumbling, 15 ml. of the solution was again applied and the tablets rolled for an additional 20 minutes. The tablets were removed and found to have a very high luster. Each tablet had an outer shiny coating.

Example 2: Conventional sugar coated chewing gum tablets of the Chiclets type are put in the tumbling barrel and the process of Example 1 is carried out. The tablets will be found to be extremely shiny.

Emulsified Wax Coatings

A method of preparing wax-coated pharmaceutical tablets is disclosed by *J.A. Biddle, Sr.; U.S. Patent 3,438,797; April 15, 1969* wherein sugar syrup coatings are applied to the tablets and while the coatings are in a tacky state a wax emulsion is applied. The tablets are then dried to obtain an unpolished wax coating and imprinted with conventional shellac-based ink indicia, if desired.

The wax emulsions are oil-in-water emulsions of waxes such as paraffin wax or carnauba wax, which are obtained by emulsification of the wax in distilled water with a suitable surfactant or a mixture or blend of surfactants. Although the preferred waxes are paraffin wax and carnauba wax, any of the commercially available, pharmaceutically acceptable waxes, such as for example beeswax, may be used. The preferred surfactants are nonionic in character, however, surfactants having anionic, cationic and ampholytic properties may also be used. Surfactants which have been found to be particularly useful in preparing the wax emulsions are a series of commercially available nonionic surfactants comprising sorbitan fatty acid esters and polyoxyethylene sorbitan fatty acid esters.

In preparing the wax emulsion, the type and amount of the surfactant used to obtain a satisfactorily stable emulsion is determined as described in *The Atlas HLB System,* Atlas Chemical Industries, Inc., 3rd Edition (1963). The HLB of an emulsifier is an expression of its hydrophile-lipophile balance, that is, the balance of the size and strength of the hydrophilic and the lipophilic groups of the emulsifier. Under the Atlas system it has also been found that oils, waxes and other materials likely to be incorporated into emulsions have an individual "required HLB." For example, the required HLB of paraffin wax is 10 and that of carnauba wax is 12. In the case of paraffin wax, therefore, this means that any emulsifier, or a blend of emulsifiers, having a combined HLB of 10, will make a more stable fluid oil-in-water paraffin emulsion than emulsifiers of any other HLB value. In this method successive smoothing and finishing coats, consisting primarily of grossing powders and coating syrups are applied to the tablets in rotary coating pans to give the tablets a smooth outer surface. After the last of several coats of syrup, each of which may contain various amounts of color, has been applied, the tablets are allowed to tumble to the point where the coating is still slightly moist. At this point the wax emulsion is then applied in a conventional manner. Only enough solution to coat all of the tablets is used, and once all of the tablets are sufficiently covered with the wax solution, as determined by visual observation, the coating pan is shut down. It is preferred to include the coloring material in the wax emulsion thus providing a final color coat.

After application of the wax coating the tablets are removed from the coating pan and placed on drying racks where they are allowed to remain until the wax coating is dry. Once the coating is thoroughly dry the wax-coated tablets may be imprinted with ink indicia in any conventional manner, it being necessary simply to cause the tablets to bear against a printing mechanism such as a roller or stamp having the desired indicia engraved therein or embossed thereon and supplied with an edible ink. For imprinting of the ink indicia on the tablets, it is preferred to use any of the various commercially available shellac-based edible ink compositions. The following example is illustrative of formulations of wax coating solutions found to be satisfactory in the process.

Example:

	Grams	Weight percent
Paraffin wax [1]	2.475	1.0
Sorbitan monostearate [2]	2.475	1.0
Polyoxyethylene sorbitan monostearate [3]	2.475	1.0
Distilled water	2.475	1.0
Simple syrup, U.S.P	237.100	96.0
Total	247.000	100.0

[1] PAROWAX (Standard Oil Company, Indiana).
[2] SPAN 60 (Atlas Chemical Industries).
[3] TWEEN 60 (ibid.).

The distilled water is charged to a beaker and heated to 130°F. on a steam heated water bath. The paraffin wax and the surfactant mixture are each charged to separate beakers and heated on a steam-heated water bath to 130°F. The surfactant mixture is then added to the melted paraffin and the mixture is mechanically stirred. The distilled water is then added to the mixture slowly with stirring, while maintaining the temperature at 130°F. The heat is then turned off and with continued agitation the paraffin wax emulsion is allowed to cool to room temperature.

In the meantime the syrup solution is charged to a beaker and heated to 120°F. While maintaining the temperature of the syrup solution at 120°F. the paraffin wax emulsion is added, with stirring, to give the final coating solution. This wax coating solution was then used in the preparation of imprinted pharmaceutical tablets following the procedure described above.

Printable Wax Coatings

A process has been developed by *H.W. Bennett; U.S. Patent 3,533,804; October 13, 1970; assigned to Miles Laboratories, Incorporated* for preparing imprintable tablets whereby ink indicia can be directly applied to an unpolished coating of wax on a tablet core. The wax is applied in an amount of 5 to 20 micrograms per tablet, the waxed surface being particularly suitable for imprinting with conventional, shellac-based printing inks.

The edible or nonedible tablet cores can be composed of a wide range of materials. The edible materials can be either food substances or pharmaceutical substances, while the nonedible materials can, for example, be test reagents, catalysts, or industrial enzyme mixtures. The primary food substance for such edible tablets are confectionary materials such as chocolate powders. The pharmaceutical cores are generally mixtures of fillers, binders, lubricants, disintegrators and active ingredients. Preferred active ingredients are multivitamin mixtures. All of these tablet cores can preferably be coated with grossing powders and sugar coating syrups to give a smooth outer coat.

A large number of these tablets can be placed in a rotatable coating pan and contacted with a warmed dilute solution of the wax in an appropriate solvent. The coating pan is immediately set in motion, and the rotation is terminated after 10 to 30 seconds to prevent the tablets from becoming polished. The wax-coated tablets are removed from the pan and marked with ink indicia by running them through conventional tablet branding machines. The unpolished state of the wax coat has been found to be receptive to conventional ink indicia with which permanent markings can be applied to the tablets. After branding, a protective coating of polished wax or shellac can be applied to the tablets.

Since a small volume of the wax solution is employed for a large number of tablets to effect a wetting of the tablets with no appreciable excess of the solution, it is considered that nearly all of the wax in the solution is deposited on the tablet surfaces since these surfaces are the most highly absorbent material present in the coating pan. The wax-coated tablets are then passed through a tablet branding machine in which they are marked with a conventional ink indicia such as the shellac-based ink.

Waxes which can be used are either the naturally occurring or the synthetic waxes. For example beeswax and carnauba wax can be employed as well as the preferred paraffin wax. Synthetic waxes such as polyethylene glycol can also be used. Suitable solvents for the natural waxes include various commercially available petroleum solvents such as Skellysolve C (essentially n-heptane), Chlorothene (a chlorohydrocarbon solvent containing methyl-chloroform) and Penolene 643 (chlorohydrocarbon solvent). The preferred solvent of these is Skellysolve C. An alcohol such as ethanol can be used as a solvent for the synthetic waxes.

Example:

Wax Solution	Amount
Paraffin wax	0.6 g.
n-Heptane	100.0 ml.

Ten thousand sugar coated tablets measuring 0.235 inch thick by 0.360 inch diameter were placed in a rotary coating pan and 10 ml. of the above wax solution when heated to 70°C. was evenly distributed thereover by tumbling the tablets for 10 seconds. The tablets were then removed while in an unpolished state and branded in a laboratory branding machine using a shellac-based ink having the composition described in U.S. Patent 3,258,347. The tablets flowed through the branding machine without chipping or breaking and the markings showed no tendency to rub off.

The ink was dried and the tablets were then given a protective polished wax coating by using a more concentrated wax solution and a longer tumbling time. The paraffin wax used was obtained under the tradename Eskar. The solvent used was Skellysolve C.

MISCELLANEOUS COATINGS

Flavor Coating

A process for adding acidulants for flavoring effects to sugar-containing confectionary products, dragees, medicinal lozenges, cores, and the like has been disclosed by *F.L. Daylor, Jr.; U.S. Patent 3,622,352; November 23, 1971; assigned to Philip Morris, Incorporated.* More particularly, the acidulants may be added to a sugar-coated product without causing inversion of the sugar coat or a resultant product that will become sticky. Nuts, chewing gum, hard candies, fruits, lozenges, dragees or medicinal tablets, cores and the like are given a candy or sugar coating by conventional procedures, as for example by drum or a rotatable vessel or pan coating using warm air or other gas to evaporate off the aqueous fraction from the sugar syrup used for coating the material. One or more coats of syrup may be applied in this fashion until the desired thickness of coating is reached. When a sufficient coating has been applied, an edible flavoring acid useful for imparting or enhancing flavor is solubilized in a nontoxic, lower alcohol of 2 to 3 carbon atoms, for example, 95% ethyl alcohol, absolute alcohol or isopropyl alcohol, selected to have little or no material amount of water present.

The acids useful for this purpose are those solid edible acids commonly used for their flavoring effects, for example, citric, tartaric, malic, fumaric, succinic, and adipic acids which remain solid at room or atmospheric temperatures and are soluble in the alcoholic solvents mentioned. Each acid should be used at or near the limit of its solubility in the alcoholic solvent, for reasons of economy and convenience. This high concentration is, of course, not an absolute requirement for the practice of the process.

The alcoholic solution of the desired acid is added to the sugar-coated air- or gas-dried product in substantially the same way as the original syrup coating was applied. After the material is completely wetted by the addition of sufficient acid solution, warm air or inert gas is then admitted to the vessel for a sufficient time until the product is dry. The application of alcoholic solution of the selected acid may be repeated after each drying step as often as necessary until the desired amount of acid coating has been applied. Suction may be applied to the coating vessel or pan during the acid solution application. The following examples will serve to illustrate the procedure in greater detail.

Example 1: In a coating pan are placed 10 lbs. of uncoated chewing gum centers. A conventional coating syrup of sugar, corn syrup, and water is applied followed by warm air to dry; this coating and drying is repeated 25 times. A solution of citric acid in 95% ethanol, in a weight ratio of 56:100, is applied while air suction is applied to the pan. This coating is dried with warm air and the acid coating is repeated four more times. After the last coat is dry, 25 additional coats of the sugar syrup are applied. A final conventional polishing and wax application completes the coating. This coating shows no signs of becoming tacky or soft on storage.

Example 2: Uncoated chewing gum centers are placed in a coating pan and a syrup of sugar, corn syrup, and water is applied followed by warm air drying. Ten coats are applied in this way. Then a solution of malic acid in 95% ethanol, weight ratio 36:100, is applied for a total of three coats, suction being applied to the pan during coating and warm air drying after each coat. A further 10 coats of sugar are applied as before. Then three coats of alcoholic malic acid are applied, followed by 10 additional sugar coats, three coats of malic acid, and 10 of sugar. A final finishing with wax and polishing give a product which has good storage stability.

Edible Ink for Pharmaceuticals

A pharmaceutically acceptable, edible ink for use on gelatin capsules, tablets, and the like has been developed by *J.R. Kane; U.S. Patent 3,475,187; October 28, 1969; assigned to Rex Laboratories, Incorporated*. This consists essentially of 5 to 20 parts by weight of a liquid dye, 0.5 to 3 parts by weight of hydroxypropylcellulose, hydroxypropylmethylcellulose or a combination of both, 2 to 10 parts by weight of alcohol, 0.001 to 1 part by weight of a surface active agent, and sufficient water to make 100 parts, all these components being of pharmaceutical grade. This ink is indelible and is not easily removed as was characteristic of prior pigmented shellac-based inks.

The above result is achieved by means of a composition containing edible liquid dyes which not only coat but impregnate the surface of the pellet and, in effect, achieve a chemical unity therewith. Furthermore, these dyes are in admixture with certain other ingredients that, although used in much smaller proportions than was heretofore the case with shellacs, supply all the viscosity and body that is required for the composition. These other ingredients comprise surface active or wetting agents such as are specifically exemplified by but not necessarily limited to polyoxyethylene sorbitan monolaurate and sorbitan monostearate, which supply the necessary viscosity, and either hydroxypropylcellulose, hydroxypropylmethylcellulose, or a combination thereof, which provide the body. Any pharmaceutically acceptable alcohol, such as ethyl, isopropyl, isoamyl, isobutyl or secondary butyl alcohol is used as a solvent, while a small amount of a pigment may be added but only for the purpose of enhancing the surface clarity of the dye. However, the proportions of such pigment must be kept very small, preferably under 3% of the total composition, and in no event more than 5%, since any greater amount would destroy or seriously reduce the indelibility factor of the composition. Water is, by far, the largest component of the composition, serving as the carrier therein. The present type of dye composition is particularly effective for use on gelatin capsules, but has also been found to be effective on polished pharmaceutical tablets and the like. The following examples are illustrative of the preparation of these coatings.

Example 1:

Components	Parts by Weight
FD&C Red #2	10.500
FD&C Blue #1	5.000
Hydroxypropylcellulose (Klucel LP)	2.250
Isopropyl alcohol	8.000
Carbon black (purified)	2.000
Polyoxyethylene sorbitan monolaurate (Tween 20)	0.002
Sorbitan monostearate (Span 60)	0.002
Distilled water	72.246

The above components are mixed at room temperature and pressure until homogeneous to form a deep black coloring agent. This coloring agent was applied to a gelatin capsule, of the type used to contain pharmaceuticals, by brushing it on the capsule under ambient temperature and pressure conditions. It was then permitted to dry in the air for 1 hour. The resultant color was permanent in that it could not be rubbed-off and could not be washed or dissolved away without destroying the capsule itself.

Example 2:

Components	Parts by Weight
FD&C Red #2	16.000
Isopropyl alcohol	6.000
Hydroxypropylcellulose LP	0.996
Sorbitan monostearate (Span 60)	0.002
Polyoxyethylene sorbitan monolaurate (Tween 20)	0.002
Distilled water	77.000

These components were mixed at room temperature and pressure until homogeneous to form a red coloring agent. All of the above coloring agents are applicable to both gelatin capsules and tablets by standard type printing mechanisms, brushing, spraying, dipping or the like.

Esterified Shellac Printing Inks

C.J. Piotrowski; U.S. Patent 3,694,237; September 26, 1972 has developed an edible ink composition for applying indicia to a capsule or tablet comprising partially esterified purified shellac, ethyl alcohol, and a coloring substance selected from edible pigments, lakes, and dyes. Conventional edible inks are made with dry shellac, ethyl alcohol, plasticizers and/or detackifiers, pigments or dyes, and solvents which give a desired drying time, say 3 minutes. As the ink ages, a process occurs wherein the acid groups of the shellac react with the ethyl alcohol to form an ethyl ester of the shellac. The presence of the shellac ester increases the drying time of the ink, and as the amount or percentage of ester increases, the drying time is increased, eventually to a point where the drying time is too long, causing offset, or pick-off, or transfer of the ink from one printed piece of tablet to another.

However, it was found that the esterified portion of the shellac actually provides an improved ink if the amount of esterification is controlled and stopped at a certain point, preferably at 24% esterified shellac solids to 76% unesterified shellac solids by weight. In fact a blend of 20 parts esterified shellac with 80 parts unesterified shellac produces a material which has excellent drying characteristics (an indication of amount of tack), better than either component.

In applying an indicia to a confectionary or pharmaceutical tablet or capsule, a process of printing is used known as offset gravure. In this method, an etched or engraved gravure cylinder is rotated through a well which contains the ink. A very thin blade wipes the excess ink from roll, leaving only the etch filled in with ink. The gravure roll contacts a rubber transfer roll which in turn contacts the piece which is being printed. Conventional inks made with unesterified shellac would build up on the transfer roll, causing the indicia to be of poor quality and unacceptable, and this usually occurred within a short period of time, for example, 20 to 30 minutes. This ink build up required stopping the printing operation so that the transfer roll could be cleaned with solvent. When the ink is old, an additional problem arises because the old ink has esterified and has very slow drying characteristics, so that the old ink after being applied to the piece is picked off onto other pieces, causing an unacceptable mark.

This improved ink, because of the partial and controlled esterification of the shellac, permits longer times between cleaning of the transfer roll, and also permits faster and easier clean-up with an appropriate solvent. The following examples of inks are given, with the ingredients being given in percent by weight.

Example 1:

	Percent
White ink:	
Esterified shellac solids (20% ester)	30.0
Ethyl alcohol 200 proof	36.7
Cellosolve	1.0
Titanium dioxide	30.0
Water	2.3

The pigment (TiO_2) to binder (esterified shellac solids) ratio is 1:1 by weight. Cellosolve is ethylene glycol monoethyl ether, and is added to improve the drying qualities of the ink.

Example 2:

	Percent
Black ink:	
Esterified shellac solids (24% ester)	34.0
Ethyl alcohol 200 proof	59.0
Channel black	6.0
Water	1.0

The pigment to binder ratio is 1:5.7.

Example 3:

	Percent
Red ink:	
Esterified shellac solids (22% ester)	30.0
Ethyl alcohol 200 proof	36.7
Cellosolve	1.0
Red iron oxide	30.0
Water	2.3

The pigment (TiO_2) to binder (esterified shellac solids) ratio is 1:1 by weight. Cellosolve is ethylene glycol monoethyl ether, and is added to improve the drying qualities of the ink.

TABLETTING LUBRICANTS

ACID LUBRICANTS

Adipic Acid Lubricant

G.C. Hoss; U.S. Patent 3,584,099; June 8, 1971; and U.S. Patent 3,506,756; April 14, 1970; both assigned to Miles Laboratories, Inc. has found that the tabletting process is improved by adding adipic acid to the composition to be subjected to compression tabletting. The acipic acid tabletting lubricant can be used with a wide range of powdered compositions to allow high speed tabletting. While various amounts of adipic acid can be mixed with such compositions depending upon the presence of ingredients which impart some lubrication and upon the tabletting speed desired, it is usually sufficient to use at least 5% adipic acid based on the total weight of the composition when no other lubricants are used. If desired, adipic acid may be used in larger amounts, approaching the total tablet weight, since it is cohesive when compressed.

The compositions which can be lubricated for tabletting with adipic acid can, for example, be any compositions which are cohesive enough when compressed to form and retain a tablet shape. Such compositions can be composed of powdered detergents, disinfectants, germicides and/or abrasives which disintegrate when placed in water to form cleaning solutions of various types. Inclusion of quaternary compounds, such as cetylpyridinium chloride, is particularly useful when cleaning tablets are to be produced.

The preferred compositions, however, are effervescent mixtures comprised of an alkali metal carbonate or bicarbonate and an acid such as malic, citric or tartaric acids which are capable of rapidly releasing carbon dioxide upon addition of water. When the carbon dioxide has been released, the solution formed is useful for its alkalizing properties when taken orally. The compositions can also include at least one therapeutic agent, water-soluble excipients, and any necessary coloring or flavoring agents, diluents, binders, or disintegrators. In such compositions the therapeutic agent may be acetylsalicylic acid, acetyl p-aminophenol or other suitable analgesic.

If necessary, binders may be added to the base composition to promote cohesion. All of such compositions are tablettable in that they are cohesive when compressed. However, without a lubricant most of such compositions can be tabletted only by hand, since they cause binding and scoring of the punches and dies of power-driven tabletting machines. In order to attain commercial production speeds, a tabletting lubricant must be employed to reduce surface friction and internal compression friction.

In effervescent tablets adipic acid provides the additional effect of taking part in the effervescent action. When the adipic acid does form part of the effervescent couple it is neutralized to a metal salt if a sufficient amount of an alkaline material is employed, and in such form is even more highly soluble than is the free adipic acid. Thus, when greater solubility than that for free adipic acid is desired, a source of alkali metal ions may be included in the pharmaceutical composition, whereby upon dissolution of the composition in water the alkali metal salt of adipic acid is formed, and any solubility limitations of adipic acid are obviated. Generally, however, this is not necessary due to the fact that the adipic acid is used in amounts low enough so that the volume of water normally used for dissolution of the tablets is sufficient to dissolve all of the adipic acid employed.

Amounts of at least about 5% adipic acid based on the total weight of the lubricated tablettable composition are generally sufficient to allow high-speed tabletting when adipic acid is used as the sole lubricant. When it is used as one of at least two tabletting lubricants, a proportionately smaller amount may be used. Amounts of about 5 to 15% adipic acid allow tabletting of effervescent mixtures at rates up to about 5,000 tablets per minute on rotary tablet machines containing 47 punch and die sets. Each punch and die set produces approximately 106 tablets per minute in such machines. On a rotary machine containing 33 punch and die sets, tablets may be compressed at a rate of 76 tablets per minute per set for a total production of about 2,500 tablets per minute.

Example: In the following example the concentrations of components are stated as weight percent of the weight of lubricated composition as tabletted.

Component	Amount, g.
Sodium bicarbonate	1,674
Citric acid (anhydrous)	1,000
Adipic acid	320
Calcium hydrogen orthophosphate	205
Magnesium oxide	4
Sodium cyclohexylsulfamate	20
Sodium saccharinate	2
Peppermint oil encapsulated in gum acacia	16

The above components were dried, reduced to 30 mesh screen size and thoroughly mixed. The adipic acid in the composition was present in a concentration of 9.8 weight percent. The resulting mixture was placed in a hopper of a hand-operated punch rotary tabletting machine from which the mixture was fed to the dies of the punch and the die sets of the machine. The compression pressure was 11 kg. The tablets produced were 0.158" thick and weighed approximately 3.2 g. each. Upon completion of the run, the tablets were found to be smooth surfaced and elegant in appearance. Upon immersing in 120 ml. of water at 25°C., a tablet quickly effervesced and dissolved to give a sparkling clear solution of pH 5.8 with no sediment.

Fumaric Acid Lubricant

P.H. Cox; U.S. Patent 3,577,491; May 4, 1971; and U.S. Patent 3,518,346; June 30, 1970; both assigned to Miles Laboratories, Incorporated has found an improvement in the process of compressing powdered tablettable compositions by mixing fumaric acid with the composition prior to compression. The fumaric acid acts as a surface lubricant and as an internal compression lubricant for the tablettable compositions. The powdered tablettable compositions lubricated with fumaric acid can be those intended for internal employment such as for alkalizing of the stomach, or intended for external use such as for general cleaning of solid surfaces.

The fumaric acid is used under the same conditions and for the same type of products as disclosed for the use of adipic acid as lubricant in U.S. Patents 3,584,099 and 3,506,756. The following examples will illustrate the process in detail. The concentrations of components are stated as weight percent of the weight of the lubricated composition as tabletted.

Example 1:

Component	Amount, g.
Sodium bicarbonate	500
Citric acid (anhydrous)	150
Fumaric acid	100

The above components were dried and reduced to 30 mesh screen size and thoroughly mixed. The fumaric acid in the composition was present in an amount of 13.3 weight percent of the weight of the mixture. The citric acid was present in an amount of 20 weight percent and the sodium bicarbonate was present in an amount of 66.6 weight percent, both based on the total weight of the mixture.

The mixture was placed in a hopper of a hand-operated punch rotary tabletting machine from which the mixture was fed to the dies of the punch and die sets of the machine. The compression pressure was set at 8 to 10 tons per square inch. The tablets produced weighed approximately 3.6 g. each. Upon completion of the run the tablets were found to be smooth surfaced and elegant in appearance. Upon dropping the same into about 100 ml. of water at room temperature, the tablets quickly effervesced and dissolved to give a sparkling clear solution with no sediment. Such a solution can be taken orally to provide an alkalizing effect in the user's stomach.

Example 2:

Component	Amount, g.
Sodium bicarbonate	500
Malic acid	150
Fumaric acid	100

The above components were dried, reduced to 30 mesh screen size and mixed. The mixed composition was then added to the hopper of a hand-operated punch rotary tabletting machine and tablets were made. Each tablet weighed approximately 3.6 g. The tablet had the same dissolving and effervescent characteristics as the tablets of Example 1.

Example 3:

Component	Amount, g.
Dicalcium phosphate dihydrate	340
Confectionery cane sugar	56.7
Gelatin, USP	3.3
Fumaric acid	100

The first three above components were mixed with the fumaric acid to make an initial mixture containing 20% fumaric acid. 200 g. of this composition were formed into placebo tablets on a single punch tabletting machine at a rate of about 125 tablets per minute. The tablets had diameters of about 0.375", thicknesses of about 0.22", and disintegrated slowly in room temperature water.

An additional 300 g. of the first three components in the same proportions as given above were then mixed with an equal amount of the initial mixture and 400 g. of the resulting mixture tabletted as above. These tablets contained 10% fumaric acid based on the total tablet weight and showed the same slow disintegration rate as the above tablets. The remaining 200 g. of the composition used for these tablets was then mixed with an additional 200 g. of the first three components in the same proportions as given above. The resulting mixture containing 5% fumaric acid was tabletted as above and the tablets exhibited similar properties.

POLYMERIC LUBRICANTS

Polyfluorocarbon Lubricants

E.A. Hotko; U.S. Patent 3,340,152; September 5, 1967; assigned to Ciba Corporation has found that polymers of the polyfluorocarbon type, i.e., the so-called polyfluorocarbons or fluorocarbon polymers, have the characteristics necessary for the lubricating agents used in manufacturing tablets. In other words, they facilitate the flow of the granulation mixture, reduce the friction between the granulation and the die during compression, prevent the compressed tablet from sticking to the face of the punches, and reduce the force necessary to eject it after compression. In addition, polymers of the polyfluorocarbon type have a sufficiently high melting point and are chemically inert; they are, therefore, compatible with tablet ingredients which are easily degraded in the presence of known lubricating material, and do not pose any physiologic and toxic problems.

Furthermore, the polymeric substances of the polyfluorocarbon type, when used as lubricating agents, affect the physical characteristics of the compressed tablet to a much smaller degree than the majority of the known lubricants. For example, the disintegration time of a tablet containing as a lubricant a polymer of the polyfluorocarbon type is smaller than that of a tablet containing a metal stearate lubricant, e.g., magnesium stearate and the like, or hydrogen castor oil. It has also been observed that, contrary to known lubricants, the disintegration time of a tablet containing, as a lubricant, a polymer of the polyfluorocarbon type is not significantly affected by various amounts of the latter. These types of lubricants also add coherent strength to the compressed tablets; this property appears to be in contrast with the effects of the known lubricating agents which tend to soften the compressed tablet.

Particularly useful as a lubricating agent is the polytetrafluoroethylene of the formula $(—CF_2—CF_2)_n$; other polyfluorocarbons capable of being used as lubricants in manufacturing tablets are the copolymer of tetrafluoroethylene and hexafluoropropylene; polyvinylidene fluoride, the copolymer of vinylidene fluoride and hexafluoropropylene, polytrifluorochloroethylene, the copolymer of vinylidene fluoride and trifluorochloroethylene, and the like.

The polymers of the polyfluorocarbon type for lubricating purposes are used in the form of powders having a particle size of from 1 to 150 microns, preferably from 1 to 25 microns. The tablets manufactured with the help of such lubricating agents have a content from 1 to 15%, preferably from 2 to 10%, of the polymers of the polyfluorocarbon type. The following examples illustrate the process.

Example 1: Tablets, each containing 0.05 g. of 2-[N-benzyl-N-(2-N,N-dimethylaminoethyl)-amino] pyridine hydrochloride as the active ingredient, and 0.01 g. of polytetrafluoroethylene of an average particle size of 5 to 10 microns, as the lubricating agent, are prepared as follows (for 5,000 tablets).

Ingredients	Grams
2-[N-benzyl-N-(2-N,N-dimethylaminoethyl)amino]-pyridine hydrochloride	250.0
Cornstarch	50.0
Lactose	650.0
Polytetrafluoroethylene	50.0
Alcohol 3A, 50%, q.s.	

The 2-[N-benzyl-N-(2-N,N-dimethylaminoethyl)-amino] pyridine hydrochloride, the cornstarch, the lactose, and the polytetrafluoroethylene are passed through a 30-mesh screen, and the powders are blended in a suitable mixer for 30 minutes. The granulate is formed by adding the alcohol (3A, 50%); the wet mass is passed through a No. 12 mesh screen and then dried at 40°C. The dried granules are broken through a 20-mesh screen and compressed into tablets weighing 0.2 g. using 10/32" standard concave punches.

Example 2: Tablets each containing 0.005 g. of methyl α-phenyl-α-(2-piperidyl)acetate hydrochloride as the physiologically active ingredient, and 0.005 g. of polytetrafluoroethylene of an average particle size of from about 5 to 10 microns as the lubricating agent, are prepared as follows (for 10,000 tablets).

Ingredients	Grams
Methyl α-phenyl-α-(2-piperidyl)acetate hydrochloride	50.0
Cornstarch	30.0
Lactose	870.0
Polytetrafluoroethylene	50.0
Alcohol 3A, 50%, q.s.	

The methyl α-phenyl-α-(2-piperidyl)acetate hydrochloride, the cornstarch, the lactose, and the polytetrafluoroethylene are passed through a 30-mesh screen and the powders are blended in a suitable mixer for 30 minutes. The granulate is formed by adding the alcohol (3A, 50%); the wet mass is passed through a No. 12 mesh screen and then dried at 40°C. The dried granules are broken through a 20-mesh screen and compressed into tablets weighing 0.1 g. using 8⁄32" standard concave punches.

Polyethylene Glycol Lubricant

It has been found by *J. Tsumura, I. Imaseki and M. Nagasawa; U.S. Patent 3,692,896; September 19, 1972; assigned to Isumura Juntendo Co., Ltd., Japan* that water-soluble tablets can be obtained by the direct compression method employing super micro particle powder of PEG (polyethylene glycol) having a particle size of less than 50μ and preferably 1 to 5μ as a lubricant.

The water-soluble main ingredients used may be, for example, water-soluble medicines such as ascorbic acid, thiamine hydrochloride, taurin, amino acids, sulpyrine, caffeine, chlorophenylamine maleate, and the like; water-soluble additives to foods such as sweeteners, i.e., dextrose, sucrose, and the like; organic acids such as citric acid, malic acid, tartaric acid, and the like; colors, flavors, preservatives, such as sodium dehydroacetate, and the like; water-soluble chemicals, such as sodium perborate, potassium cyanide, and the like; water-soluble agricultural chemicals, such as sodium pentachlorophenylamate, kasugamycin, glasticidin S and the like. These ingredients are used alone or in a suitable combination, and they are used in a form of a powder for compression.

The super micro particle powder of PEG having particle size of less than 50μ can only be obtained by puverizing PEG with supersonic air current jet mill, which pulverizes a material by jetting or impacting of mixed particle current employing supersonic air current. Using a conventional mill such as ball mill, pulverizer, micro mill, and the like, it is difficult to obtain PEG powder of super micro particles, and even if a special pulverizing method is used, PEG obtained is of at most only in a level of about 100 mesh (about 140μ).

The excellent lubricating effect of the super micro particle powder of PEG having particle size of less than 50μ compared with coarsely powdered PEG can be seen from the following experimental results. In the experiment, a single punching tablet machine of only the one side compression type is used and the rate of the pressure transmitted to the lower punch by compressing only with the upper punch while the lower punch is fixed, is shown in the following expression (R):

transmission value R = (pressure of lower punch/pressure of upper punch) x 100

Also, the ejection force to push out the molded tablet from the die by the lower punch is measured and these are compared. When the value R is more than 85, the direct compression method may be used and the lower the rejection force will be, the more effective the lubricating action will be. By using polyethylene glycol having a particle size of 1 to 10 microns, and preferably 1 to 5 microns, as lubricant, excellent water-soluble tablets can be prepared over long periods of time using only small amounts of polyethylene glycol, under the conditions of R>85 and an ejection force of less than 70 kg. The powder and formula used in the experiment are as follows:

Sodium bicarbonate (150 mesh)	95 to 99.75%
PEG 6000 (having particles sizes shown in the table below)	5 to 0.25%

The tablet is molded in diameter of 20 mm. and thickness of 5 mm. with the upper punch pressure of 2,000 kg. Results are shown in detail in the table below.

Particle Size	PEG Added (%)	R (%)	Ejection Force (kg)
	1	70.2	420
200μ	3	74.3	310
	5	78.1	250
	10	79.3	210
	1	85.2	170
50μ	2	88.7	150
	3	90.3	120
	5	93.3	105
	1	92.3	90
10μ	2	95.9	70
	3	96.4	60
	1	94.5	80
7μ	2	96.0	60
	3	96.0	50
	0.5	88.7	70
5μ	1	97.0	60
	2	96.3	50
	3	96.0	30
	0.5	90.6	65
3μ	1	96.4	50
	2	97.0	45
	0.2	89.1	65
1μ	0.5	93.5	60
	1	96.7	30
	2	97.0	25

As can be seen from the table, super micro particle powders of PEG having particle size of less than 50μ are particularly excellent in lubricating effect in direct compression method compared with the coarsely powdered PEG. A better understanding of the process will be attained from the following example. Percent means percent by weight.

Example: 30% ascorbic acid, 69% lactose powder and 1% PEG 6000 powder (having particle size of about 5μ) are mixed together homogeneously and compressed by rotary tablet machine to form tablets of 1 gram each in weight. After compressing of 5,000 tablets continuously, nothing unusual was observed in the operation of the tablet machine and in tablets obtained. Thus, white and lustrous surfaced tablets are obtained. When the tablet thus obtained is dropped into water, it dissolves quickly to form a clear solution. When ascorbic acid is processed by wet granulation method into tablets, it deteriorates, whereas when it is processed into tablets by this method, it does not deteriorate.

OILS AS LUBRICANTS

Encapsulated Lubricant Oils

A tabletting lubricant comprising an encapsulated oil is disclosed by *A.I. Dines and W.G. Brown; U.S. Patent 3,619,462; November 9, 1971; and U.S. Patent 3,513,345; June 30, 1970; both assigned to Miles Laboratories, Inc.* The lubricant comprises dry-mixable particles each having a core containing a lubricating oil and a coating of an oil-insoluble film-forming substance. The lubricant acts as both a punch face lubricant and as a diewall lubricant for the tablettable materials. The powdered materials lubricated with this lubricant can be those intended for ingestion, such as for alkalizing of the stomach, or those intended for external use, such as for the general cleaning of solid surfaces.

While various amounts of the lubricant can be mixed with such materials, depending upon the presence of other ingredients which impart lubrication and depending upon the tabletting speed desired, it is usually sufficient to use about 0.5% of the lubricant based on the weight of the lubricated tablettable material. If desired, the lubricant can be used in large amounts, approaching the limit of about 50% of the total tablet weight, at which point excess lubricating oil is evident on the tablet surface which is generally undesirable. Preferably, less than 5% of the lubricant is employed.

The coated oil particles have average diameters of 1 to 50 microns. The amount of the film-forming substance used is less than that necessary to coat the oil particles with a continuous thick, resinous coat. The use of a minimal workable amount of the film-forming material with respect to the oil is preferred, but is not critical. However, the relatively thin coating thus produced appears to allow improved lubrication.

A primary advantage of this tabletting lubricant is its dry-mixable character which renders it easily mixed and homogenized with various powdered tablettable materials. This characteristic may be defined as the ability of the lubricant to be homogeneously mixed with dry powders as if it were itself a completely dry powder. This characteristic does not imply that the particles alone are completely free-flowing, but rather than when mixed with at least an equal weight of a dry powder for tabletting the mixture is free-flowing. When the lubricant particles are dispersed in water no surface scum is produced and the solution produced is uniform.

The tablettable materials which can be lubricated with the coated oil particles can be any materials which are cohesive enough when compressed to form and retain a tablet shape. Such materials can, for example, be disinfectants, germicides or oral hygienic compositions, which disintegrate when placed in water to form solutions of various types.

Various therapeutic compositions can also be tabletted by use of the coated oil particles. Such compositions can be composed of at least one therapeutic agent, a water-soluble excipient, and any necessary coloring agents, flavoring agents, diluents, binders or disintegrators. If necessary, binders may be added to the tablettable composition to promote cohesion. Also compositions for the production of effervescent tablets for producing flavored beverages can be lubricated by the coated oil lubricant.

The preferred lubricant particles are made by spray drying an emulsion formed from a mixture of a heat and air (oxygen) stable refined vegetable oil having a viscosity of 120 to 140 cps and a starch gum solution. The emulsion is dried by spraying it into an air stream maintained at 150° to 265°C., which leaves the spray dryer at a temperature of about 110°±5°C. The resulting coated oil particles have a moisture content of 2 to 4 weight percent, are dry-mixable with powdered materials, and provide lubrication for the same upon tabletting. These and other aspects of the process will be apparent from the following example. The concentrations of components are stated as weight percent of the weight of the lubricated material as tabletted.

Example:

Emulsion Components	Weight, g.	Weight, %
Gum acacia	1,600	20
Peanut oil	400	5
Deionized water	6,000	75

A solution of the gum acacia was made by adding the deionized water. The emulsion was formed by mixing the peanut oil with this solution in a laboratory blender at room temperature. The emulsion was dried in a standard spray dryer having an atomizing wheel centrally disposed in the upper portion of the drying chamber, an air inlet port equipped with a heater spaced directly below the atomizing wheel, and an outlet port at the bottom of the chamber for removing the particles and the air. The emulsion was fed through a conduit tube from a holding tank to the atomizing wheel and the coated oil particles were collected by a cyclone separator connected to the outlet port. The dryer used was a Necro-Niro Portable Spray Dryer.

The emulsion was used at about room temperature and was placed in the holding tank and agitated until it was fed to the atomizing wheel. The inlet air temperature was maintained at 220° to 230°C. and its flow through the chamber was at a rate sufficient to reduce the moisture of the dried lubricant particles to about 2 to 4% by weight. The exit air temperature was 70° to 80°C. The atomizing wheel was rotated at about 40,000 rpm by supplying air to a connected drive turbine at a pressure of 5.8 to 6.2 kg./cm.^{2}

The weight of the coated oil particles collected at the bottom of the spray dryer was 1,880 grams, indicating a weight loss of 76.5% based on the emulsion weight. The dried particles had a moisture content of 4.45% (determined by toluene distillation) due to the retention of bound and partially bound water by the gum acacia. The moisture was further lowered to about 4% by drying the particles in a forced air oven at about 50°C. for 16 hours. The weight ratio of gum acacia to the oil in these particles was about 4:1. The spray-dried coated oil particles were then used to provide lubrication for effervescent beverage tablets of the following formulation.

Tablet Formulation		Weight, g.
Coated oil particles		819.0
Citric acid (anhydrous)		4,368.0
Sodium bicarbonate		2,910.0
Cherry flavoring		45.0
FD&C Red No. 2		56.1
Tartaric acid		330.0
Ascorbic acid		30.0
Sodium cyclohexylsulfamate		342.0
Sodium saccharin		84.0
	Total	8,984.1

The lubricated timetable composition was prepared by separately drying all components except the citric acid and then mixing the coated oil particles with sodium bicarbonate and cherry flavoring. The remainder of the components were then blended with this premix and the formulation tabletted at a commercial rate on a single punch tabletting machine with the result that good lubrication was achieved. The tablets were one inch in diameter and were compressed to a hardness of about 3 to 3.5 kg. as measured by a Stokes hardness tester. The average tablet weight was about 3 grams for a total of nearly 3,000 tablets.

Another smaller batch of the above formulation was prepared with similar coated oil particles except that no drying of the components was carried out. The formulation was likewise tabletted on a single-punch press at a commercial rate to an average hardness of about 3.9 kg. The tablets were one inch in diameter and an average of 0.156 inches thick. During tabletting, good flow of the formulation from the hopper into the die cavity was experienced. The formulation contained 9% by weight of the coated oil particles for a total of 273 mg. on the basis of the individual tablet weight.

A number of these tablets were dissolved in water at about 3° to 5°C. with the result that the average disintegration time was about 150 seconds. Upon dissolution the tablets produced a cherry-flavored effervescent beverage. The oil content in these tablets was about 54.6 mg. oil per tablet.

It was significant that the lubricant particles provided adequate lubrication for the effervescent beverage formulations which could only have been tabletted by hand, if at all, in the absence of the coated oil particles. Further, the coating of the oil particles with the film-forming gum acacia rendered them dry-mixable, in which condition they could be directly mixed with the other dry ingredients of the formulation and tabletted without difficulty.

Encapsulated Oil-Siloxane Polymer Mixtures

T.L. Welsh and G.R. Tomaich; U.S. Patent 3,518,344; June 30, 1970; assigned to Miles Laboratories, Inc. have developed an improved tabletting lubricant comprising, in combination, a siloxane polymer and dry-mixable particles of a lubricating oil coated with an oil-insoluble film-forming substance. The lubricant acts as both a punch face lubricant and as a diewall lubricant for the tablettable materials. The powdered tablettable materials lubricated with the above lubricant can be those intended for general cleaning of solid surfaces or those intended for therapeutic use.

The siloxane polymer can be any of the siloxanes having a viscosity of 250 to 12,500 cp., plus or minus 5%, and having the unit formula:

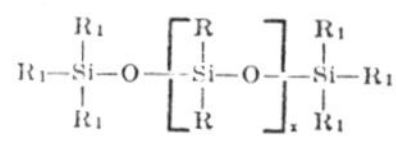

where each R can be hydrogen, an alkyl, an aryl, an aralkyl, or an alkaryl group; each R_1 can be any of these groups except hydrogen; where either of the R groups of the unit formula can be the same or different groups; and where any of the R_1 groups can be the same or different groups. Mixtures of the siloxanes are also usable. The preferred polymers are the linear dialkyl polysiloxanes.

Examples of usable polysiloxanes are polymers of dihydrogen siloxane, methyl hydrogen siloxane, dimethyl siloxane, propyl hydrogen siloxane, dipropyl siloxane, phenyl hydrogen siloxane, benzyl hydrogen siloxane, tolyl hydrogen siloxane, and mixtures of dimethyl siloxane and methyl hydrogen siloxane. All of these siloxane polymers have terminal groups in which R_1 of the formula can be an alkyl, an alkaryl, or an aralkyl group, or combinations thereof.

The coated oil particles have average diameters of 1 to 50 microns. The amount of the film-forming substance used is less than that necessary to entirely coat the oil particles with a continuous thick, resinous coat. The use of a minimal workable amount of the film-forming material with respect to the oil is preferred, but is not critical. However, the relatively thin coating thus produced appears to allow improved lubrication.

The primary advantages of this combination tabletting lubricant are that the lubricant is nearly free-flowing and that it imparts good surface lubrication properties to tablettable materials lubricated. The inclusion of the combination lubricant into tablettable materials prior to compression aids the flow of these materials into the dies of tabletting machines and, upon compression and subsequent ejection of the tablettable materials, aids in maintaining the punch and die surfaces free from any retained materials which would otherwise, if allowed to build up, cause poor tabletting characteristics.

These and other aspects of the lubricant system will be apparent from the following example. The concentrations of the components are stated as weight percents of the weight of the lubricated material as tabletted.

Example:

Emulsion Components	Weight, lbs.	Weight, %
Starch gum	100	30.7
Refined vegetable oil	50	15.3
Polydimethyl siloxane	11	3.4
Deionized water	165±1.7	50.6
Total	326±1.7	100.0

The starch gum was a stable corn dextrin having the following characteristics: viscosity – 120 to 140 cp.; particle size – 98% of the powder passes through a 40-mesh screen, U.S.

Standard; and color – light tan. This dextrin can be obtained under the trade name Nadex 772.

The vegetable oil had good heat and air stability and was resistant to rancidification. The major fatty acid moieties were: palmitic, 8 to 10%; stearic, 2 to 4%; oleic, 43 to 47%; elaidic, 39 to 43%; and linoleic, 1 to 3%. A vegetable oil of this description can be obtained under the trade name Durkex 500. The polydimethyl siloxane had a viscosity of 350 cp. ±15%, a molecular weight in the range of 15,000 to 16,000 with recurring polydimethyl siloxane units terminated by trimethyl siloxane groups.

Four batches of the above emulsion were made and spray dried. The starch gum of each batch was added to the water and the polydimethyl siloxane was added to the vegetable oil. The oil mixture was added to the gum solution with agitation in order to produce a homogeneous emulsion.

Each emulsion batch was then spray dried in a large spray dryer having a drop distance of 18 feet from the emulsion outlet to the exit port. This dryer had an atomizing wheel centrally disposed in the upper portion of the drying chamber, an air inlet port for heated air spaced directly below the atomizing wheel, and an outlet port at the bottom of the chamber for removing the dried oil particles and the air. The emulsion batches were fed through a conduit tube from a holding tank to the atomizing wheel and the bulk of the coated oil particles were collected at the outlet port. The fines were removed by a cyclone separator connected to the exit air stream and added to the main body of the particles.

The air inlet temperature was maintained at about 266°C. with the equilibrium moisture content at that temperature. The air flow rate through the chamber was held at a rate sufficient to reduce the moisture of the lubricant particles to 2 weight percent. The exit air temperature was 102°C. A total drying time of six hours was required to dry the four emulsion batches. The 52 lb. weight loss was distributed in the following manner: 20 lbs. moisture loss in the 400 lbs. of starch gum in going from an initial 7 to 2% moisture, 15 lbs. particles loss due to incomplete recovery, and 17 lbs. loss from first batch put through the dryer.

This dried combination lubricant was dry-mixable with powdered tablettable materials and was found to be stable and easily shipped in sealed containers. This spray dried lubricant was used as component (3) to lubricate mouthwash tablets compressed from the following formulation.

Tablet Formulation	Weight, g.
(1) Sodium bicarbonate	2,220.0
(2) Citric acid (anhydrous)	1,742.0
(3) Coated lubricant particles	75.0
(4) Flavoring (powdered)	100.0
(5) Dye, blue lake	0.9
(6) Sodium cyclohexylsulfamate	20.0
(7) Sodium saccharin	2.0
(8) Cetyldimethylbenzylammonium chloride	10.0
Total	4,169.9

The powdered components were mixed in the order of their decreasing amounts, i.e., components Nos. 1, 2, 4, 3, 6, 8, 7 and 5. The dry tablettable mixture was then tabletted on a single punch machine fitted with one-inch diameter punches. The tablets were 0.2" thick and showed a hardness of about 3 to 4 kg. on a Stokes hardness tester. They dissolved in an average time of 42 seconds at 23°C.

The coated lubricant particles provided excellent lubrication for these mouthwash tablets as shown by stability tests for hardness and disintegration time which were conducted on the tablets.

CONTROLLED RELEASE LUBRICANT FOR VETERINARY BOLUS

A process has been developed by *A.B. Rednick and S.J. Tucker; U.S. Patent 3,507,952; April 21, 1970; assigned to Smith Kline & French Laboratories* which provides a sustained release veterinary bolus which can be administered to food producing ruminants for therapeutic effect several weeks before slaughtering and in which the medicament present will be essentially clear of the animal tissues at the time of slaughtering.

It has been unexpectedly discovered that when a lubricant is employed in the manufacture of the bolus in certain critical percentage ranges that a definite predictable sustained release pattern is achieved. In order to achieve this sustained release pattern of the therapeutic substance, the lubricant material should be present from 1 to 3.5% by weight of the total solids. The use of these critical amounts of lubricant permits for the disintegration of the bolus within approximately ten days, and virtual clearance of the medicament from the animal tissues in approximately three weeks.

In vitro testing of sulfamethazine bolus containing various amounts of magnesium stearate lubricant has shown that when the lubricant is present up to 0.5%, all of the sulfamethazine is released in two hours. This release is much too rapid for sustained release medication. When the magnesium stearate is present in 4% or more, it was found that only 32% of the sulfamethazine is released from the bolus in four hours with an apparent leveling off of the release. This rate of release would be much too slow to give the necessary blood levels for proper sustained release treatment of the animal. The critical range of the magnesium stearate present in the bolus was found to be from 1 to 3.5%.

The critical lubricant can be any of the common tablet water-insoluble lubricants such as, for example, magnesium stearate, sodium stearate, calcium stearate, powdered stearic acid, talc, paraffin, cocoa butter, graphite, lycopodium or combinations thereof. The preferred lubricants are fatty acid derived, especially the stearates such as magnesium stearate, sodium stearate, calcium stearate and stearic acid.

This process is useful with any solid medicament which it is desired to provide in sustained release form. The medicament may be in the form of a base, salt or ester, and may be soluble or insoluble. For example, the medicament may be a sulfonamide derivative such as sulfamethazine or sulfathiazine, a tranquilizer such as chlorpromazine, an antibiotic such as chloramphenicol, tetracycline or penicillin, an anthelmintic such as piperazine phosphate, an antibloat agent such as organopolysiloxanes, hormone growth supplements such as stilbestrol, vitamins and furazolidone.

Exemplary of the dense fillers which may be used as a matrix are iron powder, calcium sulfate, portland cement, plaster of paris, magnesium oxychloride cement, zinc oxychloride cement, zinc oxyiodide cement, or mixtures thereof. Most advantageously the dense filler will be iron powder. The filler will be present from about 5 to 95% by weight of the total solids. Preferably the filler will be present from about 25 to 75%.

If binders are necessary for adequate cohesiveness of the bolus, natural gums and gum constituents such as acacia, tragacanth, agar and pectin may be used. Further examples would be cellulose esters, polyvinylpyrrolidone and proteinaceous material such as gelatin, casein and zein.

Example 1:

Ingredients	Grams/Bolus
Sulfamethazine	22.5
Reduced iron	11.25
Magnesium stearate	0.70
Gelatin solution 10%	

The sulfamethazine and iron are mixed and then wetted with the 10% gelatin solution. The wetted powders are passed through a No. 6 screen and dried at 120°F. overnight. The dried granules are then passed through a No. 14 screen and mixed with the magnesium stearate. The boluses are then compressed using cylindrical-dome shaped punches and dies. The finished bolus weighs 35.15 grams.

Example 2:

Ingredients	Grams/Bolus
Furazolidone	3.640
Reduced iron	3.640
Calcium sulfate dihydrate	5.000
Magnesium stearate	0.400
Polyvinylpyrrolidone solution (5% in 50/50 methanol-water)	

The furazolidone, iron and calcium sulfate dihydrate powders are mixed and granulated with the polyvinylpyrrolidone solution. The wetted powders are passed through a No. 6 screen and dried overnight at 120°F. The dried granules are passed through a No. 14 screen and mixed with the magnesium stearate. The mixture is then compressed into boluses using oval-shaped punches and dies. The finished tablet weighs 12.8 grams.

II. TABLETTING SPECIFIC MATERIALS

ANTIMICROBIAL AGENTS

PENICILLIN COMPOUNDS

6-Aminopenicillanic Acid Derivatives

P. Baumann and M. Zimmerman; U.S. Patent 3,354,145; November 21, 1967; assigned to Geigy Chemical Corporation have found that, surprisingly, penicillins of the formula:

(1)

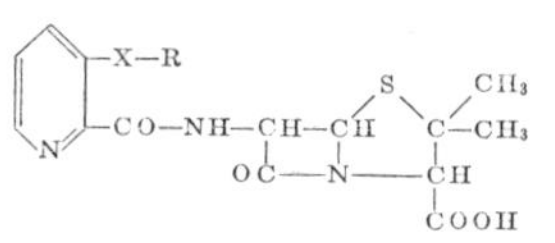

where X is oxygen or sulfur and R is a straight-chain alkyl or alkenyl radical having at most 4 carbon atoms, and their salts with inorganic and organic bases have excellent antibacterial activity against gram positive bacteria. These penicillins are also active against strains of *Staphylococcus aureus* which produce penicillinase and against which benzylpenicillin is inactive. These penicillins are substantially stable to the influence of mineral acid and can thus be administered not only parenterally but as such or, in the form of their pharmaceutically acceptable salts, also orally.

Compounds of Formula (1) in which R–X– is alkoxy of 2 to 4 carbon atoms are particularly effective against highly-resistant *Staphylococcus aureus* strains. They have 100 times greater bacteriostatic activity than the known 2-pyridylpenicillin.

The penicillins of Formula (1) and their salts are produced in a known manner; in the working up and in the formation of their salts, allowance should be made for hybrid ion properties of the end products. 6-aminopenicillanic acid or a salt therof is reacted with a compound introducing the radical of an acid of the Formula (2):

(2)

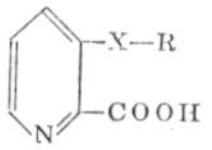

where X and R have the meanings given above and, if desired, the resulting compound of Formula (1) is converted into a salt with an inorganic or organic base.

Dosage units for peroral administration preferably contain between 10 to 90% of the acid of Formula (1) or its nontoxic salt as active ingredient. They are produced by combining the active ingredient with, e.g., solid, pulverulent carriers such as lactose, sucrose, sorbitol, mannitol; starches such as potato starch, maize starch or amylopectin; also laminaria powder or citrus pulp powder; cellulose derivatives or gelatin, optionally with the addition of lubricants such as magnesium or calcium stearate or polyethylene glycols (Carbowax) of suitable molecular weights, to form tablets or dragee (sugar-coated tablet) cores.

The latter are coated, e.g., with concentrated sugar solutions which can also contain, e.g., gum arabic, talcum and/or titanium dioxide, or with a lacquer dissolved in easily volatile organic solvents or mixtures of solvents. Dyestuffs can be added to these coatings, e.g., to distinguish between varying dosages of active substance. The following examples illustrate the production of tablets and dragees.

Example 1: 250 grams of 3-ethoxy-2-piperidylpenicillin, as in free acid form are mixed with 175.80 grams of lactose and 169.70 grams of potato starch, the mixture is moistened with an alcoholic solution of 10 grams of stearic acid and granulated through a sieve. After drying, 160 grams of potato starch, 200 grams of talcum, 2.50 grams of magnesium stearate and 32 grams of colloidal silica are mixed in and the mixture is pressed into about 10,000 tablets each weighing 100 mg. and containing 25 mg. of active substance. If desired, the tablets can be grooved for better adaptation of the dosage. Similarly, tablets are prepared in which the above active substance in free acid form is replaced by the same amount of its sodium salt or potassium salt.

Example 2: A granulate is produced from 250 grams of 3-methoxy-2-pyridylpenicillin, 175.90 grams of lactose and the alcoholic solution of 10 grams of stearic acid. After drying, it is mixed with 56.60 grams of colloidal silica, 165 grams of talcum, 20 grams of potato starch and 2.50 grams of magnesium stearate and the mixture is pressed into 10,000 dragee cores. These are then coated with a concentrated syrup of 502.28 grams of crystallized sucrose, 6 grams of shellac, 10 grams of gum arabic, 0.22 gram of dyestuff and 1.5 grams of titanium dioxide and dried. The dragees obtained each weigh 120 mg. and contain 25 mg. of active substance.

Palatable Isoxazolylpenicillin Tablets

Some of the penicillins and in particular the isoxazolyl series of penicillins, e.g., oxacillin, cloxacillin, dicloxacillin and flucloxacillin as well as nafcillin and to some extent ampicillin and hetacillin have an extremely bitter taste. The taste has been difficult to mask by the mere addition of flavoring or sweetening agents.

A palatable formulation for oral administration has been developed by *A.P. Granatek; B.C. Nunning, N.G. Athanas, R.L. Dana, E.S. Granatek and R.G. Daoust; U.S. Patent 3,549,746; December 22, 1970; assigned to Bristol-Myers Company* by coating particles of these penicillins with ethylcellulose and a wax.

These compositions are not only palatable but the penicillin is readily absorbed. The penicillin contained in the compositions is absorbed from the human gastrointestinal tract upon oral administration, substantially at the same rate as from the compositions containing the uncoated penicillin.

The waxes useful in the coatings with ethylcellulose are the water insoluble pharmaceutically acceptable waxes including paraffin wax, ozokerite wax, ceresin wax, Utah wax, montan wax, carnauba wax, Japan wax, bayberry wax, sugar cane wax, beeswax, shellac wax, spermaceti wax, Castorwax (hydrogenated castor oil), and the like. A single wax or mixture of waxes can be used. A preferred wax is spermaceti wax and a preferred mixture is spermaceti wax and Castorwax.

Example 1: Spray coated ethylcellulose-spermaceti-sodium dicloxacillin is prepared from 250.0 grams of sodium dicloxacillin, micronized, 250.0 grams of ethylcellulose (viscosity 100 cps.), 500.0 grams spermaceti wax and 15.0 liters of methylene chloride in the following manner.

Dissolve the spermaceti wax in 8 liters of methylene chloride in a 20 liter glass or stainless steel container with the aid of a mixer (e.g., a Lightnin mixer). No heat is required. Add the ethylcellulose in small portions while maintaining agitation. Stir until a clear and relatively viscous solution is obtained. Sodium dicloxacillin is then added in small portions while maintaining agitation. A milky white suspension will result. Strain the solution obtained to remove any particulate contaminants. The remainder of the methylene chloride (7 liters) is added with agitation and complete dispersion of the sodium dicloxacillin is effected.

The Nerco-Niro Laboratory model spray dryer is readied as follows and assembled completely before starting except for the atomizer. Turn the electric heater to setting number 2 or 3 until the inlet air gauge reads around 130°C. When equilibrium is reached the inner air gauge will read 115° to 120°C. and the outlet air gauge will read 50° to 55°C.

Install the turbine atomizer in its proper position over a Teflon gasket and feed compressed air until the atomizer gauge reads 6 kg./cm.^{2}. At this point maximum compressed air pressure is in use (90 to 100 lbs.) and the turbine is turning at a rate of 40,000 rpm. Allow five minutes for equilibrium in the chamber before liquid feeding is commenced.

Start liquid feed to the turbine from a 2 liter separatory funnel connected to the turbine by a short piece of Teflon tubing and feed at a rate of 60 to 80 ml. per minute. Monitor the operation to maintain the following drying conditions throughout the entire operation: inlet air 115° to 120°C. and outlet air 60° to 70°C. Stop the atomizer and turn the electric heater to position M (exhaust fan). Allow 5 minutes in this position before lifting cover. Lift cover with the aid of the hydraulic lift and collect product from the walls.

The product is not expected to stick to the walls of the chamber other than by electrostatic forces. Dry the product in a vacuum oven overnight at room temperature. The methylene chloride residue is less than 0.5%. The free flowing sodium dicloxacillin product is passed through a 40 mesh screen and collected.

Example 2: Sodium dicloxacillin monohydrate tablets are prepared from 62.5 mg., 125 mg. or 250 mg. activity per tablet of sodium dicloxacillin (ethylcellulose, spermaceti spray coated from Example 1), 41.5 to 100 mg. of Carbowax 6000, micropulverized and a sufficient quantity of magnesium stearate, U.S.P. Blend the sodium dicloxacillin, the Carbowax and magnesium stearate in a suitable mixer. Tablet by direct compression to a suitable hardness.

TETRACYCLINE FORMULATIONS

Tetracycline Cyclohexyl Sulfamate

A tetracycline derivative without the unpleasant taste of tetracycline or known tetracycline derivatives has been prepared by *J.R. Boissier and G.A. Combes; U.S. Patent 3,299,124; January 17, 1967; Ste. Industrielle pour la Fabrication des Antibiotiques (SIFA), France.* This derivative can be obtained by reacting cyclohexyl sulfamic acid with tetracycline base in organic liquid medium which is inert towards the starting products, and isolating the tetracycline cyclohexyl sulfamate formed.

In a preferred method of carrying out this process cyclohexyl sulfamic acid is reacted in solution in an alcohol of low molecular weight, either on the tetracycline base in solution in the same solvent (in which case it is advantageous to work with substantially stoichiometric quantities of the starting products dissolved in tepid ethyl alcohol), or on the tetracycline base in suspension in acetone. It is then possible to precipitate the tetracycline cyclohexyl sulfamate formed by adding ethyl or isopropyl ether and drying the product which is obtained in vacuo, if desired with the aid of a substance which absorbs the water vapor, such as phosphorus pentoxide.

As a medicament, the derivative may be used as the active principle of solid or liquid pharmaceutical compositions intended for administration by the usual means, but intended more particularly for oral administration or for the treatment of the buccal cavity. Various excipients generally employed in preparations may be used, for example talc, starch, magnesium stearate, hexoses, aqueous or nonaqueous vehicles and emulsifiers.

The pharmaceutical compositions may be of various types, but in addition to the forms administered perorally, such as compressed tablets, syrups and powders, the new derivative can be used in pharmaceutical forms adapted to the local antibiotic treatment of the buccal cavity, which forms have hitherto been difficult to obtain because of the bad taste of the tetracycline. This is the reason why tetracycline cyclohexyl sulfamate is of very great utility for the preparation of such forms as lozenges, pastilles, gums, aerosols, liquids for gargles and mouthwashes.

Tetracycline cyclohexyl sulfamate can be associated in the medicament compositions with various substances, provided that they are pharmaceutically compatible. These substances can comprise other active principles and/or ordinary excipients, but it has been found that its association with an alkali metal hexametaphosphate is particularly favorable.

When administering a mixture of tetracycline cyclohexyl sulfamate and alkali hexametaphosphate, by the digestive tract, a much higher antibiotic level is obtained in the blood than when the antibiotic is administered alone.

Example 1: Compressed tablets were produced which corresponded to the following composition: Tetracycline cyclohexyl sulfamate, 250 mg.; excipient, sufficient to make one compressed tablet comprising 400 mg.

Example 2: Lozenges were produced which corresponded to the following composition: Tetracycline cyclohexyl sulfamate, 20 mg.; excipient, sufficient to make one completed lozenge of 1 gram.

Example 3: Sugar-coated compressed tablets were prepared which corresponded to the following composition: Tetracycline cyclohexyl sulfamate, 250 mg. and sodium hexametaphosphate, 160 mg.; excipient, sufficient to make one sugar-coated compressed tablet.

Tetracycline-Enzyme Tablets

In the case of some antibiotics, and in particular of tetracycline and its derivatives, it has been shown (Pindell et col., *J. Pharm. Exp. Ther.,* April 1959, pp. 287/294) that the amount of tetracycline in the blood is greater and more lasting where the antibiotic is liberated in the hydrochloric stomachic medium than where it is liberated in the intestinal medium, where it is destroyed by hydrolysis by the action of the intestinal enzymes.

Conversely it is desirable to liberate anti-inflammatory proteolytic enzymes of the trypsin or chymotrypsin type only in the intestinal medium, where they then develop their optimum activity. It is evident that in the case of an association of these two types of constituents, if the two constituents are administered in the form of an enteric pill, then, the enzyme would indeed enjoy optimum conditions for action, the tetracycline, however, would be administered under unfavorable conditions.

To overcome this problem *J. Montandraud; U.S. Patent 3,424,839; January 28, 1969; assigned to Societe Generale de Recherches et d'Applications Scientifiques Sogeras, France* has prepared a chymotrypsin and tetracycline oral tablet by first pressing 50,000 Armour units of chymotrypsin admixed with suitable dry granulation excipients into a central core tablet form. The core is then enteric-coated and then covered all around with 250 mg. of tetracycline admixed with suitable granulation excipients. The tablet is effective for obtaining increased chymotrypsin-tetracycline anti-inflammatory and anti-infection efficacy in pre- and/or postoperative surgical patients.

As coating materials one can use gluten, acetophthalic resins, and cationic acrylic polymerizates such as Eudragit. Pills of this kind may be charged with 2,000 to 100,000 Armour units of enzymes, e.g., chymotrypsin, with 50 to 500 mg. of antibiotics, e.g., tetracycline, the preferred ratio being 50,000 Armour units of chymotrypsin for 250 mg. of tetracycline, the dose of such pills being of the order of 4 to 8 daily.

Example: The central core has 50,000 Armour units of chymotrypsin which are thoroughly mixed with 20 mg. mannitol, 1 mg. magnesium stearate and about 80 mg. talc. The mixture is dry-granulated and pressed into tablets. In a turbine apparatus there is first applied to the tablets a coating of gum arabic (from an alcoholic solution), then 19 layers of cellulose acetophthalate (from an acetonic solution).

The outer layer has 250 mg. of tetracycline hydrochloride, 35 mg. mannitol, 20 mg. sorbitol, 3 mg. carboxymethylcellulose, 7 mg. magnesium stearate and 35 mg. talc which are thoroughly mixed, granulated and pressed all around the coated core, until tablets or pills weighing 450 mg. are obtained. Such tablets can be used as such or after sugar coating.

The administration of these materials in the form of these double nucleus pills ensures a more effective and lasting action of the antibiotic than that observed where the same doses of the same antibiotic are administered by the usual methods.

The therapeutic action of the product has been studied on 57 surgical patients from which the following results were obtained: 21 excellent, or 36.8%; 24 good, or 42.2%; 12 average, or 21%; 0 nil, or 0%.

Monoalkyl Fumarates of Oxytetracyclines

A.E. Timreck and H.W. Raaf; U.S. Patent 3,595,904; July 27, 1971; assigned to Pfizer Inc. have found that monoalkyl fumarate derivatives of medicaments having basic or quaternary nitrogen atoms have a bland taste and are useful in sustained release preparations.

The monoalkyl fumaric acids having from 14 to 18 carbon atoms in the alkyl group are preferred. More particularly, monostearyl fumaric acid is most suitable. The advantage of these derivatives is that they exhibit very low water solubilities but dissociate or dissolve easily in acidic media such as the digestive fluids. Their limited aqueous solubility makes them particularly useful as dosage forms for the administration of the constituent medicaments. For example, they are useful in oral dosage forms such as tablets, chewable tablets and suspensions. Because of their relatively bland taste these dosage forms may be prepared without the use of excessive quantities of flavorants or sweeteners even where the medicament, as such, has an unpleasant taste.

The compounds are also useful as the active component of suppositories and depot injectables. As injectables, they provide a dosage form which dissociates easily, is harmless to the body and possesses sustained release characteristics. Sustained release characteristics are also provided where these compounds are used in oral dosage forms or suppositories.

The suitable medicaments include a number of vitamins, antibiotics, and central nervous system regulators, among others. More particularly, thiamine, riboflavin; oxytetracycline, tetracycline, polymyxin, triacetyloleandomycin, neomycin, 6-deoxy-6-demethyl-6-methylene-5-oxytetracycline, α-6-deoxy-5-oxytetracycline, streptomycin; caffeine, oxyphencyclimine, amphetamine, hydroxyzine, meclizine and ephedrine have been found to be suited for use in this process.

The processes for producing these derivatives involve reacting in solution, the appropriate medicament or its acid addition salt with a monoalkyl fumaric acid or a salt thereof, preferably an alkali metal salt. A precipitate of the monoalkyl fumarate of the medicament is formed and may be separated from the mother liquors by filtration, decantation or other suitable means. The precipitate, which may be washed, is then stored in a manner which will preserve it from decomposition. The tabletting of oxytetracycline stearyl fumarates is shown in the following example.

Example: A dosage form was formed which consisted of the following materials:

	Mg./Tablet
Oxytetracycline stearyl fumarate	260.91
Sorbitol	300.00
Glycine	200.00
Sodium cyclamate	20.00
Sodium saccharin	2.00
FD&C Red No. 3, Lake	10.00
FD&C Red No. 2, Lake	2.00
Dry Imitation Cherry No. 11582	10.00
Dry Imitation Cherry No. 55	3.00
Magnesium stearate	24.00

These ingredients were formed into tablets and the tablets were exposed to Modified Gastric Fluid with a pH of 1.2 at a temperature of 37°C. 20% dissolution of the whole tablets occurred after one hour of exposure to the Modified Gastric Fluid. Coarsely ground tablets evidenced 93% dissolution after one hour of exposure and finely ground tablets were completely dissolved after ten minutes of exposure to the Modified Gastric Fluid medium.

ANTIVIRAL AGENTS

Cycloalkylamines

R.J. Stedman; U.S. Patent 3,355,355; November 28, 1967; assigned to Smith Kline & French Laboratories has disclosed antiviral compositions containing as an active ingredient a cycloalkylamine of the following structure:

$$\underbrace{\overbrace{(CH_2)_n\ CH}}NRR'$$

where n is 6 to 11, and R and R' are each hydrogen, lower alkyl, lower alkenyl, lower acyl, hydroxy lower alkyl, dilower alkylamino lower alkyl, phenyl lower alkyl, hydroxy, amino, carbamoyl, thiocarbamoyl, amidino, or, when taken together with the nitrogen atom to which they are attached, form a heterocyclic ring, with the proviso that when one of R or R' is hydroxy, amino, carbamoyl, thiocarbamoyl, or amidino, the other is hydrogen or lower alkyl. A preferred group of compounds possess the following structure:

$$\underbrace{\overbrace{(CH_2)_7\ CH}}NRR'$$

where R and R' are as defined above.

These compounds may be used in the form of their pharmaceutically acceptable, nontoxic acid addition salts, such as the hydrochloride, sulfate, nitrate, hydrobromide, citrate, pamoate, maleate, cyclohexylsulfamate, acetate, tartrate, and succinate.

The cycloalkylamine compositions may be used to prevent or treat a wide variety of infections caused by viruses. Exemplary of these viruses are myxoviruses such as influenza A and A-2, swine influenza, parainfluenza 1, and Newcastle disease virus, poxviruses such as vaccinia and variola, Herpes viruses such as varicella (zoster) and pseudorabies, and picornaviruses such as rhinovirus.

The compositions may be used to prevent or treat viral infections in a variety of mammal and bird hosts or subjects. They are, for example, useful for preventing or treating Newcastle disease, swine influenza, or shipping fever. The active components described above may also be used to prevent or counteract viral infections of laboratory animals such as mice, ferrets, rats, etc.

The compositions are administered to a subject or host, either to prevent or treat a viral infection, by a variety of routes, including orally, by injection, or with the use of an inhaler or aerosol in effective, but nontoxic, doses, for example, about 0.5 to 700 mg., preferably 25 to 500 mg. of the active component when in tablet or capsule form, and 0.5 to 10 mg. when in an inhaler or aerosol. From 1 to 6 dosage units containing effective, nontoxic quantities of the active component may be administered daily.

Oral dosage forms can be in the form of tablets, capsules, troches or lozenges. In a tablet, the active antiviral component is generally incorporated in a solid carrier. Among the acceptable solid carriers are lactose, sucrose, magnesium stearate, stearic acid, starch, terra alba, talc, calcium phosphate, gelatin, agar, pectin, and acacia. A time delay material such as glyceryl monostearate or glyceryl distearate, alone or with a wax, may also be included. The tablet may be coated with materials such as methyl acrylate, methyl methacrylate, or shellac in order to form an enteric coating. The active antiviral component may be present in the composition in an amount of 1 to 95%, although 25 to 75% is the preferred amount.

Example 1: An antiviral tablet has the following components:

	Milligrams
Cyclooctylamine hydrochloride	100
Magnesium stearate	2.5
Starch	15
Terra alba	150
Granulate with syrup or gelatin (5% solution)	
terra alba q.s. ad	300

The tablet is ingested.

Example 2: An antiviral sustained release tablet has the following components:

	Milligrams
Cyclooctylamine hydrochloride	300
Sugar pellets	100
Calcium sulfate	20
Coating materials:	
Glyceryl monostearate	5
Microcrystalline wax	15
Glyceryl distearate	45
Gelatin (5% solution)	

The tablet is ingested.

Hydroxyalkyladenines with Hydroxypyrazolopyrimidines

A method of maintaining the antiviral activity of N^6-(hydroxyalkyl)adenines while reducing their toxicity has been developed by *J.E. Gray, G.E. Underwood and K.M. Mann; U.S. Patent 3,300,380; January 24, 1967; assigned to The Upjohn Company.* Unexpectedly, therapy combining N^6-(hydroxymethyl)adenine or N^6-(2-hydroxyethyl)adenine with 4-hydroxypyrazolo(3,4-d)pyrimidine has been found to provide unimpaired antiviral efficacy with significantly diminished toxicity.

Pharmaceutical compositions containing these ingredients, based on activity demonstrated against representative viruses, alter favorably the course of viral diseases in mammals caused by respiratory viruses such as Coe virus. Benefits from treatment of mammals and birds derive from reduction of virus titers, interference with a secondary viral effect with consequent shortening of the illness, prevention of infection by a regimen of prophylactic medication, and interference with the metabolism of the host cell to decrease virus synthesis.

Suitable oral dosage forms include tablets, pills, capsules, granules, powders, oral solutions or suspensions and the like. For preparing solid compositions such as tablets, the active ingredient is mixed with conventional tabletting ingredients or pharmaceutical carriers such as cornstarch, lactose, dicalcium phosphate, terra alba (calcium sulfate), talc, stearic acid, magnesium stearate, gums and functionally similar materials serving as lubricating agents, granulating agents, pharmaceutical diluents or carriers.

The tablets or pills of these compositions can be laminated or otherwise compounded to provide a dosage form affording the advantages of prolonged, delayed or predetermined successive action of the enclosed medication. For example, the tablet or pill can comprise an inner dosage and an outer dosage component, the latter being in the form of an envelope enclosing the former. The two components can be separated by an enteric layer which serves to resist disintegration until the desired site of release is encountered. A variety of materials can be used for such enteric layers or coatings, these materials including a number of polymeric acids or mixtures of polymeric acids with, for example, shellac, shellac and cetyl alcohol, cellulose acetate phthalate, and the like.

Advantageously, a coating consisting essentially of gelatin and styrene-maleic acid copolymer, deposited on the particles by a process of phase separation, such as by coacervation, can be employed as the encapsulating material capable of affording sustained release of the enclosed medication. The following examples will illustrate the formation of solid dosage forms.

Example 1: Tablets — One thousand tablets for oral use, each containing 250 mg. of N^6-(2-hydroxyethyl)adenine and 25 mg. of 4-hydroxypyrazolo(3,4-d)pyrimidine, are prepared from the following ingredients:

	Grams
N^6-(2-hydroxyethyl)adenine	250
4-hydroxypyrazolo(3,4-d)pyrimidine	25
Starch, USP	20
Talc, USP	15
Calcium stearate	2

The powdered primary ingredients are granulated with a 4% w./v. aqueous solution of methylcellulose, 1,500 cps., USP. To the dried granules is added a mixture of the remainder of the ingredients. The final mixture is compressed into tablets of proper weight.

Example 2: Veterinary Bolus — Ten thousand boluses, each containing 5 grams of N^6-(2-hydroxyethyl)adenine and 2.5 grams of 4-hydroxypyrazolo(3,4-d)pyrimidine, are prepared from the following ingredients:

	Grams
N^6-(2-hydroxyethyl)adenine	50,000
4-hydroxypyrazolo(3,4-d)pyrimidine	25,000
Lactose	250,000

The ingredients are blended and granulated with syrup-starch paste, and q.s. mineral oil is added. The granulation is then dried, lubricated with starch, talc and calcium stearate powders, and compressed with a 1½" x 11/16" die.

Live Virus Immunization Tablets

A process is disclosed by *H. Tint; U.S. Patents 3,608,030, September 21, 1971 and 3,458,621,*

July 29, 1969; both assigned to American Home Products Corporation for preparing an oral dosage-form suitable for the immunization of the intestinal tract with live virus preparations. This comprises mixing live virus with a pharmaceutically acceptable excipient, compressing the resulting mixture into a coherent tablet, compressing a pharmaceutically acceptable excipient about the tablet in an encasing layer to form a coherent shell having a wall thickness of at least 0.03 inches, and finally completely covering the tablet with an enteric coating. This oral dosage-form avoides an undesirable release of live virus in the buccal cavity or the upper intestinal tract, which may result in direct infection in the upper respiratory areas.

The successful production of an oral dosage-form by this process, is surprising in view of the supposition that there would be significant heat destruction of the virus during the double pressing of the tablet form. Surprisingly, this has been found not to occur. The following example illustrates the press-coated tablet dosage-form, and mode of preparation, in greater detail.

Example: Preparation of Lyophilized Virus — 6,000 ml. of a lot of adenovirus type IV, identified as OPL No. 10, were filtered in accordance with standard procedures. The following additives were then mixed into the filtered lot:

Component	Amount
20% skim milk autoclaved at 10 lbs. for 10 minutes	1,500 ml.
5% gelatin USP, autoclaved at 15 lbs. for 15 minutes	120 ml.
5% human serum albumin	72 ml.

The resultant virus-containing mixture was then subjected to lyophilization by the known tray-dried techniques to give 344 grams total weight lyophilized material. Thus, 1 ml. of the original virus fluid was present in each 57.3 mg. of lyophilized material.

Preparation of Dosage-Form Lots — 334.25 grams of lyophilized solids obtained above, and representing 5,833 cc original adenovirus type IV fluid, were blended with a mixture containing 350 grams of microcrystalline cellulose, 4.4 grams magnesium stearate and 885.4 g. lactose.

459 grams of the mixture obtained above were compressed in standard tabletting apparatus to yield 5,100 tablets, each weighing 90 mg. and having cylindrical dimensions equivalent to 0.250 inches diameter and 0.113 inches high. (Each tablet contained 19.1 mg. of lyophilized solid, or the equivalent of one-third cc of the original fluid.)

Of the 5,100 tablets obtained above, 2,500 were subsequently press-coated by compressing about each tablet a mixture comprising 288.7 mg. of lactose, 0.9 mg. magnesium stearate, and 72.4 mg. microcrystalline cellulose to yield 2,500 press-coated (or tablet within a tablet) tablets, each weighing 452 mg. and having cylindrical dimensions equivalent to 0.375 inches in diameter and 0.212 inches high. An enteric coating solution was prepared by admixing a batch having the following composition: 10% cellulose acetate hydrogen phthalate, 0.25% castor oil, 44.75% acetone and 45% absolute ethanol.

The 2,600 nonpress-coated tablets were coated by using conventional pan coating techniques which comprised keeping the tablets dipped in the coating composition for 2 hours at room temperatures. Each tablet was coated with approximately 6 mg. (dried weight) enteric coating material.

The 2,500 press-coated tablets were similarly coated by using the same conventional pan-coating techniques utilized for the nonpress-coated tablets above. Each of these tablets was coated with approximately 25 mg. (dried weight) enteric coating material. Prior to use, the tablets were stored at 5°C.

The superior results in antibodies titer obtained with the use of the press-coated dosage form of this process was demonstrated by a comparison of serologic data as given in the table below. The table gives the neutralizing antibody responses following administration of live type 4 adenovirus contained in enteric-coated tablets.

Type tablet	Initial neutralizing antibody titer	Number men	Number with 4-fold rise in neutralizing antibody [1]: 11 days	Number with 4-fold rise in neutralizing antibody [1]: 15 days	Geometric mean titer: 11 days	Geometric mean titer: 15 days
Press coated	<4	13	13 (100)	13 (100)	19.8	115.4
	4 or>	11	4 (36)	7 (64)	16.0	141.1
Non-press coated	<4	20	10 (50)	14 (70)	10.6	26.2
	4 or >	4	1 (25)	1 (25)	32	>256

[1] Values in parentheses are percentages.

ANTIFUNGAL COMPOSITIONS

Substituted Benzo-1,3-Oxazinediones

K. Hasspacher; U.S. Patent 3,355,453; November 28, 1967; assigned to Boehringer Ingelheim GmbH, Germany has disclosed pharmaceutically active N-substituted benzo-1,3-oxazine-diones-(2,4) of the formula:

(1)

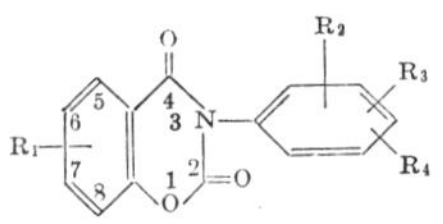

where R_1 and R_2 which may be identical or different are chlorine or bromine, R_3 is hydrogen, chlorine, or bromine, and R_4 is hydrogen, chlorine, bromine or nitro. The compounds covered by Formula (1) above, have useful properties. More particularly, they exhibit excellent antimicrobial and fungicidal activities and are in this respect surprisingly superior to structurally related known compounds.

In addition, the compounds exhibit excellent cestocidal activities, i.e., the ability to kill cestoids (tapeworms). Moreover, they have a very low toxicity toward warm-blooded animals, a very good skin compatibility and an excellent stability against oxidation, heavy metals and exposure to light. Particularly remarkable is their effectiveness against staphylococci and streptococci as well as against fungi, such as Epidermophyton.

Still further, these compounds exhibit molluscacidal and gastropodacidal activities. In this respect they are especially effective against the small water snails which are hosts of Schistosoma parasites, the trematodes which cause schistosomiasis. Structurally related known compounds are for practical purposes completely devoid of this activity. These compounds may be prepared by a variety of methods, one of which can be illustrated by the preparation of 3-(2'-chloro-4'-nitrophenyl)-6-bromobenzo-1,3-oxazinedione-(2,4), MP 253°C., of the formula:

(2)

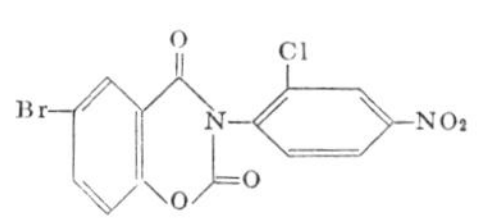

from 5-bromo-salicylic acid, 2-chloro-4-nitroaniline and chloroformic acid methyl ester in the presence of an acid-binding agent at room temperature with cooling.

Example 1: The tablets are compounded from the following ingredients:

	Parts
3-(2'-chloro-4'-nitrophenyl)-6-bromobenzo-1,3-oxazinedione-(2,4)	200.0
Lactose	100.0
Soluble starch	16.7
Glycerin	4.0
Potato starch	65.0
Talcum	12.0
Magnesium stearate	2.3
Total	400.0

The above ingredients are mixed with each other, the mixture is homogeneously blended and is then pressed into tablets weighing 400 mg. each. Each tablet contains 200 mg. of the active ingredient.

Example 2: The tablets prepared in accordance with Example 1 are coated in the customary manner with a thin candy shell consisting essentially of talcum and sugar, and the coated tablets are polished with beeswax.

Griseofulvol

J. Lassman; U.S. Patent 3,392,175; July 9, 1968; assigned to Glaxo Group Limited, England has prepared active derivatives of griseofulvin by metal hydride reduction. These compounds have the formula:

(1)

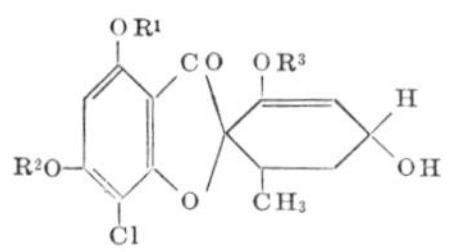

where R^1 and R^2 are alkyl groups, and R^3 is an alkyl or alkenyl group. The compounds of the above formula may also be substituted in the 3'-position, e.g., by halogen atoms, alkyl groups etc.

These compounds have in vivo biological activity akin to that of the corresponding 4'-oxo compounds, but in general possess little antifungal action in vitro. Thus some of the compounds are particularly useful for internal administration to man and animals for the treatment of various fungal conditions, particularly those fungal conditions for which grisofulvin is known to be useful. The compounds of Formula (1), however, possess the advantage of a greater water solubility than the corresponding 4'-keto compounds, thus facilitating the preparation of various pharmaceutical formulations. The compounds are also well absorbed by virtue of their solubility.

Preferred compounds are those in which R^1 is a methyl group, R^2 is a lower alkyl group, i.e., an alkyl group having 1 to 4 carbon atoms, e.g., a methyl, ethyl, propyl or isopropyl group, and R^3 is a lower alkyl group, e.g., methyl. One compound of particular interest is 7-chloro-4'-hydroxy-6'-methyl-4,6,2'-trimethoxygris-2'-en-3-one which has in vivo substantially the antifugal activity of griseofulvin itself but is substantially more water-soluble.

The compounds of Formula (1) are prepared by the reduction of compounds of the formula shown on the next page.

(2) 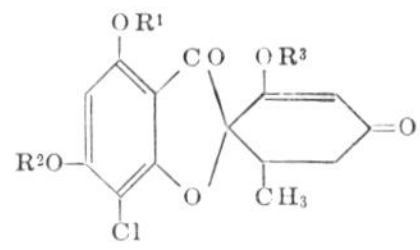

A metal hydride reducing agent is used. Suitable reducing agents are the alkali metal and alkaline earth metal hydrides, the complex alkali metal and alkaline earth metal borohydrides and aluminum hydrides. Each of such substances which are very satisfactory are sodium borohydride, potassium borohydride, calcium borohydride and lithium aluminum hydride.

The reaction is conveniently carried out in the presence of an inert solvent medium, the nature of which will depend upon the reducing agent used. In the case of borohydrides the solvent medium may in general be aqueous or nonaqueous, suitable solvent media being for example, dioxan, aqueous dioxan, tetrahydrofuran, aqueous tetrahydrofuran, methanol, aqueous methanol, ethanol, aqueous ethanol etc. However more reactive hydrides, e.g., the aluminum hydrides, in general require the use of nonhydroxylic solvents, e.g., anhydrous ether, tetrahydrofuran and dioxan. The reaction may be conveniently carried out at temperatures of from 0° to 100°C.

For administration to man or animals the compounds may be presented for oral administration in solid form, for example as tablets, pills, capsules, granules, powders, etc. Oral liquid preparations of aqueous or oily nature may also be prepared, including such flavoring, sweetening, dispersing and/or coloring agents as may be required. The compounds may also be presented in suppository form together with a suppository base.

For injection the compounds may be dissolved or dispersed in a sterile parenterally acceptable liquid which may be of an oily or aqueous nature. For administration to animals the compounds may be admixed with an animal feed or presented as a concentrate (together with an inert diluent) for admixture to an animal feed, or as a drench. The following example shows the preparation of tablets for internal administration.

Example:

	Mg.
Griseofulvol	250
Starch	24
Aerosil compositum	3
Alginic acid	20
Magnesium stearate	3

Griseofulvol (7-chloro-4'-hydroxy-6'-methyl-4,6,2'-trimethoxygris-2'-ene-3-one) is milled and blended with the alginic acid, *Aerosil compositum,* and most of the starch. The remaining starch is used in the form of starch paste as a granulating medium. The tablets may be prepared in the conventional manner, the magnesium stearate being added to the dried granules, before compression, as a lubricating medium.

The tablets may be uncoated, or sugar-coated, or they may be compressed coated, using an inert material, such as lactose or sugar for outer coating. The tablets may also be film coated.

MEDICINES FOR PAIN, FEVER AND INFLAMMATIONS

ASPIRIN TABLETTING

Aluminum Aspirin Films in Sustained Release Tablets

A process developed by *W.E. Gaunt; U.S. Patent 3,350,270; October 31, 1967; assigned to Leeds-Dixon Laboratories, Inc.* uses chloroform or methylene chloride solutions of aluminum acetylsalicylate in the preparation of sustained release tablets. On evaporation of the chloroform or methylene chloride solutions, the aluminum aspirin does not crystallize out but stays in solution during evaporation and is left as a brilliant, shining, glistening continuous film. This film is insoluble in water just as the aluminum aspirin originally used had been water-insoluble and is quite brittle.

The properties of the aluminum aspirin film can be modified by incroporating into the solvent solution of aluminum aspirin a film-forming polymer such as polyvinylpyrrolidone, polyvinyl alcohol, carboxypolymethylene, ethylcellulose, methylcellulose, hydroxyethylcellulose, polyvinyl acetate, etc. Using such polymers in films of aluminum aspirin, modify its water-solubility characteristics and makes the films more continuous and less brittle. It has also been found possible to modify the aluminum aspirin film by incorporating small amounts of surface active agents such as polyoxyethylene sorbitol monooleate and dioctyl sodium sulfosuccinate, etc.

By taking advantage of the unique characteristics of aluminum aspirin it has been found possible to make a stable sustained release aspirin tablet where part of the therapeutic content of the tablet is contributed by the material used in effecting the sustained release property. This process has also been found applicable to the preparation of therapeutic agents such as meprobamate, nicotinic acid, phenacetin, acetaminophenol, the sulfa drugs, aluminum hydroxide and other water-insoluble antacids, tetracycline and the water-insoluble penicillin salts, all being drugs required in high doses. It is also applicable to combinations of drugs such as, for example, meprobamate with pentaerythritol tetranitrate.

Sustained release tablets containing as much as 800 mg. of therapeutic agent, but still being readily swallowed have been made and others containing over 90% of therapeutic material available to the body at a controlled rate have also been prepared.

Example 1: 15 grams of aluminum aspirin is dissolved in 150 ml. of methylene chloride. This solution is added to 415 grams of acetylsalicylic acid, the whole being mixed to a smooth cream. The solvent is removed by air drying and the resulting drug mass screened through a 20 mesh sieve to provide a uniform granulation. After adding 2% of powdered hydrogenated vegetable oils as a lubricant, the granulation is compressed into a tablet having sustained release characteristics but containing 98% of the therapeutically active component. On exposure to simulated gastric fluids for 1 hour and thereafter to simulated intestinal fluids using the USP tablet disintegration equipment, this preparation gave the following release data.

Nature of Exposure	Total Time	Cumulative, Percent Release
Gastric for 1 hour	1	22
Intestinal for 1 hour	2	55
Intestinal for 2 hours	3	73
Intestinal for 3 hours	4	82
Intestinal for 4 hours	5	95

Example 2: 30 grams of aluminum aspirin and 30 grams of polyvinylpyrrolidone are dissolved in 300 ml. of methylene chloride. This solution is added to 300 grams of powdered aspirin and the whole mixed to a smooth, cream-like consistency. The solvent is then removed by evaporation and the dried mass is broken into granules to which magnesium stearate and talc were added for lubrication during subsequent compression of the powdered mixture into tablets, each of which contains 87.5% of therapeutic material which dissolved slowly upon exposure to artificial gastric and intestinal fluids as follows.

Nature of Exposure	Total Time	Cumulative, Percent Release
1 hr. (artificial gastric fluid)	1	21.8
2 hrs. (artificial intestinal fluid)	3	50.0
4 hrs. (artificial intestinal fluid)	5	69.2

Ethylcellulose Encapsulated Aspirin for Sustained Release

A method of making eight hour aspirin tablets has been developed by *W.M. Holliday, M. Berdick, S.A. Bell and G.C. Kiritsis; U.S. Patent 3,488,418; January 6, 1970; and U.S. Patent 3,524,910; August 18, 1970; both assigned to Sterling Drug Inc.* This analgesic preparation comprises ethylcellulose encapsulated particles of acetylsalicylic acid where the relative thickness of the ethylcellulose layer to the acetylsalicylic acid layer is such that substantially all of the encapsulated acetylsalicylic acid will be gradually released into the blood by a diffusion mechanism over a period of four hours upon oral administration, which surprisingly affords eight hours of analgesic relief.

Typical tablets of sustained release aspirin are made from 95% by weight encapsulated aspirin and 5% by weight tabletting excipients such as microcrystalline cellulose, guar gum, talc (USP), cornstarch (USP) employed in such combination and tabletted under such conditions that the thin walls of the encapsulated aspirin granules are not cracked or smashed. The composition must provide a tablet that will withstand storage and shipping without chipping or breaking, but will disintegrate quickly and easily when wetted by saliva or gastric fluid, to give discrete particles of encapsulated aspirin.

Tablets of sustained release aspirin can be made to contain any convenient dose of aspirin. Typical adult tablets contain 5, 7.5 or 10 grains of aspirin, the latter being about the largest that can be easily swallowed by most people. Children's tablets can typically contain 2.5 grains of aspirin.

The encapsulated aspirin used in this method consists of individual granules, or aggregates of particles of aspirin which have been coated with a thin wall of ethylcellulose built to the desired thickness by programmed control of cooling rate and agitation rate and employing in the production of the encapsulated aspirin a weight ratio of aspirin core material to ethylcellulose shell material in the range of 22:1 to 50:1. In forming tablets, conventional tabletting equipment may be used if precautions are taken to avoid breaking the encapsulated particles. One of the most important precautions is to select the optimum particle shape of encapsulated aspirin. Many commercially available forms of aspirin are crystalline rods having a ratio of length to thickness as high as 5:1. Such elongated rods are easily broken when subjected to tabletting pressures. Particles that will effectively resist breaking when subjected to tabletting pressures are those where their greatest dimension is not more than twice their second dimension, and not more than four times their smallest dimension. It is preferable to use particles of aspirin that have been formed from compacted crystals of aspirin, since such particles have less tendency to change their release rate after being subjected to the pressure of the tabletting operation. The ethylcellulose used in encapsulation has an ethoxyl content of 49.1% by weight, and a viscosity of 103 to 108 centipoises as a 5% by weight solution in a 20% alcohol-toluene solvent.

Example 1: This encapsulation makes use of a low molecular weight polyethylene resin having a viscosity in the range of 7,500 to 10,000 cp. at 150°C., such as Epolene C-10 (Tennessee Eastman Chemical Co.) to maintain the wall material solution as a separate phase. The intended ratio of core material to capsule wall material is 35:1. Into a suitable vessel, there are introduced with agitation: 500 lbs. of a 2% by weight solution of the low molecular weight polyethylene resin in cyclohexane; 1,135 ml. of acetic anhydride; 3 lbs. of the ethylcellulose; and 105 lbs. of the acetylsalicylic acid; to form a system which is heated to 80°C. and agitated sufficiently to produce minute liquid entities of ethylcellulose-cyclohexane solution dispersed among particles of aspirin.

Cooling and agitation are carried on, the individually coated aspirin particles are recovered and washed for purification, and then dried. The capsules produced in this example are substantially 96.4% aspirin, and release substantially 61% of their aspirin content when agitated in simulated gastric fluid at 37°C. for 1 hour, and may be used for preparing dosage forms.

Example 2: The following composition was mixed, using conventional pharmaceutical processing equipment.

	Weight		
	Batch (kg.)	Per tablet (mg.)	Percent
Encapsulated aspirin of Ex. 1 (96.4% acetylsalicylic acid)	25.896	664	93.13
Avicel (microcrystalline cellulose)	1.365	35	4.91
Cornstarch	0.390	10	1.40
Guar Gum	0.156	4	0.56
Total	27.807	713	100.00

This mixture was tabletted on a conventional pharmaceutical rotary tabletting machine, using capsule shaped punches (length 0.627 in., width 0.286 in.) yielding tablets having a thickness of substantially 0.259 in., a weight of substantially 713 mg., a hardness of substantially 12.5 kg. by a Stokes tablet hardness tester, and a disintegration time of less than 45 seconds in distilled water at 37°C. The tablets assayed 10.0 grains acetylsalicylic acid per tablet, contained 0.05% salicylic acid, and released substantially 68% of their aspirin when agitated in simulated gastric fluid at 37°C. for 1 hour.

Dual Release Aspirin Tablets

A dual release aspirin of 8 to 12 hours duration has been prepared by *E.H. Gans and H.M. Apelian; U.S. Patent 3,388,041; June 11, 1968; assigned to Richardson-Merrell Inc.* In this process a mixture of hydroxypropylmethylcellulose and ethylcellulose in an organic solvent is used as the binder for the sustained release layer of the tablet. A standard aspirin formulation is used for the rapid release layer. The advantages shown by the sustained release portion on the two-ply aspirin tablet laminate are achieved by the use of a cellulosic ether derivative which is hydrophilic and organic solvent-soluble, in combination with a cellulosic ether derivative which is hydrophobic and organic solvent-soluble. A suitable hydrophilic organic solvent-soluble cellulosic ether derivative is the propylene glycol ether of methylcellulose. Typical is the commercial blend of hydroxypropylmethylcellulose NF (The Dow Chemical Company). This material is characterized as containing both methoxy and propylene glycol ether groups substituted on the anhydroglucose units of the basic repeating cellulosic structure. This derivative is produced by the reactions of alkali cellulose first with methyl chloride, then with propylene oxide. Suitable hydrophobic organic solvent-soluble cellulosic ether derivative are the thermoplastic ethyl ethers of cellulose which result from the interaction of ethyl chloride with alkali cellulose. Ethylcellulose is produced commercially under the trade name Ethocel.

In a preferred two-ply tablet construction, the total tablet weight will range between 650 and 720 mg. In the sustained release layer of the tablet, between 5 and 6 grams of aspirin are preferred and between 1.75 and 14 mg. total weight of the two cellulosic derivatives. In the rapid release layer of the tablet, between 4.4 and 4.8 grains of aspirin are preferred and between 2.0 and 45 mg. of starch or other rapid release excipient. If desired, a dye may be included in either of the two layers in order to advertise the two-layer construction of the tablet.

Example: The following is the preparation of sustained release granulation for 200,000 tablets. In preparing the tablet composition, 6 liters of SD alcohol is weighed into a suitable size container equipped with a high speed, explosion proof propeller stirrer. Hydroxypropylmethylcellulose (0.352 kg.) and ethylcellulose (0.352 kg.) are mixed together. This excipient combination is slowly added to the alcohol with high speed stirring and mixed for 30 minutes to obtain a uniform suspension free of lumps. Additional alcohol is added to the suspension until the total weight of the suspension is 5.7 kg. The solution, when dried, forms a clear film.

The aspirin (70 kg.) is placed in a granulator and granulation is accomplished with the granulating solution prepared above. The wet granulation is passed through an oscillating granulator with a No. 4 screen. The granulation is spread on trays and dried until the volatile content is less than 1.0%. The granulation is then passed through a No. 16 screen in the oscillating granulator and talc (0.70 kg.) is added and blended in.

The preparation of rapid release granulation for 200,000 tablets is as follows. The aspirin (60 kg.), starch (5.76 kg.), and FD&C No. 3 (40 grams) are placed in a mixer and passed through a Fitzpatrick mill using impact forward, No. 00 screen and medium speed. This powder mixture is transferred to a slugging press and the resulting slugs are reduced to small granules by passage through an oscillating granulator with a No. 16 mesh screen.

A layer press is used to produce tablets at the rate of several hundred per minute or as high as several thousand per minute depending on which of the layer-press machines is employed. The dies are filled with sustained release layer material to a weight of 357 mg. and the layer-tamping compression pressure is adjusted so that a layer is compressed to a smooth upper surface.

The dies containing the sustained release layers are filled with rapid release granulation to form a rapid release layer weight of 329 mg. The layers are compressed together to obtain good bonding and sharp demarcation between the layers and to give a fracture pressure of 8 to 12 kg. (Stokes Tester). For preparation of tablets consisting solely of the sustained release granulation, the usual tablet production method is employed.

Tablets, when prepared by the procedure just described, will, when swallowed, release approximately the normal dose of 5 grains of aspirin almost immediately. The sustained release portion of the tablet does not disintegrate immediately because of the protective action of the cellulosic derivatives which form a film or coating over the aspirin particles. This coating, being composed of hydrophilic and hydrophobic materials, will slowly disintegrate and release the aspirin at a rate slower than that at which the aspirin would normally be dissolved. As a result of the protective action of the cellulosic derivatives, the aspirin in this part of the tablet is released at a rate to maintain therapeutic levels of the salicylate in the blood stream over a period of 8 to 12 hours.

Milk Buffered Aspirin

Individuals having weak stomachs or an ulcer condition are advised against taking aspirin, since aspirin acts as an irritant and often aggravates the condition. When aspirin has been combined with various buffering agents, present compounds of this class do not alleviate or minimize stomach bleeding.

A.H. Lamb; U.S. Patent 3,608,064; September 21, 1971 has developed a formulation where aspirin is mixed with powdered milk. When first introduced into the stomach, the milk provides a natural alkaline barrier which minimizes the possible effects of aspirin and, also, provides nutritional value.

The term "powdered milk" refers to milk from which substantially all water has been removed, the remaining milk solids being either a fine powder or small crystals having a moisture content of not more than 5%. The term "powdered aspirin" includes aspirin in granular or powder form. In one method, a substantially homogenous mixture is formed of powdered aspirin and powdered milk and the mixture is placed into conventional gelatin capsules. Preferably, the powdered milk comprises at least 50% of the mixture.

In another method the above mixture is formed into a tablet in a conventional tablet-making machine. For example, as shown in Figure 10.1a, an appropriate quantity of the mixture **10** is placed into a mold **11** and compressed by means of a plunger **12** to produce a generally disc-like tablet. A pressure of the order of 2 to 5 tons/square inch applied to the plunger results in a tablet having a crush strength of 10 to 20 psi, the higher crush strength corresponding to the higher pressure. By applying such pressure in the formation of the tablet, the tablet has a thin, smooth, shiny outer surface, presenting a semiglazed appearance. This surface, which may be likened to a mild case hardening, is of such homogeneity and density as to constitute an envelope forming an effective moisture barrier to prevent tablet deterioration prior to its consumption.

Referring to Figure 10.1a, instead of loading the mold with a mixture of granular aspirin and powdered milk, a lower layer of powdered milk is formed in the mold, then a layer of granular aspirin and then a top layer of powdered milk. The resulting tablet will have a cross-sectional appearance as shown in Figure 10.1b, that is, a layer of compressed aspirin **14** sandwiched between the layers **15** and **16** of compressed powdered milk.

Another form of the tablet can be made where a previously compressed tablet of aspirin is encased within a shell of compressed, powdered milk. To form such tablet the mold has a larger cross-sectional diameter than the compressed aspirin tablet. A layer of powdered milk is first placed into the mold. The aspirin tablet then is centered upon such layer, after which the mold is filled to an appropriate level with the powdered milk.

FIGURE 10.1: MILK BUFFERED ASPIRIN TABLETS

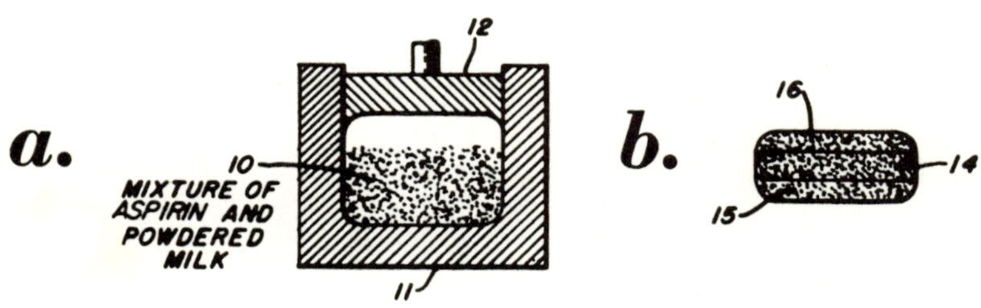

Source: A.H. Lamb; U.S. Patent 3,608,064; September 21, 1971

Aspirin-Pectin Compositions

Sustained release aspirin formulations which minimize the gastrointestinal distress caused by aspirin have been prepared by *W.A. Bender; U.S. Patent 3,485,920; December 23, 1969; assigned to General Foods Corporation.* This comprises an analgesic composition containing aspirin and pectin where the aspirin/pectin ratio may be from 1 to 2 to 1 to 15, by weight. The composition may be administered to warm blooded animals in palatable, controlled dosage form to afford, for example, temporary relief of minor aches and pains resulting from the common cold or flu.

Any one of various pectins and mixtures, may be used in these compositions. As previously mentioned, the amount of pectin, on a weight basis, may range from 15 to 1 to 2 to 1 parts of aspirin. Certain pectins such as citrus and apple pectins have been reported by D.W. Wooley of Rockefeller Institute and associates in 1947 to 1949 to have antiviral activity and such pectins are quite suitable in the aspirin-pectin composition. Preferably, a dispersible pectin is used when the aspirin-pectin composition is to be dissolved in water as a means of administering the composition to host warm blooded animals, including humans.

The aspirin-pectin composition may be prepared as troches or lozenges. In such form, the composition may be used locally for temporary relief of minor sore throat pain due to colds or the flu. The aspirin and pectin may be combined and further reduced to a powder, admixed with other ingredients and then compressed into troches having the desired size and shape on a tablet press. Lozenges may be prepared by admixing aspirin and pectin with a liquid binder such as corn syrup, sugar syrup, honey or the like, together with flavor, color, edible acid, additional sweetener, and similar conventional lozenge ingredients and then cast.

The size and shape of the troches and lozenges are dependent upon the time of release intended for the aspirin and pectin components. Thus, local therapy as well as therapy by sustained release thereby providing absorption with a minimum amount of gastrointestinal distress may be achieved by using the aspirin-pectin composition in such form.

Example: An aspirin-pectin throat lozenge is prepared by blending and later casting the following.

Ingredients	Grams/Lozenge	Percentage
Sugar, granulated	1.8585	74.34
Corn syrup (81.1%)	0.3820	15.28
Pectin	0.1500	6.00
Aspirin, USP (1.25 grains)	0.0810	3.24
Citric acid	0.0240	0.96
Flavor, lemon	0.0040	0.16
Color, FD&C Yellow #5	0.0005	0.02
	2.5000	100.00

The lozenge as formulated may be used as needed by adult humans for temporary relief of minor sore throat due to colds by allowing the lozenge to dissolve slowly in the mouth. For children (ages 6 to 12), one lozenge as needed for temporary relief of minor sore throat due to colds may be taken and repeated every half hour as needed up to 10 lozenges per day.

OTHER ANALGESIC COMPOUNDS

Tertiary Aniline Analgesics

H. Zellner; U.S. Patent 3,300,532; January 24, 1967; assigned to Donau-Pharmazie GmbH, Austria has prepared compounds of the following Formula (1) and Formula (2) which have valuable pharmaceutical properties

(1) 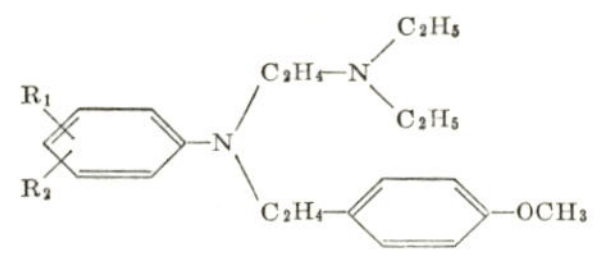

where R_1 and R_2 are hydrogen and/or methoxy, at least one being methoxy.

(2) 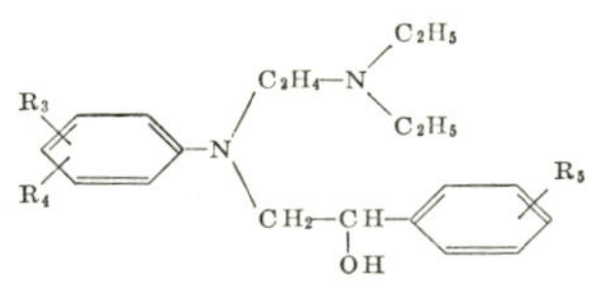

In the above Formula (2), R_3 and R_4 are hydrogen, halogen, especially chlorine, and/or methoxy, while R_5 is hydrogen or methoxy. These compounds are prepared by a reduction of the corresponding anilide. For example, N-(β-diethylaminoethyl)-N-[β-(p-methoxyphenyl)ethyl]-p-anisidine is obtained by the reduction of N-(β-diethylaminoethyl)-N-(p-methoxyphenylacetyl)-p-methoxyaniline with lithium aluminum hydride.

Compounds of Formula (1) have an analgesic effect without any inhibiting effect upon respiration and the autonomic nervous system while compounds of Formula (2) also exhibit local anesthetic activity and retard blood coagulation. The preferred and most effective compounds according to Formula (1) are N-(β-diethylaminoethyl)-N-[β-(p-methoxyphenyl)ethyl]-p-anisidine and N-(β-diethylaminoethyl)-N-[β-(p-methoxyphenyl)ethyl]-m-anisidine. The preferred and most effective compound according to Formula (2) is N-(β-diethylaminoethyl)-N-(β-hydroxy-β-phenylethyl)-2,5-dichloroaniline.

These tertiary anilines and their acid addition salts can be administered orally, parenterally or in the form of suppositories. The compounds may also be administered in powder form, preferably enclosed in gelatin capsules. Oral administration in liquid form, such as in the form of emulsions, suspensions, sirups and the like is also possible. The following examples illustrate the pharmaceutical preparations.

Example 1: Tablets – The following two ingredients are intimately mixed with each other:

	Grams
N-(β-diethylaminoethyl)-N-[β-(p-methoxyphenyl)ethyl]-p-anisidine	75
Colloidal silica (Aerosil)	56

After mixing, the following substances are added:

	Grams
Cornstarch	99
Milk sugar	120
Magnesium stearate	2
Gelatin	1.5
Cocoa butter	1.5

The resulting mixture is compressed to 1,000 tablets, each tablet weighing about 355 mg. and containing about 75 mg. of the analgesic tertiary aniline compound.

Example 2: Dragées – The tablets obtained according to Example 1 are sugar coated by rotating in a coating pan with sugar solution. Sugar-coating is repeated until each dragée has attained a weight of about 500 mg.

Indenylacetic Acid Esters

A series of substituted acyloxyalkyl indenylacetates have been disclosed by *K. Peister, M. Sletzinger and D.F. Hinkley; U.S. Patent 3,720,774; March 13, 1973; assigned to Merck & Co., Inc.* These compounds are useful as in vivo cleavable, long-lasting antiinflammatory and analgesic agents. Also included are processes for preparing these compounds and the tabletting of these compounds. Specifically these compounds have the following formula:

(1)

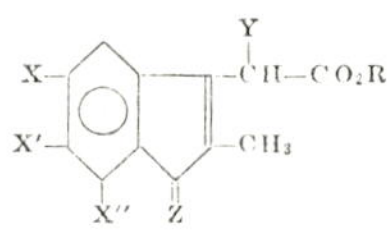

where X is lower alkoxy or halo; X' is hydrogen or halo; X" is hydrogen or halo; Y is hydrogen or lower alkyl; Z is p-methylsulfinylbenzylidenyl; and R is an acyloxyalkyl function of the formula

$$\begin{array}{l}-CH-O-B \\ \;\;\,| \\ \;\;\,A\end{array}$$

where A is hydrogen, lower alkyl, halo lower alkyl, or aryl; and B is an acyl group. In preferred compounds, X is halo, X' is hydrogen, Y is hydrogen, Z is p-methylsulfinylbenzylidenyl; A is hydrogen or lower alkyl; and B is acetyl, pivaloyl or benzoyl.

The compounds of Formula (1) can be used to treat inflammation by reducing inflammation and relieving pain in such diseases as rheumatoid arthritis, osteoarthritis, gout, infectious arthritis and rheumatic fever. These compounds are particularly useful because they are cleavable in vivo over an extended period of time and their action is lasting.

Several forms of these therapeutic compositions can be used. For example, if a solid carrier is used, the compositions may take the form of tablets, capsules, powders, troches or lozenges, prepared by standard pharmaceutical techniques. If a liquid carrier is used, the preparation may be in the form of a soft gelatin capsule, a syrup, an aqueous solution or a liquid suspension.

Suppositories may be prepared in a conventional manner by mixing the compounds with a suitable nonirritating excipient which is solid at room temperature, but liquid at the rectal temperature. Gels and lotions for topical application may be prepared in conventional manners. Advantageously, the compositions will contain the active ingredient in an amount of 0.1 to 50 mg. per kilogram body weight per day (5 mg. to 3.5 grams per patient per day), preferably from 1 to 15 mg./kg. body weight per day (50 mg. to 1 gram per patient per day).

The compounds of Formula (1) may be prepared by several methods. For example, the sodium salt of the preferred indenylacetic acids may be reacted with the desired acyloxyalkyl halide. Alternatively, the free acid or the silver salt may be reacted with p-formaldehyde to produce the chloromethyl derivative of the indenylacetic acid. This compound is then reacted with an acid having the desired acyl group. The following examples show preparation of tablets from these active ingredients.

Example 1: A mixture of 250 parts of pivaloyloxymethyl 6-fluoro-5-methoxy-2-methyl-1-(p-methylsulfinylbenzylidene)-3-indenyl acetate and 25 parts of lactose is granulated with suitable water and to this is added 100 parts of maize starch. The mass is passed through a 16 mesh screen. The granules are dried below 60°C. The dry granules are passed through a 16 mesh screen and mixed with 3.8 parts of magnesium stearate. They are then compressed into tablets suitable for oral administration as an anti-inflammatory.

Example 2: A mixture of 250 parts of benzoyloxymethyl 5-fluoro-2-methyl-1-(p-methylsulfinylbenzylidene)-3-indenyl acetate, 200 parts of maize starch and 30 parts of alginic acid is mixed with a sufficient quantity of a 10% aqueous paste of maize starch and granulated. The granules are dried in a current of warm air and the dry granules are then passed through a 16 mesh screen, mixed with 6 parts of magnesium stearate and compressed into tablet form to obtain tablets suitable for oral administration.

ANTIPYRETIC AND COLD TABLETS

Dihydropyridobenzodiazepines

G. Schmidt; U.S. Patent 3,321,473; May 23, 1967; assigned to Boehringer Ingelheim GmbH, Germany has prepared substitution products of 5,6-dihydro-11H-pyrido[2,3-b] [1,4] benzodiazepines and their acid addition salts. These compounds have the formula

(1)

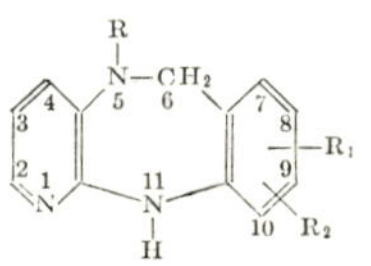

where R is hydrogen, or a straight or branched alkyl which may have a halogen, hydroxyl, lower alkoxy or basic substituent of the formula $-NR_3R_4$ where R_3 and R_4, which may be identical or different are lower alkyl or, together with the adjacent nitrogen atom, form a basic heterocyclic ring attached thereto, or a cycloalkyl or an aralkyl whose aromatic moiety may have one or more halogen, lower alkyl or lower alkoxy substituents attached, and R_1 and R_2, which may be identical or different are hydrogen or halogen, lower alkyl or lower alkoxy substituents, and their nontoxic pharmacologically acceptable acid addition salts. These compounds may be prepared by reducing a 5,6-dihydro-6-oxo-11H-pyrido-[2,3-b] [1,4] benzodiazepine of the formula

(2)

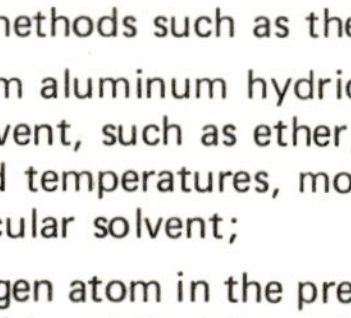

where R, R_1 and R_2 have the same meanings as in Formula (1). The reduction may be accomplished by a number of known methods such as the following.

(a) Reduction with lithium aluminum hydride in the presence of an inert, anhydrous organic solvent, such as ether, tetrahydrofuran or dioxane, at moderately elevated temperatures, most advantageously at the boiling point of the particular solvent;

(b) Reduction with hydrogen atom in the presence of a catalyst, especially a copper-chromium oxide catalyst, in an inert organic solvent, such as dioxane, at a temperature between 100° and 250°C. and a pressure between 100 and 250 atm. gauge; or

(c) Reduction with an alkali metal in an absolute lower alkanol, especially ethanol, by the Bouveault-Blanc method [*Compt. Rend.* 136, 1676 (1903)].

The compounds of Formula (1) and their nontoxic acid addition salts exhibit antitussive, antipyretic, antiphlogistic, and bronchial secretion-promoting activities in animals. Moreover, those compounds of the Formula (1) where R is a basic substituent and their nontoxic acid addition salts also exhibit antihistaminic activities and antagonize the sedative activity of reserpine in animals.

For therapeutic purposes these compounds are administered perorally or parenterally as active ingredients in dosage units consisting essentially of an inert, physiologically compatible carrier and one dosage unit of the active ingredient, such as tablets, coated pills, syrups, solutions, suspensions, suppositories, hypodermic solutions, and the like. One dosage unit of the compounds is from 30 to 100 mg., preferably 50 mg. The following example illustrates tablet formation. The parts are by weight unless otherwise specified.

Example: Coated Pills – The pill core composition is compounded from the following ingredients.

	Parts by Weight
5,8-dimethyl-5,6-dihydro-11H-pyrido[2,3-b]-[1,4]-benzodiazepine hydrochloride	50.0
Secondary calcium phosphate	130.0
Cornstarch	26.0
Polyvinylpyrrolidone	10.0
Tartaric acid	2.0
Talcum	10.0
Magnesium stearate	2.0
	230.0

The compounding procedure follows. The pyridobenzodiazepine is thoroughly mixed with the calcium phosphate and the cornstarch, the mixture moistened with an aqueous 20% solution of the polyvinylpyrrolidone which also has the tartaric acid dissolved therein, and the moist mass granulated by passing it through a 1.5 mm. mesh screen. The granulate is dried at 45°C., again passed through the screen and is then mixed with the talcum and the magnesium stearate.

The mixture is subsequently pressed into 230 mg. pill cores, which are coated with a thin shell consisting essentially of sugar and talcum. The coated pills are finally polished with beeswax. Each pill core weighs approximately 300 mg. and contains 50 mg. of the active ingredient.

Aminohalobenzylamines

Compounds having useful pharmacodynamic properties have been prepared by *J. Keck; U.S. Patent 3,336,308; August 15, 1967; assigned to Boehringer Ingelheim GmbH, Germany.* More particularly, they exhibit an excellent secretolytic activity (increase bronchial secretions) with extremely low toxicity and cough-suppressing, monoaminooxidase-inhibiting and antipyretic activities. These compounds are aminohalobenzylamines having formulas

(1)

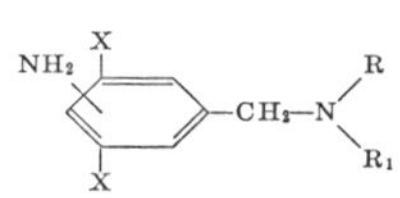

(2)

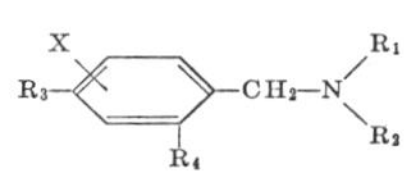

where X is chlorine or bromine, R is hydrogen, lower alkyl, hydroxy lower alkyl, halo lower alkyl, lower alkenyl, cycloalkyl, aralkyl or aryl; R_1 and R_2 are lower alkyl, lower alkenyl, cycloalkyl, aralkyl, hydroxy lower alkyl, halo lower alkyl, pyridyl lower alkyl, or aryl; and R and R_1, and R_1 and R_2 when taken together with the nitrogen atom form a heterocyclic such as pyrrolidino, piperidino, piperazino, hexamethylene imino, and R_1 and R_2 together with the nitrogen atom also form a heterocyclic selected from lower alkyl-morpholino and morpholino, and R_3 and R_4 are different and are hydrogen, $-NH_2$, or their nontoxic pharmacologically acceptable acid addition salts. These compounds may be prepared by methods which are well-known for the synthesis of other halogenated amino benzylamines such as:

(a) clorination or bromination of aminobenzylamines;

(b) reaction of halonitrobenzylamines;

(c) reaction of dihalodiacylaminobenzyl halides with amines; or

(d) reduction of aminohalobenzamides.

The dosage unit of these compounds is from 1 to 100 mg. depending upon the desired activity. Thus, the effective individual dose for increasing bronchial secretion is from 0.5 to 10 mg., preferably 2 to 4.0 mg., while the effective antitussive dose is 10 to 100 mg., preferably 25 to 50 mg. The compounds can be administered perorally or parenterally in the form of tablets, coated pills, syrups, aerosols, solutions, suspensions, suppositories, etc. The following examples show tablet formation from a compound of Formula (1).

Example 1: Tablets – The tablets are compounded from the following ingredients.

	Parts by Weight
N-(2-amino-3,5-dibromobenzyl)-N-methyl-cyclohexylamine hydrochloride	2.0
Lactose	60.0
Potato starch, dry	43.0
Soluble starch	4.0
Magnesium stearate	1.0
	110.0

The compounding procedure is as follows. The active ingredient and the lactose are thoroughly blended and mixed with the potato starch, and this mixture is granulated by moistening it with an aqueous 20% solution of the soluble starch, and passing the moistened mixture through a 1 mm. mesh screen. The moist granulate is then dried at 40°C., again passed through the screen and finally mixed with the magnesium stearate. The resulting mixture is then pressed into tablets weighing 110 mg. each.

Example 2: Coated Pills – The tablets obtained in the preceding example are provided with a thin shell consisting essentially of sugar and talcum in the customary manner. The coated pills thus obtained are then polished with beeswax. Each coated pill weighs about 170 mg. and contains 4.0 mg. of the active ingredient.

Chewable Cold Tablets

Chewable tablets which have no medicinal aftertaste have been developed by *B. Idson and M.S. Weiss; U.S. Patent 3,567,819; March 2, 1971; assigned to Hoffmann-La Roche Inc.* These contain aspirin (acetylsalicylic acid) as the analgesic-antipyretic and the decongestant, phenylpropanolamine hydrochloride (2-amino-1-phenyl-1-propanol hydrochloride).

In addition to the problems of taste and stability inherent in compounding preparations containing aspirin, the choice of phenylpropanolamine hydrochloride as the decongestant created a problem of chemical incompatibility. Also, the taste of phenylpropanolamine hydrochloride added to that of aspirin produces an extremely bitter product with an unpleasant aftertaste. These problems are resolved by the combination of using unique flavor-masking techniques and the incorporation of the active ingredients into a three-layered tablet which effectively negates the problem of chemical incompatibility of aspirin and phenylpropanolamine hydrochloride as each is incorporated in a separate layer of the tablet and these layers are separated by a placebo layer. The problem of the objectionable taste of the phenylpropanolamine hydrochloride is resolved by reacting it with a complex magnesium aluminum silicate compound as, for example, a product known as Veegum.

Example: One thousand trilayered chewable tablets are prepared in the following manner.

Layer 1 – 6.31 grams of phenylpropanolamine hydrochloride were dissolved with gentle heat (45° to 50°C.) in a mixture of 24.0 ml. isopropyl alcohol and 6.0 ml. distilled water. After solution, 0.30 ml. of blended fruit liquid flavoring were blended into the solution. 35.0 grams of Veegum F were added, mixed in a suitable mixer and dried on paper lined trays for 2 hours at 43°C. The resulting granules were then mixed in a suitable mixer for 10 minutes at medium speed with 67.9 grams of an excipient mixture of sucrose, mannitol and artificial sweeteners, 13.0 grams of pregelatinized cornstarch, 6.0 grams of starch (corn) and 0.22 gram FD&C Red No. 3 Lake.

The mixture was then passed through a Fitzpatrick Comminuting Machine utilizing a No. 1 screen, knives forward. The granules were granulated with distilled water until they became suitably wet. The wet granules were then dried overnight at 43°C. The dry granules were mixed with 2.0 grams talc, 4.0 grams fully hydrogenated cottonseed oil and 14.0 grams spray dried fruit flavors and passed through a Fitzpatrick Comminuting Machine at medium speed utilizing a No. 1B screen. The resulting granules were blended until homogeneous.

Layer 2 – 24.0 grams of confectionary grade sucrose, 5.0 grams of pregelatinized cornstarch, 40.5 grams of mannitol and 7.0 grams of starch (corn) were combined in a mixer and wet granulated with distilled water. The wet granules were passed through a Fitzpatrick Comminuting Machine, at medium speed and utilizing a No. 6 screen, knives forward. The granules were then dried at 43°C. for 12 hours. The dry granules were combined with 2.0 grams fully hydrogenated cottonseed oil and a sufficient amount of powdered anise flavor and passed through a Fitzpatrick Comminuting Machine, running at medium speed, utilizing a No. 1B screen with knives forward. The resultant granules were blended in a suitable mixer until homogeneous and stored in polyethylene bags until the tablets were compressed.

Layer 3 – 81.0 grams of aspirin as an aspirin-cornstarch granulation and 10.0 grams talc were blended in a suitable blender until homogeneous. The resultant granules were stored in polyethylene bags until the tablets were compressed.

Formation of Tablets – A Manesty Layer Press equipped with 11/32 inch flat faced beveled edge punches was used to form the layers which were in turn compressed to form the finished tablets. The approximate weight of a single tablet is 343 mg. being made up of 150 milligrams of Layer 1; 80 mg. of Layer 2; and 113 mg. of Layer 3. The finished tablets contain approximately 1.25 grains (81 mg.) aspirin and 6.25 mg. phenylpropanolamine hydrochloride.

ANTI-INFLAMMATORY PREPARATIONS

Enzyme-Adrenal Glucocorticoid Blends

The use of steroids to produce systemic anti-inflammatory effects has been very beneficial, but at the same time has been accompanied by side effects which often are very serious. By way of example, the oral use of cortico steroids for absorption from the digestive tract to produce systemic anti-inflammatory effects has resulted in an insufficiency of adrenal output at times of stress, such as, surgery, etc., and has been followed by serious consequences. If it were possible to reduce the level of steroids so as to avoid side effects while at the same time maintaining the desired anti-inflammatory, etc., effects, a substantial advance would be made.

H.J. Antonides; U.S. Patent 3,324,002; June 6, 1967; assigned to Armour Pharmaceutical

Company has found that the use of enzymes in combination with steroids enables the steroids to be employed at a reduced level, while the combined anti-inflammatory effect is maintained at the desired level and with the substantial absence of side effects. By way of illustration, an oral preparation in tablet form comprising 1.25 mg. of prednisolone and an enzyme having a proteolytic activity of 50,000 AU, and administered at a dosage of two tablets four times daily (10 mg. prednisolone total daily), was found to be the equivalent of 20 to 30 mg. of prednisolone per day in anti-inflammatory effect.

Any anti-inflammatory enzyme material may be employed, such as those derived from animal, plant and bacterial sources. Examples of the enzymes of animal origin are the pancreatic enzymes, including trypsin, chymotrypsin, etc., collagenase, etc. Examples of enzymes derived from plants are papain, bromelin and ficin. Proteases are examples of suitable enzymes from both animal and plant origin. Examples of bacterial enzymes are streptokinase, streptodornase, etc. Trypsin, chymotrypsin or combinations thereof are preferred.

Anti-inflammatory steroid substances, their qualities, characteristics, uses and dosages are well-known. Examples of such are cortisone, hydrocortisone, hydrocortamate, prednisone, prednisolone, triamcinolone, dexamethasone, methyl prednisolone, paramethasone, betamethasone and fluorocortisone.

Since the use of these steroids is well-known and the dosages employed on a daily basis are well understood, it will be sufficient to indicate ranges of potencies of the enzyme component of the preparation for use with such common dosages. As previously indicated, it is possible when using this combination to obtain the same response while using a significantly reduced amount of steroid. The range of potencies of the enzyme component is not critical and may vary widely.

For example, potencies may vary from 1,000 to 250,000 AU/tablet or other dose of the preparation consisting of the steroid and the enzyme. Preferably, the range of potencies of the enzyme component is from 10,000 to 100,000 AU. The term "AU" or "Armour Unit" is obtained by a modification of the Anson hemoglobin method. One Armour Unit of proteolytic activity is that amount which, upon incubation with the hemoglobin substrate, as directed in the method of assay, will release a quantity of phenolic substances which when reacted with Folin-Ciocalteau Phenol Reagent, will result in the formation of a colored solution of equal intensity to that produced from the reaction of 1 mcg. of tyrosine with Folin-Ciocalteau Phenol Reagent.

The enzyme and steroid may be prepared as a tablet, and preferably with a base or carrier material. The carrier may comprise a readily soluble base consisting of, for example, magnesium stearate, sorbitol and mannitol. Other carriers or bases may consist of lactose and magnesium stearate, lactose and polyethylene glycol, or other suitable base material employed for tablet components, such as, dicalcium phosphate, starch, sugar, acacia, gelatin, etc.

Example 1: Enteric coated compressed tablets were prepared for oral administration using conventional techniques, and had the following composition.

Trypsin and/or chymotrypsin	50,000 AU
Prednisolone	1.25 mg.
Magnesium stearate	1.0 mg.
Polyethylene glycol 4000	5.0 mg.
Sorbitol	50.0 mg.
Mannitol (q.s.)	120.0 mg.
Enteric coating, e.g., cellulose acetate phthalate	

Example 2: Enteric compressed tablets were prepared for oral administration using known techniques and had the following composition.

Gastric resistant trypsin and/or chymotrypsin granules	50,000 AU
Prednisolone	1.25 mg.

(continued)

Magnesium stearate	2.0 mg.
Lactose, to make	200.0 mg.

The following table summarizes clinical results with respect to anti-inflammatory activity results obtained from oral administration of the formulation of Example 1 to 128 patients.

Diagnosis	Number Patients	Results							
		Excellent	Percent	Good	Percent	Fair	Percent	Poor	Percent
Abscess	1	1	100	0	......	0	......	0	......
Arthritis, osteo	23	19	83	4	17	0	......	0	......
Arthritis, traumatic	9	3	33	4	44	1	11	1	11
Asthma	9	6	67	3	33	0	......	0	......
Bursitis	19	13	68	6	32	0	......	0	......
Cellulitis	14	14	100	0	......	0	......	0	......
Eczema	15	12	80	3	20	0	......	0	......
Ophthalmology	12	5	42	5	42	1	8	1	8
Thrombophlebitis	4	2	50	2	50	0	......	0	......
Trauma and Contusion	16	12	75	4	25	0	......	0	......
Ulcerative Colitis	5	4	80	1	20	0	......	0	......
Urticaria	1	1	100	0	......	0	......	0	......
Totals	128	92	72	32	25	2	1.5	2	1.5

5H-Dibenz[b,f] Azepine-4-Carboxylic Acid Derivatives

5H-dibenz[b,f] azepine-4-carboxylic acids, the 10,11-dihydro and other substituted derivatives have been developed by *N. Gruenfeld; U.S. Patent 3,624,072; November 30, 1971; assigned to Geigy Chemical Corporation* as anti-inflammatory agents. They can be prepared among other ways, through treatment of the appropriate 4,5-oxalyl-5H-dibenz[b,f] azepine with aqueous base followed by hydrogen peroxide. Esterification, N-acylation and/or amidation can optionally follow. Typical examples are 3-methoxy-10,11-dihydro-5H-dibenz[b,f] azepine-4-carboxylic acid and 3,7-dichloro-5H-dibenz[b,f] azepine-4-carboxylic acid. These compounds can be shown by the following formula

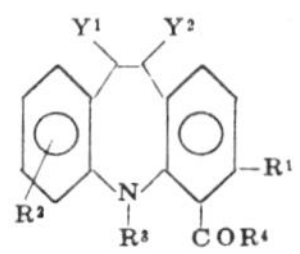

where R^1 is hydrogen, methoxy or chloro; R^2 is hydrogen, chloro or methyl; R^3 is hydrogen, (lower)alkanoyl, benzoyl or chlorobenzoyl; R^4 is hydroxy, amino, (lower)alkoxy, or di(lower)alkylamino(lower)alkoxy; and Y^1 and Y^2 taken separately are each hydrogen or taken together are a carbon-carbon bond. The nontoxic pharmaceutically acceptable alkali metal, alkaline earth metal and organic amine salts of the compounds of Formula (1) where R^4 is hydroxy and to the pharmaceutically acceptable acid addition salts of the compounds of Formula (1) where R^4 is di(lower)alkylamino(lower)alkoxy are also included in the process.

These compounds are anti-inflammatory agents and can be shown to demonstrate activity in classical anti-inflammatory laboratory models such as the carrageenin test, the turbidity test, the Whitehouse screen and the established adjuvant arthritis assay. The compounds also exhibit antipyretic and analgesic properties.

The 5H-dibenz[b,f] azepine derivatives are administered parenterally or orally to achieve an anti-inflammatory effect, in any of the usual pharmaceutical forms. These include solid and liquid unit oral dosage forms such as tablets, capsules, powders, suspensions, solutions, syrups and the like, including sustained release preparations, and fluid injectable forms such as sterile solutions and suspensions. Tablets are made by preparing a powder mixture, granulating or slugging, adding a lubricant and disintegrant and pressing into tablets.

A powder mixture is prepared by mixing the compound, suitably comminuted, with a diluent or base such as starch, sucrose, kaolin, dicalcium phosphate and the like. The powder mixture can be granulated by wetting with a binder such as syrup, starch paste, acacia mucilage or solutions of cellulosic or polymeric materials and forcing through a screen. As an alternative to granulating, the powder mixture can be run through the tablet machine and the resulting imperfectly formed slugs broken into granules. The granules can be lubricated to prevent sticking to the tablet-forming dies by means of the addition of stearic acid, a stearate salt, talc or mineral oil.

The lubricated mixture is then compressed into tablets. The medicaments can also be combined with free-flowing inert carriers and compressed into tablets directly without going through the granulating or slugging steps. A protective coating consisting of a sealing coat of shellac, a coating of sugar or polymeric material and a polish coating of wax can be provided. Dyestuffs can be added to these coatings to distinguish different unit dosages.

Example 1:

Ingredient	Quantity/Tablet
5H-dibenz[b,f]azepine-4-carboxylic acid	25 mg.
Cornstarch USP	130 mg.
Lactose	160 mg.
Cab-O-Sil M-5 colloidal silica	4 mg.
Gelatin USP	5 mg.
Magnesium Stearate USP	1 mg.

The foregoing ingredients are thoroughly mixed and pressed into tablets suitable for oral administration of 25 mg. of active ingredient. The tablets may be scored to permit administration of fractional doses.

Example 2:

Ingredients	Grams
β-Diethylaminoethyl 10,11-dihydro-5H-dibenz[b,f]azepine-4-carboxylate hydrochloride	100.0
Lactose	80.0
Cornstarch	70.0
Soluble starch	15.0
Magnesium stearate	5.0
	270.0

The first three ingredients are thoroughly mixed, granulated with an aqueous solution of the soluble starch, dried, mixed with magnesium stearate and pressed into 270.0 mg. tablet cores. Each tablet core contains 100.0 mg. of the active substance and is sugar coated according to the usual art practices. Color may be added to the coating.

Furanoside Tablets

A process of manufacturing a free-flowing granular material from a liquid or oily furanoside has been developed by *G. Mueller; U.S. Patent 3,594,474; July 20, 1971; assigned to Ciba Corporation.* The furanosides, such as ethyl-3,5,6-tri-O-benzyl-D-glucofuranoside and ethyl-3-O-propyl-5,6-di-O-para-chlorobenzyl-D-glucofuranoside have properties which inhibit inflammatory and allergy reactions and show other therapeutic activity. However, their oily nature and unpleasant taste have made formulation in liquid or capsule form difficult.

It has been found that a free-flowing granular material which can easily be processed into solid oral administration forms can be obtained if an oily or liquid therapeutically usable glucofuranoside or other oily or liquid therapeutically usable furanosides are mixed with a film-forming agent and a lower alkanol such as methanol, isopropanol or primarily ethanol, worked into a plastic mass with magnesium trisilicate, if desired together with a further adsorbent such as colloidal silica or cellulose, especially microcrystalline cellulose, and the mass granulated while drying, for example, with warm air. As film-forming agents there are preferably used those which also act as binding agents, especially shellac, polyacrylic or methacrylic derivatives, especially their esters, carbowaxes, polyvinyl derivatives such as polyvinyl alcohols or their esters, or primarily polyvinylpyrrolidones. Further possible film-forming agents are alcohol-soluble or water-soluble cellulose derivatives, especially cellulose acetate-phthalate, hydroxypropylmethylcellulose, ethylcellulose, ethylhydroxyethylcellulose, hydroxypropylcellulose or carboxymethylcellulose.

The process is preferably effected by dissolving the film-forming agent in the lower alkanol, working up the furanoside with this solution, and working up this solution with the magnesium trisilicate and optionally the adsorbent to give a plastic mass, and drying and granulating the latter in the usual manner. When working up the solution of the furanoside with magnesium trisilicate, the sugar is adsorbed on the latter.

The film-forming agent is preferably used in a concentration of 0.2 to 20, primarily 2 to 4 parts by weight relative to 10 parts by weight of furanoside. The magnesium trisilicate is used in an amount which permits adsorption of the furanoside, especially in a concentration of 5 to 20, primarily about 10 to 12, parts by weight relative to 10 parts by weight of furanoside. The further adsorbent is used in an amount of 1 to 20, primarily 4 to 6, parts by weight relative to 10 parts by weight of furanoside.

The granular material obtainable by the process is characterized by containing an oily or liquid, therapeutically usable furanoside adsorbed on magnesium trisilicate and if desired on a further adsorbent, and a film-forming agent. This granular material is stable for prolonged periods even at a higher temperature, for example 60°C., and can be easily processed into any desired oral administration form. This granular material is used for the manufacture of solid oral administration forms such as tablets, push-fit capsules or primarily dragées.

Example: Composition of the Granular Material – 10 parts by weight of ethyl-3,5,6-tri-O-benzyl-D-glucofuranoside (Glyvenol), 10 parts by weight of magnesium trisilicate, 5 parts by weight of colloidal silica and 2.5 parts by weight of polyvinylpyrrolidone.

Manufacture of the Granular Material – The PVP is dissolved in a fourfold amount of alcohol and mixed with the Glyvenol. This solution is processed into a paste with the magnesium trisilicate in a suitable apparatus and is kneaded with colloidal silica to give a plastic mass. It is then granulated and dried in the usual manner.

Manufacture of Dragées – 5.45 parts by weight of granular material are mixed with 2.0 parts by weight of starch, 1.7 parts by weight of talc and 0.3 part by weight of magnesium stearate and processed into pressed blanks weighing 585 mg. and containing 200 mg. of ethyl-3,5,6-tri-O-benzyl-D-glucofuranoside. In order to hide the bad taste, the pressed blanks are, after coating with a protective lacquer, converted into dragées with sugar in the usual manner.

NEUROLOGICAL PREPARATIONS

ANTIDEPRESSANTS

Propargylamine Formulations

Propargylamine and its acid addition salts at well tolerated dosage cause a striking elevation in tissue norepinephrine levels and also possess significant antireserpine activity. For example, propargylamine hydrochloride administered to rats at a dose of 40 mg./kg. daily for 4 days by the intraperitoneal route elevates the norepinephrine level beyond control levels by as much as 130% in the heart and 185% in the brain, in accordance with the assay procedure described in *Acta Phys. Scand.*, vol. 118, Sup. 33, page 45 (1955).

According to the methods disclosed by *E.F. Elslager; U.S. Patent 3,297,527; January 10, 1967; assigned to Parke Davis & Company* pharmaceutical compositions are produced by formulating the free base propargylamine or its physiologically acceptable acid addition salts in dosage unit form. Such compositions are constituted with pharmaceutical carriers or diluents. In view of the oral activity of propargylamine and its salts, dosage unit forms for oral administration are particularly suitable, such as tablets, powders, capsules, solutions and suspensions in which the propargylamine compound is incorporated with carrier or diluent.

In general, the daily oral dosage range, calculated as propargylamine free base content, is about 10 to 250 mg./kg. of body weight, in single or divided doses; and the dosage is continued until the condition under treatment is relieved. In the preparation of dosage units such as tablets or capsules, the quantity of medicament furnished by each dosage unit is selected so that the proper dose can be reached by administering one or a reasonable number of the dosage units. For convenience of manufacture and ease of administration, it is preferable that such dosage forms contain at least 2.5 mg. or more, up to 125 mg., of the propargylamine compound (calculated as free base) per unit.

Propargylamine salts are obtained by mixing an ether or acetone solution of one equivalent of the respective acid (one-half equivalent for dibasic acids) with the propargylamine solution and isolating the resulting crystalline salt product. The following example illustrates the preparation of the tablet form of this drug.

Example: The formula for 5 mg. tablets was as follows: propargylamine hydrochloride, 5 g.; sugar with 3% starch, powdered, 165 g.; milk sugar, USP, powder, 165 g.; solution A (acacia solution), q.s.; cornstarch, sifted, 30 g.; talc, sifted, 10 g.; magnesium stearate USP,

3 grams. Blend the propargylamine hydrochloride, powdered sugar, and milk sugar in a twin shell blender. Wet granulate the powder blend with solution A. Finish granulating with distilled water, if necessary. Screen the wet granulation through a No. 6 stainless steel screen. Dry overnight at 120° to 130°F. Reduce the dried granulation through a No. 14 stainless steel screen. Blend in the cornstarch, talc and magnesium stearate. Compress the blend on a rotary tabletting machine using 13⁄32" concave punches. Yield, approximately 1,000 tablets each containing 5 mg. of propargylamine hydrochloride.

Other salts of propargylamine can be substituted for the hydrochloride in this formulation. An alternative materials list for making 1,000-lot capsules by this procedure, each containing 50 mg. of propargylamine p-toluenesulfonate is the following: propargylamine p-toluenesulfonate, 50 g.; dibasic calcium phosphate, 140 g.; milk sugar, USP, powder, 140 g.; 10% w./w. polyvinylpyrrolidone solution, q.s.; cornstarch, sifter, 40 g.; talc, sifted, 10 g.; magnesium stearate, USP, 3 g.

2-Amino-4-Methyl-6-Methoxy-1,3,5-Triazine

According to *T. Yui and Y. Takeo; U.S. Patent 3,296,074; January 3, 1967; assigned to Takeda Chemical Industries, Ltd., Japan* 2-amino-4-methyl-6-methoxy-1,3,5-triazine and its pharmaceutically acceptable salts show a remarkable and consistent therapeutic effect in the treatment of neuroses and psychoses without undesirable side-effects. The compound can be synthesized in a variety of ways, for example: ring closure condensation between guanyl-O-methylisourea and acetic acid esters in the presence of basic substance; reaction of sodium salt of N,N'-dicyanoacetamidine with hydrogen chloride in dry methanol; reaction between N-cyanoacetoimidoether and methylisourea in the presence of a basic substance; reaction between 2-amino-4-halo-6-methyl-1,3,5-triazine and methanol in the presence of a basic substance; and reaction between 2-methyl-4,6-dimethoxy-1,3,5-triazine and ammonia under elevated pressure, whereby one of the two methoxy groups in the former is replaced by amino.

Administration of 2-amino-4-methyl-6-methoxy-1,3,5-triazine to patients suffering from chronic schizophrenia in an amount of 20 to 100 mg./day causes a remarkable therapeutic effect, relief of autism, acceleration of volition, improvement of depressive state and activation of volitive behavior. Administration of the compound in larger doses than 100 mg. per day causes at times temporary decrease of urine volume, which reverts to normal state soon after reduction of dose or cessation of administration. Clinical tests were as follows.

Thirty-two hospitalized, schizophrenic patients with autism and involutional syndromes were selected for clinical study of 2-amino-4-methyl-6-methoxy-1,3,5-triazine with daily oral dosage ranging from 40 to 120 mg. for 60 to 140 days. Of the total group, 29 patients had chronic schizophrenic syndromes which had developed more than 2 years before and resulted nearly in dissociation of personality. They never respond to any other psychotherapeutic drugs. Three other patients were comparatively acute type. After about 20 to 30 days of treatment, 14 of the 29 chronic patients exhibited slight emotional excitement and became volitional and regained rapport with the psychiatrist.

Even after about 2 months of treatment, 6 of the above improved patients continued to progress favorably, but some syndromes of 6 other patients tended to deteriorate. Fifteen patients did not respond to treatment at all. One female patient of the 3 acute ones became volitional and began to speak to the psychiatrist especially about her own psychic problems. After about 20 days of treatment with 40 mg. daily, the patient became active in her facial expression and in working, e.g., in lace-making, and thus became easy to subject to psychotherapy. The other two acute type patients did not respond to treatment.

Side effects were of no major importance; blood pressure levels, urine volume and composition, red and white cell counts did not change significantly during all the periods of treatment in all cases, but a little decrease of hemoglobin content was seen only in some cases. Three cases tested here showed slight (quantitatively insignificant) decrease in basal metabolic rate (BMR) and protein-bound iodine (PBI).

The following example shows the preparation of tablets of this compound.

	Per Tablet, mg.
2-amino-4-methyl-6-methoxy-1,3,5-triazine	20
Lactose	80
Cornstarch	38
Magnesium stearate	2
Total	140

They are processed into tablet form in known manner and, if desired, the tablets may further be coated with sugar, e.g., powdered sugar, to enhance palatability.

Substituted 9,10-Dihydro-9,10-Ethanoanthracenes

H. Schröter and D.A. Prins; U.S. Patent 3,422,104; January 14, 1969; assigned to Geigy Chemical Corporation have found that compounds of 9,10-dihydro-9,10-ethanoanthracene, substituted in 11-position by a straight or branched chain alkylene of 1 to 5 carbon atoms substituted by amino, substituted amino, polymethyleneimino, morpholino, or piperazino are useful spasmolytic, antidepressant and antiemetic agents. Examples of these compounds are 11-dimethylaminomethyl-9,10-dihydro-9,10-ethanoanthracene, 11-morpholinomethyl-9,10-ethanoanthracene, 4-chloro-11-methylaminomethyl-9,10-dihydro-9,10-ethanoanthracene, and 4-(9',10'-dihydro-9',10'-ethanoanthracene-11'-methyl)piperazine-(1)-ethanol.

These compounds, for example, are prepared by first reacting the anthracene or substituted anthracene with acrylonitrile or substituted acrylonitrile to form an 11-cyano-9,10-dihydro 9,10-ethanoanthrocene which is then converted to the 11-aminomethyl groups. The 11-aminomethyl group is then converted by known methods to the various derivatives.

To produce tablets and like dosage units for oral application, the active substances or their pharmaceutically acceptable salts are combined, e.g., with solid pulverulent carriers such as talcum, lactose, saccharose, sorbitol, mannite; starches such as potato starch, cornstarch or amylopectin; cellulose derivatives or gelatin, possibly with the addition of lubricants such as magnesium or calcium stearate or polyethylene oxides of suitable molecular weights (Carbowax) and disintegrating agents such as, e.g., alginic acid, laminaria powder or citrus pulp powder, to form tablets or dragee cores. Preferred compositions contain 10 to 50 mg. of active compound per tablet, and consist essentially of:

	Parts by Weight
Active compound	250.0
Lactose	100.0 to 200.0
Potato starch or cornstarch	150.0 to 360.0
Stearic acid	8.0 to 20.0
Talcum	100.0 to 200.0
Magnesium stearate	2.5 to 10.0
Colloidal silicon oxide	10.0 to 35.0
Ethanol, q.s.	

Compositions in the form of dragees cores having the same content of active ingredients consist essentially of:

	Parts by Weight
Active compound	250.0
Lactose	100.0 to 200.0
Stearic acid	8.0 to 20.0
Potato starch	10.0 to 50.0
Talcum	60.0 to 200.0

(continued)

		Parts by Weight
	Magnesium stearate	2.5 to 10.0
	Colloidal silicon oxide	5.0 to 60.0
	Ethanol, q.s.	

The quantum satis (q.s.) for 250 parts of active ingredient in 1,000 grams of the solid part of the tablet or dragee core material amounts to about 90 parts by volume of ethanol.

Example 1: To produce 10,000 tablets each containing 25 mg. of 11-methylaminomethyl-9,10-dihydro-9,10-ethanoanthracene hydrochloride the following components are used:

(1)	Active substance	250.0 g.
	Lactose	175.8 g.
	Potato starch	169.7 g.
(2)	Stearic acid	10.0 g.
	Ethanol (about 90 ml.), q.s.	
(3)	Potato starch	160.0 g.
	Talcum	200.0 g.
	Magnesium stearate	2.5 g.
	Colloidal silicon oxide	32.0 g.
		1,000.0 g.

The substances (1) are well mixed and moistened with the granulating solution (2). The granulated mass is passed through a sieve having 49 to 64 meshes per sq. cm. The moist granulate is then dried for about 12 hours at about 20°C. The dried granulate is again passed through a sieve of the same mesh number and then intimately mixed with the substances (3). The resulting mass is then pressed into tablets of 100 mg., containing 25 mg. of active substance each.

Example 2: To produce 10,000 dragees containing each 25 mg. of 4-(9',10'-ethanoanthracene-11'-methyl)piperazine-(1)-ethanol, the following components are used:

(1)	Active substance	250.0 g.
	Lactose	175.9 g.
(2)	Stearic acid	10.0 g.
	Ethanol (about 90 ml.), q.s.	
(3)	Potato starch	20.0 g.
	Talcum	165.0 g.
	Magnesium stearate	2.5 g.
	Colloidal silicon oxide	56.6 g.
		680.0 g.

The substances (1) are well mixed and moistened with the granulating solution (2). The moistened mass is granulated through a sieve having 49 to 64 meshes per sq. cm. The moist granulate is then dried for about 12 hours at about 20°C. and then passed again through a sieve of the same mesh number. The dried granulate is then initmately mixed with the substances (3) and the resulting mass is compressed into cores of a weight of 68 mg. containing each 25 mg. of the aforesaid active substance. The production of the dragees is then completed in a conventional manner by applying to the cores a conventional coating solution. In this manner, dragees having each a total weight (i.e., core plus coating) of about 100 mg. and containing 25 mg. of active substance are obtained.

Lithium Salts

The use of lithium salts in the treatment of manic states, and in particular as a prophylaxis in recurrent manic-depressive or depressive illness, has been known for several years. Unfortunately, lithium is quickly absorbed and excreted, so to maintain therapeutic plasma levels, the salt must be administered 3 to 4 times a day. This is not only inconvenient but also dangerous since lithium tends to accumulate in the body and produces severe side effects at blood levels only a little higher than the therapeutic levels. Cases of severe lithium poisoning have been frequently reported.

A.J. Coppen and J.-P. Metral; U.S. Patent 3,641,236; February 8, 1972; assigned to Delandale Laboratories Limited, England have provided a lithium-containing therapeutic composition which need be taken not more than once daily, and which is capable of maintaining a therapeutic blood level of lithium throughout the 24 hours. In one form, the pharmaceutical composition comprises: a powdered lithium salt; a sustained release agent comprising a mixture of glyceryl mono-, di- and triesters of one or more C_{16}–C_{18} straight chain saturated fatty acids; and other innocuous compound materials.

Preferably, the sustained release agent is present in 51 to 61 parts by weight per 100 parts by weight of therapeutically available lithium. The lithium salt is preferably lithium carbonate. The other innocuous compounds may include a filler such as mannitol, a binding agent such as gum acacia, and a lubricant such as magnesium stearate. The composition may be in a form of tablets comprising a compressed mixture which includes a lubricant and particles of a dried, granulated mixture of binding agent, sustained release material, filler and lithium salt.

The sustained release agent will normally be prepared from a mixture of fatty acids. It is important that the mixture contains principally C_{16}–C_{18} straight chain saturated fatty acids. In practice, since acids are normally obtained from natural sources, the mixture will contain principally palmitic and stearic acids, and small amounts of other acids outside the stated range will inevitably be present. It is to be understood in the definition of the sustained release agent that minor amounts of such other acid radicals may be present in quantities which do not significantly effect the function of the sustained release agent. Delayed release lithium carbonate tablets are made to the following formula:

	Parts by Weight
Lithium carbonate	100
Mannitol	16.5
Precirol	9.75
Gum acacia	10
Magnesium stearate	1.25

Precirol is a trade name for a mixture of glycerol mono-, di- and tripalmitostearate esters manufactured by Messrs. Gattefosse in France. It is prepared from palmitostearic acids having the approximate composition by weight: stearic acid 46.5%, palmitic acid 51%, lauric acid 2%, and traces of myristic and oleic acids. The final ester composition by weight is monoester 12 to 17%, diester 43 to 47% and triester 35 to 44%, there being less than 1% free glycerol. The tablets are manufactured in the following way. The mannitol is sieved on a 25 mesh screen (AFNOR – Association Francaise de Normalisation). The sieved mannitol is mixed in a heated tank at about 68°C. with powdered lithium carbonate of pharmaceutical quality (BPC – 1949).

An alcholic solution of Precirol is prepared by dissolving 39 grams of Precirol in every 170 ml. of 96°C. alcohol and bringing the temperature of the solution to about 70°C. and is then poured onto the powdered mixture of mannitol and lithium carbonate at about 68°C., and mixed. An aqueous solution of gum acacia is prepared with 1 part by weight of gum acacia to 2 parts by volume of water, and poured onto the mixture, and the whole mass is kneaded. The mass is then dried at 40°C. by evaporation, e.g., in an Aeromatic drier. It is then granulated on a number 10 screen (mesh 2 mm.; wire diameter 0.7 mm.) and dried for a further 5 minutes. The dry mass is then further granulated on a number 16 screen (mesh 1.19 mm.; wire diameter 0.5 mm.). The magnesium stearate is added to the dry granulate and mixed. The mixture is then compressed into tablets on a rotary machine with flat, cup-shaped, and rod-shaped punches. Each tablet should have a weight of about 550 mg. and contain 400 mg. of lithium carbonate and 39 mg. of Precirol. These tablets can be administered once daily to obtain a sustained therapeutic level of lithium in the blood plasma throughout the 24 hour period.

SEDATIVES AND TRANQUILIZERS

Combined Sedative-Muscle Relaxant Steroid

The method has been developed by *W.J. Wechter; U.S. Patent 3,316,146; April 25, 1967; assigned to The Upjohn Company* using compositions comprising 3α-hydroxy-5β-pregnane-11,20-dione 20-cyclic (ethylene acetal), for inducing sedation and muscular relaxation, and inhibiting the glutamic dehydrogenase enzyme system. The principal active ingredient is 3α-hydroxy-5β-pregnane-11,20-dione 20-cyclic (ethylene acetal) represented by the formula:

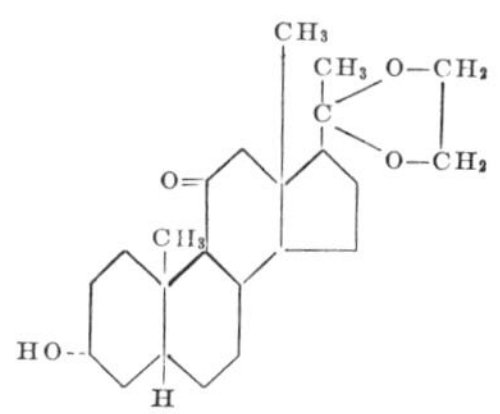

The compound can be prepared by known methods as, for example, described in U.S. Patent 2,824,871. The compositions are presented for oral administration to animals in solid and liquid unit dosage forms, such as tablets, capsules, powders, granules, syrups, elixirs, and the like, containing suitable quantities of 3α-hydroxy-5β-pregnane-11,20-dione 20-cyclic (ethylene acetal).

Tablets are made by preparing a powder mixture, granulating or slugging, adding a lubricant and pressing into tablets. The powder mixture is prepared by mixing the 3α-hydroxy-5β-pregnane-11,20-dione 20-cyclic (ethylene acetal), suitably comminuted, with a diluent or base such as starch, sucrose, kaolin, dicalcium phosphate and the like. The powder mixture can be granulated by wetting with a binder such as syrup, starch paste or acacia mucilage and forcing through a screen. As an alternative to granulating, the powder mixture can be slugged, i.e., run through the tablet machine and the resulting imperfectly formed tablets broken into pieces (slugs). The slugs can be lubricated to prevent sticking to the tablet forming dies by means of the addition of stearic acid, a stearate salt, talc or mineral oil. The lubricating mixture is then compressed into tablets.

Advantageously, the tablet can be provided with a protective coating consisting of a sealing coat of shellac, a coating of sugar and methylcellulose, and a polish coating of carnauba wax. The amount of compound of 3α-hydroxy-5β-pregnane-11,20-dione 20-cyclic (ethylene acetal) to be administered depends on the species, age, weight, subject, and the particular condition to be treated. A dose of from about 1 to about 10 mg./kg. of body weight can be used.

3α-hydroxy-5β-pregnane-11,20-dione 20-cyclic (ethylene acetal) is an orally and parenterally active steroid, i.e., it is systematically absorbed when administered orally and parenterally, having muscle relaxant and sedative-hypnotic properties. The compound is essentially devoid of hormonal effects. The central nervous system depressant properties are exemplified by depression of motor activity and potentiation of hexobarbital-induced sleep. Small doses produce muscle-relaxant effects with moderate depression whereas larger doses produce a progressive depression leading to deep hypnosis.

Example: 1,000 tablets for oral administration, each containing 100 mg. of 3α-hydroxy-5β-pregnane-11,20-dione 20-cyclic (ethylene acetal), are prepared from the following types and amounts of ingredients:

3α-hydroxy-5β-pregnane-11,20-dione 20-cyclic (ethylene acetal)	100 g.
Calcium carbonate	100 g.
Cornstarch	65 g.
Magnesium stearate	15 g.

The ingredients are thoroughly mixed and slugged. The slugs are broken down by forcing through a screen. The resulting granules are then compressed into tablets, each tablet containing 100 mg. of 3α-hydroxy-5β-pregnane-11,20-dione 20-cyclic (ethylene acetal).

Following the foregoing procedure, tablets are prepared containing 3α-hydroxy-5β-pregnane-11,20-dione 20-cyclic (ethylene acetal) in 25 mg., 50 mg. and 75 mg. amounts by substituting 25, 50 and 75 gram amounts of 3α-hydroxy-5β-pregnane-11,20-dione 20-cyclic (ethylene acetal) for the 100 gram amount of the example.

2-Alkoxy-2-Formyl-Δ^2-Steroids

A method of preparing 3-alkoxy-2-formyl-Δ^2-steroids from the corresponding 2-unsubstituted steroids has been developed by *J.P. Dusza, J.P. Joseph and S. Bernstein; U.S. Patent 3,415,852; December 10, 1968; assigned to American Cyanamid Company.* The products are physiologically active in warm-blooded animals as central nervous system depressants.

Among the starting materials useful in the process are, cholestan-3-one; 17β-hydroxy-17α-methylandrostan-3-one; 17β-hydroxy-17α-propylandrostan-3-one; 17β-hydroxyandrostan-3-one; 17β-formyloxyandrostan-3-one; 17β-acetoxyandrostan-3-one; 17β-propionoxyandrostan-3-one and the like.

The process consists of reacting the appropriate steroid, in solution or suspension with tri(lower)alkylorthoformate. Ordinarily, the reaction is carried out by adding an excess of a strong acid such as aqueous perchloric acid (e.g., 72% perchloric acid) or concentrated fluoroboric acid with stirring. Usually, the reaction proceeds satisfactorily at room temperature, but the mixture may be heated gently. In general, the reaction may be carried out at a temperature within the range of 15° to 75°C. for a period of from 10 minutes to 2 hours. Stirring is continued for 40 to 60 minutes. The reaction mixture is neutralized with an excess of a saturated sodium bicarbonate or other acid acceptor solution.

The aqueous layer is discarded after the product has been extracted with methylene chloride. The methylene chloride is then washed with a saturated saline solution and dried over sodium sulfate. Concentration of the dried extract in a round-bottomed flask on a rotary evaporator ordinarily produces an oily residue from which the product may be precipitated. Purification of the steroid can usually be achieved by direct recrystallization from appropriate solvents such as methanol or acetone-hexane mixture, or by column chromatography on magnesium silicate.

The compounds are physiologically active in warm-blooded animals as central nervous system depressants. They are therefore useful in the field of hypnotics, tranquilizers and the like. The compounds are active in antagonizing the phenyl-p-quinone (PPQ) "writhing" syndrome. The compounds were tested by a modification of the method described by E. Siegmund et al. *Proc. Soc. Exptl. Biol. Med.,* 95, 729 (1957). Briefly, the test is described as follows: Two mice are administered the test compound, orally, 30 minutes prior to the intraperitoneal injection of 1 mg./kg. phenyl-p-quinone. Fifteen minutes later the mice are observed for a period of 3 minutes and the total number of characteristic writhing episodes for both animals is counted and recorded. The mean number of writhes exhibited by 21 pairs of control animals (dosed orally with 2% starch) was 29. For these purposes any compound that reduces the incidence of writhing to 18 or less (2 standard deviations from historical control) is considered a possible active lead. To confirm activity the test is repeated in another pair of mice. If the incidence of writhing is again reduced to 18 or less, the compound is considered active in the PPQ test as a central nervous system depressant, otherwise the compound is rejected.

These compounds can be administered as tablets, pills, capsules, powders, granules, parenteral solutions or suspensions, oral solutions or suspensions and the like. A total daily dose of 5 to 250 mg. may be given singly or in divided doses. For preparing solid compositions such as tablets, the principal active ingredient is mixed with conventional tabletting ingredients, such as cornstarch, lactose, sucrose, sorbitol, talc, stearic acid, magnesium stearate, dicalcium phosphate, gums, and similar materials as pharmaceutical diluents or carriers. The tablets or pills can be laminated or otherwise compounded to provide a dosage form affording prolonged or delayed action or predetermined successive action of the enclosed medication.

For example, the tablet or pill can comprise an inner dosage and an outer dosage component, the latter being in the form of an envelope over the former. The two components can be separated by an enteric layer which serves to resist disintegration in the stomach and permits the inner component to pass intact into the duodenum or to be delayed in release. A variety of materials can be used for such enteric layers or coatings, such materials including a number of polymeric acids or mixtures of polymeric acids with such materials as shellac, shellac and cetyl alcohol, cellulose acetate and the like.

5-Phenylpyrrolidine-2,4-Diones

C.M. Hofmann and S.R. Safir; U.S. Patent 3,317,390; May 2, 1967; assigned to American Cyanamid Company have developed substituted 5-phenylpyrrolidine-2,4-diones having central nervous system depressant activity. These compounds may be illustrated by the following formula:

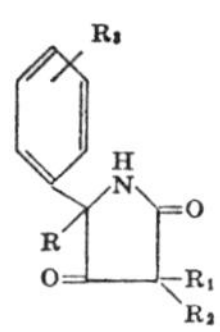

where R and R_1 are lower alkyl and R_2 and R_3 are hydrogen or lower alkyl. The active components in which either R_1 or R_2 or both are lower alkyl may be prepared by reacting a 2-amino-2-phenyl(or lower alkylphenyl)alkanamide with an α-alkylacetoacetic ester in an inert solvent such as boiling toluene, xylene, or mesitylene. The resulting 2-(α-alkylacetoacetamido)-2-phenyl(or lower alkylphenyl)alkanamide may be treated with an acid such as polyphosphoric or sulfuric acid at temperatures of 50° to 100°C. for 15 minutes to 2 hours or so, followed by treatment with an alcohol such as methanol or ethanol, to give the corresponding 2-(α-alkylacetoacetamido)-2-phenyl-(or lower alkylphenyl)-alkanoic esters. These are cyclized with an aqueous alkali metal hydroxide or an alcoholic alkali metal alkoxide at temperatures of 50° to 100°C.

The resulting 3,5-substituted-5-phenyl-(or lower alkylphenyl)-pyrrolidine-2,4-diones may be further alkylated with lower alkyl halides, such as methyl iodide, ethyl bromide or the like, in a suitable solvent, as, for example, ethanol, in the presence of an alkali metal alkoxide, as for example, sodium methoxide at temperatures of 25° to 80°C. In the case where R_1 is lower alkyl and the lower alkyl halide is ethyl iodide a small amount of O-ethylated product is obtained also.

These compounds are physiologically active in warm-blooded animals as central nervous system depressants. They may be used as sedatives, hypnotics or tranquilizers. The dosage will depend on the route of administration, age, weight, and condition of the warm-blooded animal. A total daily dose of from 10 to 1,000 mg. given singly or in divided dosage several times daily embraces the effective range of treatment of most conditions for which the compounds are useful. These compounds can be given in unit dosage form such as tablets, pills, capsules, powders, granules, sterile solutions or suspensions, and the like. The following example shows the preparation of tablets from such material.

Example: 1,000 tablets each containing 100 mg. of 3,5-diethyl-3-methyl-5-phenylpyrrolidine-2,4-dione are prepared from the following ingredients: 3,5-diethyl-3-methyl-5-phenylpyrrolidine-2,4-dione, 100 grams; lactose, 50 grams; starch, 50 grams; calcium stearate, 10 grams; talc, 10 grams. The finely powdered ingredients are mixed thoroughly and then tabletted by a slugging procedure.

Substituted Ureas

V.J. Bauer and H.P. Dalalian; U.S. Patent 3,332,975; July 25, 1967; assigned to American Cyanamid Company have prepared mono- and disubstituted ureas useful as depressants. These compounds may be represented by the following formula:

$$R^1{-}O{-}\overset{H}{\underset{|}{N}}{-}\overset{O}{\underset{\|}{C}}{-}\overset{H}{\underset{|}{N}}{-}R$$

where R is hydrogen, lower alkyl, lower alkenyl, phenyl, cycloalkyl or naphthyl and R^1 is phenyl, lower alkylphenyl or chlorophenyl. Lower alkyl includes those having 1 to 4 carbon atoms and additionally lower alkenyl has one double bond. These compounds are, in general, crystalline solids slightly soluble in water but soluble in dilute aqueous bases, such as, sodium hydroxide, potassium hydroxide or sodium carbonate. These compounds are likewise soluble in organic solvents, such as, for example acetone or ether.

The compounds are preferably prepared by reacting a salt of an aryloxyamine, such as phenoxyamine hydrochloride, with a salt of cyanic acid, such as, potassium cyanate, to prepare the monosubstituted ureas. A further method can be used wherein an aryloxy amine, such as phenoxyamine, is reacted with a lower alkyl, lower alkenyl, phenyl, cycloalkyl or naphthyl isocyanate to produce disubstituted ureas. The reaction is usually carried out at about room temperature in solvents such as water or ether. The reaction is completed in a matter of minutes to several hours. The reactions described above may be illustrated as follows:

$$(1)\qquad R^1{-}O{-}NH_2\cdot HCl + KCNO \longrightarrow R^1{-}O{-}NH\overset{O}{\overset{\|}{C}}NH_2$$

$$(2)\qquad R^1{-}O{-}NH_2 + RNCO \longrightarrow R^1{-}O{-}NH\overset{O}{\overset{\|}{C}}NHR$$

where R and R^1 are as described previously. These are physiologically active in warm-blooded animals as central nervous system depressants. This activity is indicative of uses in the field of hypnotics, tranquilizers and the like. The dosage of these compounds will depend on the route of administration, age, weight, and condition of the warm-blooded animal. A total daily dose of 10 to 1,000 mg. given once or in divided dosage several times daily is the effective range of treatment of most conditions for which the compounds are useful.

Examples of suitable oral unit dosage forms of these compounds are tablets, capsules, pills, powder packets, granules, wafers, cachets, ampules, vials and the like. The following example illustrates the preparation of tablets from a disubstituted urea.

Example: 1,000 tablets each containing 100 mg. of 1-n-butyl-3-phenoxyurea are prepared from the following ingredients:

1-n-butyl-3-phenoxyurea	100 g.
Lactose	50 g.
Starch	50 g.
Calcium stearate	10 g.
Talc	10 g.

The finely powdered ingredients are mixed thoroughly and then tabletted by a slugging procedure.

MISCELLANEOUS CONTROL DRUGS

Halophenyl Amino Alkanones as Appetite Supressants

Weight reducing compounds which do not cause an increase in blood pressure have been synthesized by *H. Siemer; U.S. Patent 3,313,687; April 11, 1967; assigned to Andreas J. Rottendorf Chemische Fabrik, Germany.* These are secondary and tertiary 1-halogen-phenyl-2-amino-alkanones represented by Formula (1)

(1) 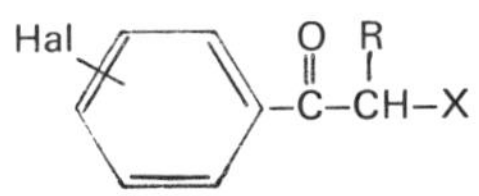

where R is a lower alkyl with 1 to 3 carbon atoms, and X is a monoalkylamino or dialkyl-amino radical, which has alkyl groups of straight or branched chains of 1 to 5 carbon atoms atoms, or a cyclic amino radical with 4 or 5 carbon atoms, e.g., a piperidino-, pyrrolidino or morpholino radical. These compounds have excellent appetite-reducing properties without causing restlessness by over-stimulation of the sympathetic nervous system or hypertension. In view of the low side effects, these compounds are very useful drugs in the treatment of obesity and particularly in preexisting hypertension. Moreover, no abuse is to be expected because of the comparatively low central stimulation, such abuse being due to the stimulating and euphoric effect of known anorexigenic agents.

The tertiary 1-halogenphenyl-2-amino-alkanones corresponding to Formula (1) where X is

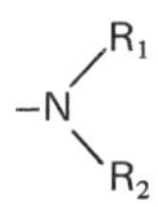

can be prepared under favorable economical and operational conditions, by reacting 1-halogenated-2-bromoalkanones with dialkylamines such as dimethylamine, diethylamine, dibutylamine, or ethylpropylamine, in the presence of a solvent, e.g., an alkanol, dioxane, or the like inert solvents and by dissolving the bromoalkanones in the dialkylamine, which is preferably used in excess, by heating to temperatures between 40° and 60°C. The reaction during which the corresponding dialkylamino hydrobromides precipitate, becomes markedly exothermic toward the end and it should be adjusted, if necessary, by cooling the reaction vessel externally, in such a manner that with the use of dialkylamines of lower boiling point, e.g., diethylamine, these amines are refluxed.

When higher boiling amines are used, the reaction temperature should preferably not exceed 80°C. After the reaction has slowed down, stirring may be continued for half an hour between 50° and 80°C. until the conversion is complete. The following pharmacological test shows that the 1-halogenphenyl-2-amino-propanone salts (compounds I to IV) distinguish favorably over the known compounds V and VI. The following compounds have been tested:

(I) 1-p-chlorophenyl-2-ethylamino-propanone HCl
(II) 1-p-chlorophenyl-2-ethylamino-propanone-nicotinate hydrochloride
(III) 1-p-chlorophenyl-2-diethylamino-propanone HCl
(IV) 1-p-chlorophenyl-2-pyrrolidino-propanone HCl
(V) d-1-phenyl-2-amino-propene sulfate
(VI) 2-phenyl-3-methyl-morpholine HCl

TABLE 1: BLOOD PRESSURE TESTS ON CATS

Compounds	Doses	Blood Pressure
I	500 μg./kg. i.v.	10 mm. Hg. decrease.
II	500 μg./kg. i.v.	22 mm. Hg. decrease.
V	50 μg./kg. i.v.	11 mm. Hg. increase.
VI	500 μg./kg. i.v.	30 mm. Hg. increase.

Method: The tests were made with female cats, (whole animals, weight between 2 and 3 kg.) in Chloralose-Urethane-Anesthesia. The drugs to be tested were injected into the femural vein in 0.9% NaCl solution at body temperatures.

TABLE 2: ACUTE TOXICITY, HYPERMOTILIZING AND ANOREXIGENIC EFFECTS

Compound	LD_{50}(s.c.)	Hypermotilizing Eff.	Anorexigenic Effect
I	280 mg./kg.	30 mg./kg. 237±83%	30 mg./kg. 90.82%
II	388 mg./kg.	30 mg./kg. 206±27%	30 mg./kg. 51.3%
III	650 mg./kg.	30 mg./kg. 256±46%	30 mg./kg. 98.2%
IV	410 mg./kg.	30 mg./kg. 208±47%	30 mg./kg. 83.3%
V	45 mg./kg.	3 mg./kg. 472±81%	10 mg./kg. 94.7%
VI	170 mg./kg.	30 mg./kg. 320±46%	30 mg./kg. 78%

In the tests tabulated in Table 2, the acute toxicity was determined on white mice (weight 20 to 22 grams). The spontaneous running urge was tested on female mice in circular cages, with the use of photo-electric recorders. Application of the compounds tested was subcutaneous. All figures are given in percentages of intrinsic hypermotility of untreated mice. The anorexigenic effect was determined in single feeding tests after oral application of the compounds to be tested. The tested animals were female Wistar rats. The following examples illustrate the preparation of tablets and dragees.

Example 1: 10,000 tablets were made as follows:

(I)	1-p-chlorophenyl-2-ethylamino-propanone HCl	300 g.
	Milk sugar	400 g.
	Potato starch	700 g.
(II)	Starch solution, 10%	500 g.
(III)	Talcum	30 g.
	Stearic acid	20 g.
	Potato starch	300 g.

(I) and (II) are granulated and dried, and thereafter mixed with (III) and compressed into tablets. The 10,000 tablets weigh 1.80 kg., the diameter of each tablet is 8 mm.; 1 tablet contains 30 mg. effective drug.

Example 2: 10,000 dragees were made as follows: 25 mg. of 1-o-bromophenyl-2-ethyl-amino-propanone were used as a core for each dragee; each core was then covered with 100 ml. Eudragit L and then coated in a conventional manner with sugar, talcum, calcium carbonate, gum arabic and sugar solution to a final weight of 350 mg./dragee. The dragees are then covered with Eudragit E. The dragee coating contains/per dragee:

Sugar	0.1275 g.
Talcum	0.0170 g.
Calcium carbonate	0.0170 g.
Gum arabic	0.0085 g.
Eudragit L	0.0012 g.
Eudragit E	0.0001 g.

For making the final dragees the sugar solution is colored with 0.0004 gram per dragee of one of the following dyestuffs: Orange 1, Red 1, Yellow 3.

4,4-Diphenylcyclohexylamines as Spasmolytic and Cholinolytic Agents

Therapeutic formulations have been developed by *R. Unger, S. Sommer, E. Schorscher and H-J. Eneakel; U.S. Patent 3,376,312; April 2, 1968; assigned to E. Merck AG, Germany* containing 4,4-diphenylcyclohexylamines. These are illustrated by Formula (1):

(1)

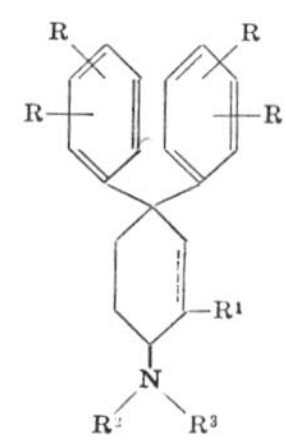

where each R can be hydrogen, alkyl of 1 to 4 carbon atoms, lower alkoxy, hydroxy, halogen such as fluorine or chlorine; and two R moieties can represent methylene dioxy; R^1 represents H, alkyl, alkenyl or alkynyl of up to 6 carbon atoms, and R^2 and R^3 each represents H, alkyl, or alkenyl of up to 8 carbon atoms, cycloalkyl of 3 to 8 carbon atoms, or aralkyl whose aliphatic portion contains 1 to 4 carbon atoms, and of which the aromatic portion is preferably unsubstituted hydrocarbon or it can be substituted in the same manner as the phenyl groups present in the 4-position, and where the residues R^2 and R^3 together with the nitrogen atom can also form a pyrrolidine or piperidine ring which is optionally substituted by a methyl or ethyl group, and the dashed line in the 2,3-position indicates the optional presence of a double bond.

These compounds possess valuable pharmacological properties, particularly exhibiting spasmolytic and cholinolytic effects. Some cause increasing flow through the coronaries, in addition; this latter effect is particularly exhibited by those compounds of the Formula (1) above in which R is H, R^1 is H or lower alkyl (up to 4 carbon atoms), R^2 and R^3 are both methyl and there is no double bond in 2,3-position.

To illustrate such effects, 1-isopropylamino-4,4-diphenyl-cyclohexane and 1-(N-methyl-N-isopropylamino)-4,4-diphenyl-cyclohexane, tested on an isolated rat intestine, exhibited approximately 9 to 10 times the spasmolytic effect of Eupaverin; where these same compounds exhibited about the same cholinolytic efficaciousness and duration of activity as atropine sulfate (tested on an isolated guinea pig intestine). This combination of a strong prolonged cholinolytic effect taken together with a strong spasmolytic activity component (the latter being present in most of the known cholinolytics to a slight degree or not at all) is considered a particular advantage. Furthermore, the substances are well-resorbed from the stomach-intestinal tract, in contradistinction to Eupaverin, as well as to known cholinolytics with quaternary nitrogen. These compounds are preferably administered to mammals in dosages between 1 and 100 mg. per dosage unit. Ampoules are considered to be a dosage unit for parenteral application. With respect to enteral application, tablets are considered unit dosages, the tablets usually being formulated with at least one carbohydrate. If a liquid is used for enteral application, a sweetened vehicle is customarily employed.

The compounds have been tested in vitro on isolated organs such as intestines, gall bladders or ureters of rats, guinea pigs or hogs. Additionally, they have been tested in vitro orally subcutaneously, intravenously and intraperitoneally on mice, rats, rabbits, cats, guinea pigs, and dogs. For clinical studies, the compounds are applied to humans orally, subcutaneously, intravenously or rectally. The following examples are such for suitable tablet preparations. The figures given are parts by weight.

Example 1: Tablets –

1-isopropylamino-4,4-diphenyl-cyclohexane hydrochloride	5
Lactose	90
Cornstarch	18
Talc	7

are thoroughly mixed. The powder obtained is processed into tablets in such a manner that each tablet contains 5 mg. of the active ingredient.

Example 2: Coated Tablets –

1-isopropylamino-4,4-diphenyl-cyclohexane hydrochloride	5
Lactose	93
Talc	2

are thoroughly mixed and processed into tablets each containing 5 mg. of the active ingredient. These tablets are coated with sugar syrup in the customary manner until the total weight of one coated tablet is 200 mg.

Nerve Regeneration by 2-Amino-1,3,3-Tricyano-2-Propene

2-amino-1,3,3-tricyano-2-propene has the structural formula $(CN)_2C{=}C(NH_2)CH_2CN$. In purified form it is a white crystalline compound with a melting point of about 172°C. It can be prepared in accordance with the methods of U.S. Patent 2,719,861.

F.S. Eberts, Jr.; U.S. Patent 3,311,539; March 28, 1967; assigned to The Upjohn Company has found that compositions containing this compound demonstrate beneficial effects in the treatment of certain neurological afflictions, for example, in nerve trauma, by hastening nerve regeneration.

By use of the ultraviolet photomicrography technique, it was demonstrated that 2-amino-1,3,3-tricyano-2-propene administered intravenously to rabbits at doses of 4 to 5 mg./kg. produces cytological changes in neuronal tissues. Tissue specimens taken 1 hour after drug injection showed marked increases in protein and nucleoprotein as determined by increased ultraviolet absorption in the cytoplasm and nucleus. This response occurred in the cells of the dorsal root ganglia, anterior horn cells of the spinal cord, Purkinje cells of the cerebellum, and pyramidal cells of the frontal cortex. While the ribonucleic acid content of neurons increased that of the associated oligodendroglia decreased. Accompanying alterations of base ratio also occurred.

The compositions have also been found to augment neuromuscular transmission. Although the mechanism of this augmentation is not thoroughly understood, it is thought that neuromuscular transmission at the motor end plate is facilitated.

It has been found that oran administration of 2-amino-1,3,3-tricyano-2-propene, results in quite rapid absorption and provides demonstrable blood levels of the active ingredient.

Toxicological studies of 2-amino-1,3,3-tricyano-2-propene have shown the following results:

	Mg./Kg.
Acute LD_{50} in mice, intraperitoneally	140
Acute LD_{50} in rats, orally	185
Acute LD_{50} in rats, intraperitoneally	75

The compositions are preferably presented for administration in unit dosage form as tablets, pills, capsules, powders, granules, sterile parenteral solutions or suspensions and the like. For preparing solid compositions such as tablets, the principal active ingredient is mixed with conventional tabletting ingredients such as cornstarch, lactose, sucrose, sorbitol, talc, stearic acid, magnesium stearate, dicalcium phosphate, gums, and functionally similar materials. The following example will illustrate the formation of tablets from the material.

Example: Tablets (125 mg.) – To prepare 1,000 tablets (125 mg.), 500 grains of talc is added to 100 grains of calcium stearate, and the resulting mixture is slugged together with 125 grams of 2-amino-1,3,3-tricyano-2-propene. The slugs are reduced to granules through a 14-mesh screen. A lactose granulation is prepared from 2,400 grains of lactose, 50 grains of starch and 50 grains of sucrose, the latter two constituting the granulating paste. The 2-amino-1,3,3-tricyano-2-propene and lactose granulations are mixed, 250 grains of talc and 100 grains of calcium stearate are added, and the resulting mixture is compressed into tablets, each tablet containing:

2-amino-1,3,3-tricyano-2-propene	125 mg.
Talc	0.75 gr.
Calcium stearate	0.2 gr.
Lactose	2.4 gr.
Starch	0.05 gr.
Sucrose	0.05 gr.

Scored tablets, each containing 200 mg. of 2-amino-1,3,3-tricyano-2-propene and prepared in like manner also provide a beneficial dosage form.

BLOOD AND CARDIOVASCULAR PREPARATIONS

ANTICOAGULANTS

Heparin Acid Salts

T.Y. Koh; U.S. Patent 3,482,014; December 2, 1969; assigned to Canada Packers Limited, Canada has found that acid salts of heparin, in contrast to the neutral salts of heparin, are absorbable through the walls of the intestinal tract to provide effective anticoagulant activity in the blood stream. The acid salts, such as sodium acid heparinate, may be orally administered as enteric pills or tablets.

Heparinic acid and the heparinic acid salts may be prepared by ion exchange methods starting with any available heparin salt, such as, the neutral sodium salt of commerce. For example, the neutral salt in aqueous solution is treated with an appropriate ion exchange resin to produce a solution of heparinic acid which can be introduced as such into the intestinal tract or first may be reacted with a calculated amount of the appropriate base to yield the desired acid salt.

Suitable ion exchange resins are commercially available. Different types of ion exchange resins and different techniques may be employed. For example, strongly acidic cationic exchange resins, such as the nuclear sulfonated ion exchange resins described in U.S. Patent 2,366,007, may be used in the hydrogen form in excess of the theoretical amount for direct production of heparinic acid from sodium heparinate solution. The acid can be reacted with any desired amount of base to provide a heparinic acid salt with a predetermined cation content. Alternatively, an aqueous solution of neutral heparinate may be contacted with the exact amount of the ion exchange resin calculated to produce the desired acid heparinate. The aqueous phase is then separated from the resin and lyophilized to give a solid product.

Example 1: An aqueous solution of 4.4 grams of neutral sodium heparinate (11.6% Na, 147 USP anticoagulant units per milligram) was mixed with 60 ml., an excess, of a strongly acidic cation exchange resin in the acid form and contact was maintained for 15 minutes. After separation of the aqueous heparinic acid phase from the resin beads by filtration, it was partially neutralized with NaOH containing 0.36 gram Na and lyophilized. There was obtained a white powdery sodium acid heparinate containing approximately 8.3% sodium and having an anticoagulant activity of 130 units per milligram.

Example 2: Sodium acid heparinate containing 8.3% Na and having a heparin activity of approximately 130 USP anticoagulant units per milligram prepared by the procedure of Example 1, is compressed into tablets, by known tabletting techniques, each containing 120 mg. of the sodium acid heparinate (i.e., 15,000 anticoagulant units). The tablets are then provided with a standard enteric coating.

Example 3: Six enteric-coated tablets, each containing 75 mg. sodium acid heparinate (108 USP anticoagulant units per milligram 8.3% Na) were fed to a dog, weighing 8 kg. Blood samples were drawn by venepuncture at intervals after feeding and the clotting time determined by the method of Mayer. The clotting time was raised to 50% above normal one hour after feeding, with the peak activity of three times the normal at 3 hours after feeding. At 4½ hours, the blood clotting time declined to approximately twice the normal. At this point, two more tablets were fed again to the dog. This maintenance dose had the effect of raising the blood clotting time to approximately twice the normal 6¾ hours after the first feeding. The results are shown as follows:

Hours After Feeding	Clotting Time
0	6'48"
1	9'12"
2	15'05"
3	18'23"
4½	11'16"
5¾	9'48"
6¾	11'50"
7¾	6'25"

Sulfone Enhanced Heparin

It was also found by *T.Y. Koh; U.S. Patent 3,510,561; May 5, 1970; assigned to Canada Packers Limited, Canada* that a composition containing a sulfone combined with heparin promotes the absorption of the heparin anticoagulant through the mucous membranes. The compositions may also contain a fatty alcohol of chain length C_{14} to C_{24} to prolong or regulate the time period of absorption of the active anticoagulant substance from the composition. The composition may be administered in the form of solids or liquids which may be incorporated in enteric-coated tablets or capsules for oral administration. Examples of the sulfones which enhance the absorption of heparin through mucous membranes are those of the formula $R_1R_2SO_2$ where R_1 and R_2 are alkyl, alkylene, aralkyl, or together form with the sulfur atom a saturated or unsaturated five or six membered ring such as in sulfolane and sulfolene. R_1 and R_2 may be the same or may be different.

The fatty alcohols of chain length C_{14} to C_{24} are exemplified by cetyl alcohol (C_{16}), stearyl alcohol (C_{18}), oleyl alcohol (C_{18}), arachidyl alcohol (C_{20}), behenyl alcohol (C_{22}) and mixtures thereof which are obtainable, for example, by reduction of corresponding fatty acids. The fatty acids themselves are ineffective. The fatty alcohols of the chain length specified may either be saturated or unsaturated, e.g., oleyl alcohol. They possess good emulsifying properties. Further, it has been found that in general, the longer the chain length of the fatty alcohol, the better the degree of enhancement of the heparin composition with respect to sustained time of absorption of the anticoagulant activity.

In anticoagulant therapy, the desired therapeutic dosage is the amount of heparin which is sufficient to double blood clotting time. For example, sufficient of the composition is administered orally in one or more tablets or capsules to double the blood clotting time as determined on a sample of withdrawn blood of the particular species of mammal undergoing treatment. If the therapeutic level is to be maintained the dosage is repeated at intervals as deemed necessary. Representative therapeutic dosages may contain, for example, 50 to 100 mg. of heparin having an activity of 100 anticoagulant μ/mg., and from 0.5 to 10 grams of the selected sulfone per 100 mg. of heparin. From 0.1 to 2 grams of fatty alcohol may be included. If water is included in the composition, the amount can vary over wide limits, e.g., from 0 to 90%.

The total daily unit of heparin for a mammal, such as a dog, may,be 50 to 1,000 mg. (based on heparin having an activity of 100 μ/mg.) in combination with 0.5 to 10 grams of the sulfone and, if desired, 0.1 to 10 grams of the fatty alcohol. Because of the well-known instability of heparin in acids, standard enteric encapsulation procedure is used to provide an enteric capsule which when swallowed will survive the acid medium of the stomach and will be dissolved in the alkaline medium of the intestine. As an example of this mode of administration, the dosage unit sufficient to double blood clotting time is given in the form of one or more enteric-coated gelatin capsules or tablets.

Example 1: 25 grams of diethyl sulfone (MP 73°C.) were dissolved in 100 ml. of water to provide a 25 gram percent solution which was adjusted by NaOH addition to a pH of 7.4. 100 mg. of heparin was then dissolved in 4 ml. of this solution. The resulting solution can be administered by injection or to mucous membranes by known routes or may be encapsulated for oral administration. For the latter, the amount of water can be decreased or omitted entirely.

Example 2: (a) 25 grams of n-propylsulfone (MP 28° to 29°C.) is mixed with 50 ml. of water and adjusted to pH 7.4 as in Example 1. From 2 to 4 ml. of the resulting suspension is mixed with 100 mg. of heparin.

(b) For encapsulation, the water in (a) may be omitted. Thus, 100 mg. of heparin are mixed with 2 grams of substantially neutral di-n-propyl sulfone warmed to liquid form. The resulting suspension is cooled to solid form, pressed into a tablet, or encapsulated in gelatin, following which the capsules are given a standard enteric coating, for example, with cellulose acetate phthalate.

VASODILATORS

Dihydrothienopyrimidines

Compounds having cardiovascular and sedative activities have been prepared by *G. Ohnacker and E. Woitun; U.S. Patent 3,318,883; May 9, 1967; assigned to Boehringer Ingelheim GmbH, Germany.* The cardiovascular activity includes both coronary vascular dilating and peripheral vascular dilating activities. These compounds are dihydrothieno[3,2-d]pyrimidines having the fomula

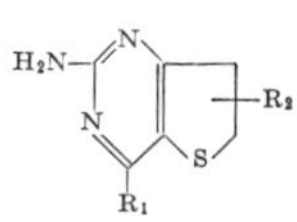

where R_1 is lower alkoxy-lower alkoxy, lower alkyl-mercapto or

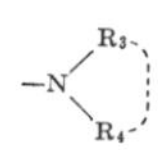

where R_3 is hydrogen, amino, lower alkyl, hydroxy-lower alkyl, lower alkoxy-lower alkyl, di(lower alkyl) amino-lower alkyl, lower alkenyl, benzyl or cyclohexyl and R_4 is hydrogen, lower alkyl or hydroxy-lower alkyl, and R_3 and R_4, together with each other and the adjacent nitrogen atom, form a basic heterocycle selected from morpholino, piperidino, pyrrolidino, 2-methyl-morpholino and N'-methyl-piperazino, and R_2 is hydrogen or methyl, and their nontoxic, pharmacologically acceptable acid addition salts. These compounds are prepared by reacting, for example, 2-amino-4-chlorodihydrothieno[3,2-d]pyrimidine with morpholine to form 2-amino-4-morpholinodihydrothieno[3,2-d]pyrimidine.

For pharmacological purposes, these compounds may be administered perorally or parenterally as active ingredients in customary dosage unit compositions. One dosage unit of these compounds is 10 to 200 mg., preferably 20 to 100 mg. Typical examples of such dosage unit compositions are tablets, coated pills, hypodermic solutions, rectal suppositories, suspensions or solutions adapted for administration per os, gelatin capsules, wafer capsules and the like. The following examples illustrate tablet dosage units comprising these compounds as active ingredients. The parts are parts by weight unless otherwise specified.

Example 1: Coated Pills – The pill cores are compounded from the following ingredients:

	Parts
2-amino-4-morpholinodihydrothieno[3,2-d] pyrimidine	25.0
Secondary calcium phosphate	75.0
Cornstarch	21.0
Gelatin	4.0
Talcum	4.0
Magnesium stearate	1.0
Total	130.0

The dihydrothieno-pyrimidine compound, the calcium phosphate and the cornstarch are admixed with each other, and the mixture is moistened with an aqueous 14% solution of the gelatin. The moist mixture is granulated by passing it through a 1.5 mm. mesh screen. The moist granulate is dried at 40°C. and is again passed through the screen. The dry granulate is admixed with the talcum and the magnesium stearate, and the mixture is pressed into 130 mg. tablets, which are then provided with a coating consisting essentially of sugar and talcum. The coated pills are then polished with beeswax. Each pill weighs 200 mg. and contains 25 mg. of the active ingredient.

Example 2: Tablets – The tablets are compounded from the following ingredients:

	Parts
2-amino-4-piperidino-7-methyldihydrothieno[3,2-d]-pyrimidine	100.0
Lactose	80.0
Potato starch, undried	10.0
Potato starch, dried	16.0
Polyvinylpyrrolidone	10.0
Colloidal silicic acid	2.0
Magnesium stearate	2.0
Total	220.0

The dihydrothieno-pyrimidine compound, the lactose and dried potato starch are admixed with each other, and the mixture is moistened with a 20% aqueous solution of the polyvinylpyrrolidone. The moistened mixture is then granulated by passing it through a 1.5 mm. mesh screen, and the moist granulate is dried at 40°C. The dry granulate is once again passed through the screen, and then the remainder of the ingredients are added and thoroughly admixed. The resulting mixture is pressed into tablets each weighing 220 mg. Each tablet contains 100 mg. of the active ingredient.

2-Oxodihydrofurylbenzo[b]furans

Furan derivatives having therapeutic properties have been prepared by *J. Schmitt; U.S. Patent 3,355,463; November 28, 1967; assigned to Etablissements Clin-Byla, France*. These are compounds having the formula:

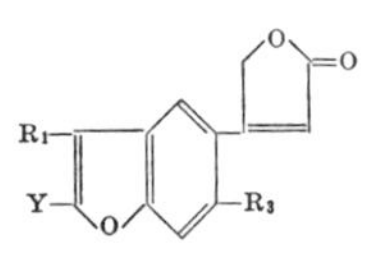

where R_1 is a lower alkyl, R_3 is hydrogen or lower alkoxy and Y is

$$R_2\text{–}\underset{\underset{\displaystyle O}{\|}}{C}\text{–} \quad \text{or} \quad R_2\text{–}\underset{\underset{\displaystyle OR_4}{|}}{CH}\text{–}$$

in which R_2 is a lower alkyl, an unsubstituted phenyl or a phenyl having in one or more substitution positions, a hydroxyl, a lower aliphatic ester, or a lower alkoxy, (including a tertiary amino-substituted alkoxy) and R_4 is hydrogen, a lower alkyl or a mono- or di-carboxylic acyl.

These compounds possess one or more of the following three types of therapeutic activity, coronary-dilatant, cardiotonic or hypotensive activity. The degree and type of activity for a particular compound depend upon the nature of the substituents. One may prepare these compounds by starting from p-methoxyphenylbutenolide, i.e., 4-(4-methoxyphenyl)-2-oxo-2,5-dihydrofuran, or from the corresponding lower alkoxy derivatives, by a three step process.

The first step gives a phenolic ketone by reaction of an acid halide, particularly the chloride, with the alkoxyphenylbutenolide in the presence of a Friedel-Crafts type of catalyst such as aluminum chloride, preferably in an appropriate diluent such as methylene chloride, dichlorethane or nitrobenzene, or alternatively in the presence of an excess of the acid halide used as the reactant. The reaction temperature may vary between room temperature and 70°C.; the time taken does not normally exceed 10 hours.

The second step consists of the condensation of the phenolic ketone with a halomethyl ketone. The reaction may be carried out in a diluent, particularly dimethyl formamide, in the presence of an alkali carbonate, for example potassium carbonate; the dimethyl formamide solubilizes the alkali salts of hydroxy ketones and permits the reaction to take place in a homogeneous medium. One may operate at temperatures between room temperature and 50°C.

The third step, the cyclization, takes place on more or less prolonged heating, e.g., on a water bath, in the presence of a mineral acid reagent, for example hydrochloric acid. One may operate without a diluent, but preferably, with a diluent such as ethyl alcohol, acetic acid or dimethyl formamide. There is often an advantage in not isolating the intermediates and consequently directly acidifying the solution containing them to cause their cyclization, with the formation of a benzofuran ring system.

These compounds may be used in therapeutic dosage units of 5 to 500 mg. in the form of tablets or in the form of a solution for intravenal or intramuscular injection (in cases where the selected compound is soluble in a pharmaceutically acceptable solvent). Examples of suitable pharmaceutical tablets are: Formulation 1 – 50 mg. of 2-(1-succinyloxyethyl)-3-methyl-5-(2-oxo-2,5-dihydro-4-furyl)benzo[b] furan and pharmaceutical excipient sufficient for a tablet. Formulation 2 – 250 mg. of [2-(3,4-dimethoxyphenyl)hydroxymethyl] -3-ethyl-5-(2-oxo-2,5-dihydro-4-furyl)benzo[b] furan and pharmaceutical excipient sufficient for a tablet.

The tablets are prepared according to the usual methods of double compression or granulation with the help of an aqueous solution of a gum or a nonaqueous solvent such as ethyl alcohol. The excipients used may be, for example, starch, talc, gum arabic, magnesium stearate or carboxymethylcellulose. The tablets may be rendered enteric by glutinization or covering with a substance resistant to the action of gastric juice such as cellulose acetophthalate with a view to preventing an action of stomach hydrochloric acid on the active principle or avoiding possible gastric disorders. The tablets may be enveloped in a sugar or other coating, which is opaque and may be colored.

DIURETICS

Substituted Sulfamylbenzoic Acids

Diuretic and saluretic preparations in dosage unit form, containing 3-butylamino-4-phenoxy-5-sulfamylbenzoic acid or a salt thereof as the active component are disclosed by *P.W. Feit; U.S. Patent 3,634,583; January 11, 1972; assigned to Lovens Kemiske Fabrik Produktionsaktieselskab, Denmark.* The dose of the diuretic is between 0.1 and 10 mg. calculated as the free acid, and may be combined with a hypotenser.

3-Butylamino-4-phenoxy-5-sulfamylbenzoic acid possesses a favorable diuretic and saluretic activity. As far as the saluretic effect is concerned, the compound causes, in particular, an excretion of sodium and of chlorine in approximately equivalent proportions, while the excretion of the potassium ion remains substantially normal, or is only slightly increased. 3-Butylamino-4-phenoxy-5-sulfamylbenzoic acid may be prepared, for example, by 3-amino-4-phenoxy-5-sulfamylbenzoic acid being butylated at the N-atom in the 3-position.

Example 1: Tablets containing free 3-butylamino-4-phenoxy-5-sulfamylbenzoic acid are as follows.

Ingredients	Grams
3-Butylamino-4-phenoxy-5-sulfamylbenzoic acid	3
Cornstarch	250
Lactose	250
Talc	25

The ingredients were mixed and screened through a 20 mesh per linear inch sieve and subsequently treated with an aqueous solution of gelatin (4%) in sufficient amount to form a granulate. The granulate was dried and broken on a 16 mesh per linear inch sieve. After addition of talc, the granulate was compressed into tablets of 180 mg. each, using 8 mm. punches and dies, to obtain 3,000 tablets, each containing 1 mg. of the free 3-butylamino-4-phenoxy-5-sulfamylbenzoic acid.

The effect of the tablets was tested as follows. Nine healthy persons each received 1 tablet corresponding to 1 mg. of the drug, after which the urinary excretion was observed for 24 hours. The average effect appears in the following table, in which is also tabulated the corresponding effects after administering fursemide in the dose of 1 tablet containing 40 mg. fursemide to the same persons.

	Hours after administration											
	Sodium (meq.)			Chloride (meq.)			Volume (ml.)			Potassium (meq.)		
Treatment	0-6	6-24	0-24	0-6	6-24	0-24	0-6	6-24	0-24	0-6	6-24	0-24
Tablets active substance	201	48	249	236	40	276	1,784	577	2,361	47	34	81
Fursemide tablets ~40 mg. active substance	215	45	260	243	33	276	1,842	587	2,429	51	29	80
Controls	57	94	151	66	80	146	387	607	994	32	33	65

Example 2: Tablets containing the potassium salt of 3-butylamino-4-phenoxy-5-sulfamylbenzoic acid are as follows.

Ingredients	Grams
3-Butylamino-4-phenoxy-5-sulfamylbenzoic acid as the potassium salt	6
Lactose	650
Cornstarch	844

The potassium salt was mixed with the other ingredients and granulated after moistening with a 10% aqueous solution of polyvinylpyrrolidone. The granulate was dried and broken on a 16 mesh per linear inch sieve. After addition of 100 grams of talc and 10 grams of magnesium stearate, and mixing, the mixture was compressed into tablets, using 10 mm. punches and dies, yielding 250 mg. tablets, each containing active substance corresponding to 1 mg. of 3-butylamino-4-phenoxy-5-sulfamylbenzoic acid.

Gradual Release Diuretic Tablets

E.A. Hotko and L. Lachman; U.S. Patent 3,456,049; July 15, 1969; assigned to Ciba Corporation have found a solid pharmaceutical excipient comprising: (a) a fatty substance, (b) alginic acid, and (c) a granulating liquid, which is suitable for pharmaceutical compositions containing at least one readily soluble component, e.g., a potassium salt, and one slightly soluble component, e.g., a diuretic benzothiadiazine.

The fatty substances used in the preparations are, for example, fats, preferably vegetable fats, or their partly or entirely hydrogenated forms; fatty acids as well as their alkaline earth and earth metal salts; natural and synthetic waxes; fatty alcohols, as well as their esters; fatty acid amides; and mixtures of these substances. These fatty substances preferably should melt in the range between 40° and 100°C. The alginic acid used is a colloidal substance, obtained from seaweeds and containing as the main constituents mannuronic and galuronic acid. It may be used in its various marketed forms.

The granulating liquid is such that forms a film insoluble in an acidic medium but soluble in an alkaline medium, such as an acidic cellulose ester, preferably a cellulose acetate phthalate or a salt or ester thereof. Other granulating liquids used are for example, aqueous solutions of a salt of carboxymethylcellulose or of alginic acid. The granulating liquid, however, may also be a solvent of the above solids only, which latter may be mixed together with the fatty substance and the alginic acid. Especially valuable are compositions that contain per unit doses a therapeutically acceptable potassium salt, preferably dipotassium tartrate or tripotassium citrate, equivalent to 500 to 1,000 mg. of potassium chloride, together with about:

(a) 10 to 50 mg. of 6-chloro-7-sulfamyl-2H-3,4-dihydro-1,2,4-benzothiadiazine-1,1-dioxide,
(b) 10 to 50 mg. of 6-trifluoromethyl-7-sulfamyl-2H-3,4-dihydro-1,2,4-benzothiadiazine-1,1-dioxide,
(c) 0.1 to 0.5 mg. of 3-cyclopentylmethyl-6-chloro-7-sulfamyl-2H-3,4-dihydro-1,2,4-benzothiadiazine-1,1-dioxide,
(d) 1.0 to 5.0 mg. of 3-(5-norbornenyl-2)-6-chloro-7-sulfamyl-2H-3,4-dihydro-1,2,4-benzothiadiazine-1,1-dioxide,
(e) 1.0 to 5.0 mg. of 2-methyl-3-chloromethyl-6-chloro-7-sulfamyl-2H-3,4-dihydro-1,2,4-benzothiadiazine-1,1-dioxide,
(f) 1.0 to 5.0 mg. of 3-dichloromethyl-6-chloro-7-sulfamyl-2H-3,4-dihydro-1,2,4-benzothiadiazine-1,1-dioxide,
(g) 1.0 to 5.0 mg. of 3-benzyl-6-trifluoromethyl-7-sulfamyl-2H-3,4-dihydro-1,2,4-benzothiadiazine-1,1-dioxide,
(h) 1.0 to 5.0 mg. of 2-methyl-3-(2,2,2-trifluoroethylmercaptomethyl)-6-chloro-7-sulfamyl-2H-3,4-dihydro-1,2,4-benzothiadiazine-1,1-dioxide,

both active components of which are embedded in a mixture comprising relative to the potassium salt 5 to 15% of the fatty substance, 3 to 15% of alginic acid and 5 to 10% of cellulose acetate phthalate or one of the above shown derivatives thereof. Following are working examples, illustrative of tablet formation. Unless otherwise indicated, all parts are by weight. All sieve sizes are U.S. Standard sieve sizes.

Example 1: Material for 8,000 tablets consists of the following ingredients.

	Grams
Mixture of hydrogenated vegetable oil melting at 60°C., particle size 325 to 400 mesh (Sterotex)	580.0

(continued)

	Grams
Alginic acid (purified grade having less than 3% ignition residue) 50 to 100 mesh	174.0
Cellulose acetate phthalate	500.0
Tripotassium citrate monohydrate, 60 to 200 mesh	5,800.0
6-Chloro-7-sulfamyl-2H-3,4-dihydro-1,2,4-benzothiadiazine-1,1-dioxide, 60 to 100 mesh	200.0
Anydrous ethanol	750.0
Anhydrous acetone	750.0

The powders, except the cellulose acetate phthalate, are screened through a 20 mesh screen and mixed in a mixer for 30 minutes. A 25% solution of the cellulose acetate phthalate in a 1:1 mixture of anhydrous ethanol and acetone is added to the powder mixture to form a granulate. After a period of mixing the wet mass is screened through a 10 mesh screen and dried in a circulating hot air oven. The dry granulate is screened again through a 10 mesh screen and compressed on a suitable tablet press into tablets each weighing 906 mg. The substances used in the following example have the analogous particle size and quality respectively.

Example 2: Material for 6,000 tablets consists of the following ingredients.

	Grams
Sterotex	238.5
Alginic acid	143.0
Cellulose acetate phthalate	500.0
Dipotassium tartrate hemihydrate	4,770.0
6-Chloro-7-sulfamyl-2H-3,4-dihydro-1,2,4-benzothiadiazine-1,1-dioxide	150.0
Anhydrous ethanol, q.s.	
Anhydrous acetone, q.s.	

The procedure is the same as described in Example 1.

CHOLESTEROL DERIVATIVES FOR HYPERCHOLESTEREMIA

It was found by *K. Irmscher, K. Brückner, J. Krämer, K.-H. Bork, R. Watzel and H.-O. Voge; U.S. Patent 3,326,758; June 20, 1967; assigned to E. Merck AG, Germany* that certain cholesterol derivatives substituted by nitrogen and/or oxygen in the side chain attached to the 17-position, have a retarding effect on the physiological synthesis of cholesterol. These compounds are also physiologically compatible, and are suitable for the treatment of hypercholesteremia. These compounds have the following formula:

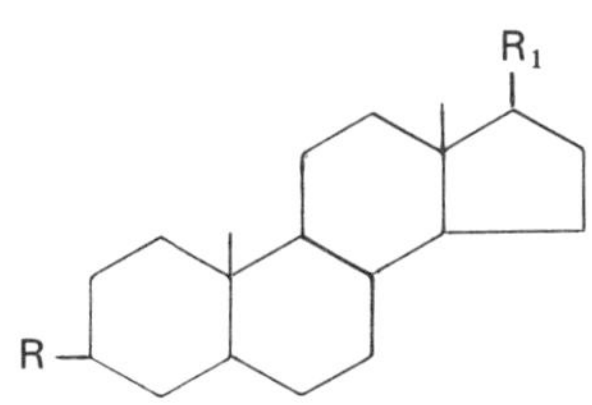

and include its 5-dehydro derivatives and its acid-addition salts where: R is any halo, preferably chloro, hydroxy-O-alkyl of 1 to 4 carbon atoms or O-acyl having 1 to 18 carbon atoms, R_1 represents any of the following:

$-CH(CH_3)-(CH_2)_{n_1}-N(R_3)-R_2$; 6 to 10 carbons

$-CH(CH_3)-(CH_2)_{n_2}-O-R_4$ 6 or 7 carbons

$$\begin{matrix} CH_3 \\ | \\ -N-(CH_2)_2-R_5, \end{matrix} \qquad \begin{matrix} CH_3 \qquad\quad R_3 \\ | \qquad\qquad | \\ -N-(CH_2)_2-N-CH_2-(CH_3)_2, \end{matrix}$$

$$\begin{matrix} CH_3 \\ | \\ -N-(CH_2)_2-O-CH-(CH_3)_2, \end{matrix} \qquad -O-(CH_2)_{n_3}-CH-(CH_3)_2,$$

$$\begin{matrix} R_3 \\ | \\ -O-(CH_2)_{n_3}-N-R_6 \end{matrix}$$

4 to 7 carbons

or

$$-O-(CH_2)_2-O-CH-(CH_3)_2$$

R_2 is methyl, ethyl, isopropyl, isobutyl, isopentyl, 1-methylpropyl, 1-ethylpropyl, 2-methylbutyl or 2-ethylbutyl; R_3 is hydrogen, methyl or ethyl; R_4 is isopropyl, isobutyl, isopentyl or dimethylaminoethyl; R_5 is isopropyl, isobutyl, 1-methylpropyl or 1-ethylpropyl; R_6 is methyl, ethyl or isopropyl; n_1 is 0, 1, 2 or 3; n_2 is 0, 1 or 2; and n_3 is 2 or 3; and where a double bond can occur in the 5-position. These compounds are prepared by numerous synthetic routes as used in steroid chemistry. The preferred compounds for this therapeutic use are:

22-oxa-25-aza-cholesterol
22-aza-cholestane-3β-ol
20-oxa-21,24-bis-nor-25-aza-cholesterol
3β-chloro-22-oxa-25-aza-5-cholestene
20-aza-24-oxa-cholestane-3β-ol
20-aza-24-oxa-cholesterol
20-oxa-21-nor-25-aza-cholestane-3β-ol
20-aza-cholestane-3β-ol
N-ethyl-26-nor-24-aza-cholestane-3β-ol
20-oxa-21,24-bis-nor-cholestane-3β-ol
22-oxa-24-nor-cholestane-3β-ol
23-oxa-24-nor-cholestane-3β-ol
22-aza-24-nor-cholestane-3β-ol
24-nor-25-aza-cholestane-3β-ol

These compounds can be employed in admixture with the usual pharmaceutical carriers. As carriers, there can be used those organic and inorganic substances which are suitable for parenteral or enteral application and which do not react with the compounds, as for example, water, vegetable oils, polyethylene glycol, gelatin, lactose, starch, magnesium stearate, talcum, etc. For enteral application, tablets, dragees or solutions can be used which can be sterilized if necessary or mixed with ancillary materials such as preservatives, stabilizers or wetting agents, or with salts for influencing the osmotic pressure, or with buffer substances. These compounds are preferably used in oral dosage units of 2 to 300 mg., but it is also possible to administer them parenterally when necessary. In the following examples the formulations relate to solid pharmaceutical compositions.

Example 1: Tablets – Each tablet contains the following ingredients.

	Milligrams
20-aza-24-oxa-cholestanol	50
Lactose	120
Cornstarch	30
Talc	2

Example 2: Dragees – The compressed cores contain the following ingredients.

	Milligrams
N-ethyl-22-aza-24-nor-cholesterol	40
Lactose	80
Potato starch	10

The cores were then coated, according to conventional methods, with a mixture of wheat starch, sugar, talc and tragacanth.

Example 3: Tablets – The following ingredients were mixed and stamped into 10,000 tablets so that the dosage unit is 10 mg./tablet.

	Kilograms
22-oxa-25-aza-cholestanol	0.100
Lactose	0.500
Cornstarch	0.200
Talc	0.150
Magnesium stearate	0.050

STEROIDAL HORMONES

ESTROGEN DEFICIENCY THERAPY

17-Ethynyl-$\Delta^{1,4}$-Androstadiene-11β,17β-Diol-3-one

It was found by *P. Destouches; U.S. Patent 3,308,025; March 7, 1967; assigned to Roussel-Uclaf, SA, France* that 17α-ethynyl-$\Delta^{1,4}$-androstadiene-11β,17β-diol-3-one in small doses of from 0.5 to 5 mg. per day has an excellent estrogenic effect in human females, especially on oral administration. This effect is completely unexpected since the compound is practically devoid of estrogenic activity when administered to laboratory animals at daily dosages of up to 200 mg. per kilogram of body weight.

17α-ethynyl-$\Delta^{1,4}$-androstadiene-11β,17β-diol-3-one is described in U.S. Patent 3,127,314, and corresponds to the formula:

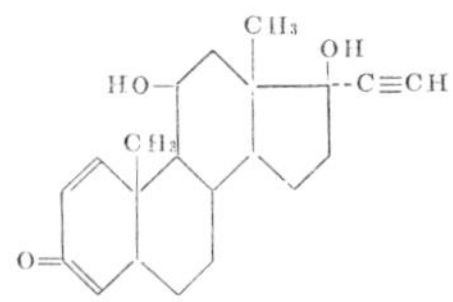

The compound is prepared by direct ethynylation of $\Delta^{1,4}$-androstadiene-3,11,17-trione without protection of the 3-keto group. The resulting 17-ethynyl-$\Delta^{1,4}$-androstadiene-17-ol-3,11-dione is converted into its 3-mono-semicarbazone, which is reduced by a mixed hydride of boron and an alkali metal or an alkaline earth metal, such as the borohydrides of lithium, sodium, potassium, or calcium. The 3-semicarbazone of 17α-ethynyl-$\Delta^{1,4}$-androstadiene-11β,17β-diol-3-one is obtained which is converted, by treatment with pyruvic acid, into 17α-ethynyl-$\Delta^{1,4}$-androstadiene-11β,17β-diol-3-one, the active estrogenic agent.

The starting material, the $\Delta^{1,4}$-androstadiene-3,11,17-trione, is readily available by treating Δ^{1}-dehydrocortisone with sodium bismuthate according to Hershberg et al (*J. Am. Chem. Soc.*), 1955, 77, 4781-4784.

Acetylene is attached to $\Delta^{1,4}$-androstadiene-3,11,17-trione according to known methods in the presence of alcoholates or amides of alkali metals or alkaline earth metals such as potassium, lithium or calcium, in an inert solvent. It is also possible to carry out the process in the presence of liquid ammonia which, upon dissolving the alkali metals, produces their amides in situ. Upon completion of the reaction, the mixture is acidified and 11-keto-17α-ethynyl-$\Delta^{1,4}$-androstadienolone is extracted by means of a solvent and purified by recrystallization. To produce the corresponding 11β-hydroxylated compound, the 3-monosemicarbazone of the 3,11-diketone is prepared and is reduced in a solvent, preferably in aqueous tetrahydrofuran.

The active compound is administered orally in the form of tablets, sugar coated pills, powders, solutions, emulsions, suspensions, or other known preparations. For tablets, sugar-coated pills and other solid forms of preparation, conventional solubilizing, binding, lubricating, disintegrating agents and other adjuvants may be used such as sugar, lactose, sorbitol, talc, starch, pectin, gelatin, gum arabic, methylcellulose, carboxymethylcellulose, yeast extracts, agar, calcium sulfate, calcium carbonate, kaolin, stearic acid, magnesium stearate, etc. The content of the active compound in such preparations may vary. Preferably the preparation should not contain less than 0.5% of the active agent. The optimum dose may vary between 0.5 and 5% by weight of the preparation.

Example 1: Preparation of Tablets – 50 g. of 17α-ethynyl-$\Delta^{1,4}$-androstadiene-11β, 17β-diol-3-one are thoroughly mixed with 26.60 g. of sugar, 957.6 g. of lactose, and 332.5 g. of starch, 13.30 g. of gelatin moistened with water, and stirred so as to obtain a solid paste, which is granulated. The resulting granules are dried in a drying oven, ground and after the addition of 20 g. of magnesium stearate, and 100 g. of talc are compressed to tablets, each weighing 150 mg. and containing 5 mg. of the active compound.

Example 2: Preparation of Tablets – 500 g. of 17α-ethynyl-$\Delta^{1,4}$-androstadiene-11β, 17β-diol-3-one, 4,000 g. of sugar, 16,100 g. of lactose, and 4,000 g. of starch are thoroughly mixed, moistened with water, and stirred to yield a solid paste, which is granulated. The resulting granules obtained are dried in a drying oven, ground and, after the addition of 400 g. of magnesium stearate, are compressed to tablets each weighing 100 mg. and containing 2 mg. of the active compound.

Clinical tests of patients undergoing menopause, suffering from neurovegetative disturbances, demonstrated that a 5 mg. tablet of 17α-ethynyl-$\Delta^{1,4}$-androstadiene-11β, 17β-diol-3-one effected relief of the symptoms and caused a change in the appearance of vaginal smears. This relief was continued by a regime of one 5 mg. tablet every five to seven days. Daily dosage of a 5 mg. tablet over a period of 15 days was likewise well tolerated with good results.

Sulfoconjugated Neutral Steriods

G.W. Oertel and K. Munzel; U.S. Patent 3,600,495; August 17, 1971; assigned to Hoffmann-La Roche Inc. have found that hormone imbalance can be favorably influenced by the oral administration of sulfoconjugated neutral steroids in gastric-juice-resistant form. This form of administration ensures a complete and physiological absorption of these conjugates by the organism.

In this manner, the disturbed hormonal equilibrium is returned to normal and the consequences of the hormone imbalance are reduced. This is achieved by the natural metabolic transformation of the sulfoconjugated neutral steroids. The preferred treatment is with a tablet dosage form characterized by a medicament nucleus containing a sulfoconjugated neutral steroid which is coated with a gastric-juice-resistant layer. As used here, the sulfoconjugated neutral steroids mean nonphenolic steroids which are esterified with sulfuric acid or with sulfuric acid derivatives, i.e., the sulfates or sulfatides of the steroids. Such nonphenolic steroids are, for example, cholesterol, C_{21}-steroids such as pregnenolone, desoxycorticosterone, progesterone (in enol form), C_{19}-steroids such as dehydro-epi-androsterone, testosterone and C_{18}-steroids such as 19-nortestosterone.

Preferred compounds are pregnenolone and dehydro-epi-androsterone in the form of the sulfate or sulfatide. Sulfates as used here include both the acidic sulfates and the mixed salts of sulfuric acid with a nontoxic pharmaceutically acceptable cation such as ammonium, sodium, potassium and calcium. In the case of the sulfatides, the alcoholic part of the ester must be derived from a nontoxic pharmaceutically acceptable monovalent or polyvalent alcohol, e.g., from glycerine or higher fatty alcohols such as palmityl or stearyl alcohol.

The administration of this composition in unit dosage form is controlled by the particular needs of the patients and by the symptoms and disease being treated as well as by the specific active substance being used. In one example, a dosage of between about 5 mg. and about 30 mg. of dehydro-epi-androsterone 3-sulfate per day has proven efficacious for influencing menopausal symptoms in controlled trial using dehydro-epi-androsterone-3-sulfate in a dosage of between 10 and 20 mg. per day. The results are given in the table below.

	Before treatment				First month				Second month				Third month			
Symptoms	Severe	Med.	Mild	ϕ	Severe	Med.	Mild	ϕ	Severe	Med.	Mild	ϕ	Severe	Med.	Mild	ϕ
Flush	41	1	6	3	12	2	27	10	9	3	16	15	7	2	19	15
Anxiety	22	0	13	16	7	3	18	23	3	3	11	26	4	2	12	25
Depression	10	1	22	18	6	1	22	31	2	1	9	31	2	0	8	33
Nervousness	23	0	17	11	10	1	22	18	8	2	17	16	7	2	13	21
Irritability	10	3	12	26	7	5	12	27	7	2	10	24	4	2	8	29
Sleeplessness	24	1	14	12	7	0	25	19	2	3	18	20	5	0	18	20
Transpiration	24	4	12	11	8	2	23	18	7	2	14	20	4	3	13	23
Headaches	13	1	11	26	5	1	11	34	2	1	10	30	3	1	6	33
Dizziness	9	16	0	26	1	2	15	33	3	1	8	31	2	1	8	32
Tachycardia	13	1	17	20	3	0	20	28	3	1	8	31	4	0	8	31
Total	189	28	124	169	66	17	186	241	46	19	121	244	42	13	113	262
Women	51				51				43				43			
Percent	37.0	5.5	24.3	33.2	12.9	3.3	36.5	47.3	10.7	4.4	28.1	56.8	9.8	3.0	26.3	60.9

The manufacture of the unit dosage form is achieved by conventional methods using conventional equipment as shown in the following example.

Example: Dragee nuclei of 75 mg. weight and a diameter of 6 mm. containing 10.0 mg. of sodium dehydro-epi-androsterone sulfate, 50.00 mg. of lactose, 13.50 mg. of cornstarch, 1.35 mg. of talc and 0.15 mg. of magnesium stearate per nucleus are formed and coated with a gastric-juice-resistant lacquer layer by using a lacquer solution consisting of 10 parts by weight of cellulose acetate phthalate, 3 parts by weight of triacetin, 10 parts by weight of ethanol and 77 parts by weight of methylene chloride. A sufficient resistance to gastric juices is ensured by application of about 25 layers. The coating amounts to about 10 mg. per nucleus. The lacquered nuclei obtained are dried at about 37°C. for 24 to 36 hours and then dredged until they have an end weight of about 150 mg.

FERTILITY CONTROL STEROLS

Hormone-Containing Veterinary Bolus

A bolus which remains in the rumeno-reticular portions of a ruminant's stomach for a fixed time has been developed by *J.C. Siegrist and M. Katz; U.S. Patent 3,535,419; October 20, 1970; assigned to Syntex Corporation, Panama.* These compositions release the therapeutic agent at a fixed rate over an extended but finite period of time; i.e., for a known and predetermined period of time which is longer than that for which the drug would be effective if administered via the usual oral route. Moreover, these compositions fully disintegrate during this time, thus permitting repeated use.

Any therapeutic agent which in veterinary practice can be administered orally may be incorporated in these compositions. Typical of these are vitamins, anthelmintics, anti-inflammatory agents, estrogenic hormones, antibloat agents, antibiotics and especially progestational agents in the synchronization of estrus.

The compositions will comprise as a first major component, one or more highly water-insoluble solid wax, fat, oil, fatty acid amide, fatty acid ester, fatty amide alcohol, or polymer; as a second major component, a high-density, nontoxic metal derivative; and as a third major component, the particular therapeutic agent to be administered. To this may be added various adjuncts to aid in processing or to modify the properties of the principal components. Thus with oils, substances such as aluminum stearate may be added to cause gelling so as to obtain a solid material.

The rate of release of the therapeutic agent and disintegration of the composition is inversely proportional, within limits, to the pressure of compression. Within the range of 100 to 5,000 lbs./in.^{2} the rate of disintegration remains relatively constant for a given pressure, however, the higher the pressure, the slower the rate. For each formulation, there is a pressure over which further increases in pressure fail to cause significant changes in the disintegration rate. Below certain pressures, insufficient cohesion is obtained and accelerated rates of disintegration are observed. A preferred pressure is in the range of from 1,500 to 4,000 lbs./in.^{2}.

The rate of release is also dependent upon the nature of the first component. Thus the use of a very high hydrophobic substance such as carnauba wax produces an extremely long-lasting composition, e.g., in the order of magnitude of 100 days, depending upon the degree of compression. Other materials, such as glyceryl monostearate, have faster rates of disintegration, e.g., 10 g. at a compression of about 4,000 lbs./in.^{2} provides a composition lasting about 30 days.

Example 1:

Ingredient	Amount, G.
Glyceryl monostearate	345
Polyethylene glycol (Carbowax 4000)	55
Barium sulfate	592
6-chloro-17α-acetoxy-$\Delta^{4,6}$-pregnadiene-3,20-dione	8

The glyceryl monostearate and polyethylene glycol are combined and melted. The 6-chloro-17α-acetoxy-$\Delta^{4,6}$-pregnadiene-3,20-dione is added and mixed and the resulting melt is employed to granulate the barium sulfate. The cooled mass is screened and 25 g. portions are compressed in a hydraulic press using a punch and die of 0.5 inch radius and 1 inch height at a pressure of 4,000 lbs./in.^{2}. There are thus obtained 40 cylinders having a density of approximately 1.9 g./cm.^{3} and containing 200 mg. of 6-chloro-17α-acetoxy-$\Delta^{4,6}$-pregnadiene-3,20-dione. Each cylinder, upon oral administration to an adult normal cow, will lodge in the rumen or reticulum and release approximately 10 mg. of steroid per day for 20 days. Estrus will follow shortly thereafter.

Example 2: Individual batches were prepared in accordance with the procedure of Example 1, using however the following proportions:

Ingredient	A	B	C
Glyceryl monostearate	160	240	320
Polyethylene glycol (Carbowax 4000)	240	160	80
Barium sulfate	600	600	600
6-chloro-17α-acetoxy-$\Delta^{4,6}$-pregnadiene-3,20-dione	7.2	7.2	7.2

These compositions were administered to two fistulated cows and were removed via the fistula and examined periodically. A had a disintegration rate of 7.20 g./day and released 85 mg. of steroid/day for 3 to 4 days; B a disintegration rate of 3.00 g./day and released 46 mg. of steroid/day for 8 to 9 days; C a disintegration rate of 1.54 g./day and released 11 mg. of steroid/day for 16 days. All compositions remained in the rumeno-recticular portions of the stomach until totally disintegrated.

Gonadotropin Antigens

A method has been found by *D. Dingwall; U.S. Patent 3,548,051; December 15, 1970; assigned to Organon Inc.* for tabletting erythrocytes used in the immunochemical determination of antigens. This is particularly useful for pregnancy tests using erythrocytes sensitized with human chorionic gonadotropin (HCG). The method for the preparation of erythrocytes suitable for immunochemical determinations of antigens comprises treating erythrocytes with one or more tanning agents, followed by sensitization with the antigen, and characterized in that the last stage of the sensitization is carried out in the presence of formaldehyde in a concentration below 2% (weight/volume) at a pH between 5.5 and 8. Of the thus treated erythrocytes the mechanical properties have improved to such a degree that they can be pressed to tablets, the erythrocytes having kept their usability as an auxiliary in immunochemical reactions after suspension of these tablets.

It was already known from U.S. Patent 3,096,250 to perform the sensitization of erythrocytes pretreated with Formalin in the presence of a Formalin solution, at a pH within 2 units of the isoelectric point of the antigen used. This means that when the antigen HCG with an isoelectric point of 2.98 is applied, sensitization must take place below pH 5, unlike the present method, in which good results are only obtained at a pH over 5.5. Yet another difference is that according to the known method a higher Formalin concentration, viz. of 2 to 8%, is applied, while this method uses a concentration below 2%, and preferably below 0.25% (weight/volume). Finally the presence of formaldehyde is required throughout the sensitization period according to the above patent, unlike the present method.

Further it has been found that excellent results are obtained with erythrocytes pretreated successively with Formalin and tannin. This method lends itself particularly well for the use of human chorionic gonadotrophin (HCG) as antigen. An HCG concentration of 10 to 50 IU/ml. is preferred. When very pure HCG is used, the concentration must be raised to about 200 IU/ml. During the sensitization with HCG, which process usually takes one or a few days, the formaldehyde is allowed to act upon the erythrocytes during the last 12 to 24 hours or thereabouts, but preferably during the last 15 hours. The temperature at which the action is optimal lies between 30° and 40°C., but preferably a temperature of 37°C. is applied.

Further it has been found that when HCG is used as antigen, the treatment always yields very good results at a pH of about 6.4. Finally a process has been found for the manufacture of tablets or other solid dosage unit forms of erythrocytes suitable for immunochemical determinations, characterized in that erythrocytes prepared by this method are mixed with the auxiliaries required for tabletting and the immunochemical determination, and next compressed to dosage unit forms.

The process is not limited to the sensitization of erythrocytes with HCG; it can also be applied in the sensitization with any antigen that can stand up to this treatment with formaldehyde. For immunochemical determinations both the powder of sensitized erythrocytes obtained, for example, after freeze-drying or spray-drying of the suspension, can be applied and the tablets compressed therefrom.

As examples of auxiliaries, the following are preferably applied in the preparation of tablets for the performance of pregnancy reactions. As fillers: saccharose, mannitol, lactose and ureum; as lubricants: boric acid, starch, Carbowax 4000 (polyethylene glycol) and magnesium stearate, as disintegration agents: starch and alginic acid.

Other ingredients are for instance substances used in the determination, such as phosphates, for example, monopotassium phosphate and disodium phosphate, serving as buffers for the suspension prepared from the tablets, further sodium chloride and a chelating agent, such as the disodium salt of ethylenediaminetetraacetic acid (EDTA) and albumin.

The required ingredients can be mixed in a dry condition with the treated erythrocytes before tabletting, but it is more advantageous to dissolve the soluble ingredients together and to dry them by spray-drying, followed by mixing with the treated erythrocytes to obtain a very homogeneous mixture and to prevent the erythrocytes from being damaged during the further treatment by coarse crystalline components of the auxiliaries. Further details of the process are to be found in the following examples.

Example 1: A suspension of sheep erythrocytes treated in a known manner with formalin and tannin was centrifuged and washed with a phosphate sodium chloride buffer of pH 6.4 and next incorporated in this buffer. To this mixture an equal volume was added of a solution of 50 IU HCG per ml. in a buffer of pH 6.4. This mixture was stored for 48 hours at 37°C., whereupon formaldehyde was added till a final concentration had been obtained of 0.25% (weight/volume) formaldehyde.

Next this mixture was stored for 15 hours at a temperature of 37°C., whereupon the erythrocytes were again centrifuged, washed with a physiological salt solution, incorporated as 10% v./v. suspension in a physiological salt solution containing 0.1% of bovine serum albumin, and stored for a few days at 0° to 4°C. After that the erythrocytes were centrifuged, washed with a physiological salt solution and freeze-dried in a known manner. The powder is a good reagent on HCG.

Example 2: 300 ml. of the suspension of erythrocytes of pH 6.4 according to Example 1 were treated with 300 ml. of a solution of HCG with 50 IU HCG per ml. at pH 7.6 and next with formaldehyde in a final concentration of 0.5%. After freeze-drying the powder was tabletted. The tablets obtained gave excellent results as a reagent in immunochemical pregnancy tests.

Example 3: By the method of Example 1 erythrocytes were sensitized with HCG in the presence of formaldehyde in a final concentration of 0.25%, and that for the last 24 hours at 30°C. After freeze-drying and compression tablets were obtained which gave excellent results as a reagent in an HCG test.

Contraceptive Formulations

R.C. Jones and R.A. Edgren; U.S. Patent 3,591,688; July 6, 1971; assigned to American Home Products Corporation has disclosed compositions comprising (a) a progestogen, specifically, a 3-cyclopentyloxy-13-polycarbonalkyl-17α-ethynyl-gona-3,5-diene-17β-ol, or 17-acylate mixed with (b) an estrogen, specifically, a 3-cyclopentyloxy-13-alkyl-17α-ethynyl-gona-1,3,5(10)-trien-17β-ol or a Δ^7-dehydro analog thereof. The compositions are used to prevent ovulation in warm-blooded ovulating vertebrates after oral administration, and because of their prolonged duration of activity, the compositions may be administered in simplified regimens, e.g., at once-a-week intervals.

It follows therefore that the use of the compositions will allow very simple regimens for oral contraception. For example, in vertebrates of the highest order, the initial tablet can be scheduled shortly after completion of menses, by way of illustration, on a Sunday, providing this does not go beyond day 7 of the usual 28 day cycle. The veterbrate then would be administered a unit dosage on the Sunday following the menses and on the subsequent 2 Sundays.

Because of the surprisingly long duration of activity of these compositions, protection is excellent during about the next week and menses will occur during the second week following the final tablet. The menses should be complete, in due course, so that tablet administration would be initiated again on the fourth Sunday following the initial tablet.

Thus, in this very simple regimen the composition would be administered on the same day of the week, three weeks in a row, skipped the next week and initiated again the following week. For convenience of administration an inert tablet (placebo) may be included in a tablet sequence which will have the effect of a skipped administration and increase the ease of the administration regimen. In addition to permitting administration on a much simplified basis, these compositions are highly effective and their use is accompanied by a minimum of side effects.

Example 1: A tablet for use in the prevention of ovulation is prepared from the ingredients as shown on the following page.

	Mg.
dl-3-cyclopentyloxy-13-ethyl-17α-ethynylgona-3,5-dien-17β-ol, acetate	5
dl-3-cyclopentyloxy-13-ethyl-17α-ethynylgona-1,3,5(10),7-tetraen-17β-ol	1
Carboxymethylcellulose (400 cp.)	15
Lactose powder	25
Redried cornstarch	25
Magnesium stearate powder	4
Calcium silicate powder, q.s.	
	200

The tablet is prepared by dissolving the steroids in benzene, mixing the solution with starch, drying the mix in a current of air, adding the remaining ingredients, mixing and compressing into slugs. The slugs are regranulated and compressed into tablets, each containing 5 mg. of the progestagen and 1 mg. of the estrogen.

Example 2: Tablets are prepared having the same composition as in Example 1, except that an equal weight, respectively, of the d-enantiomorph of the progestogen, d-3-cyclopentyloxy-13-ethyl-17α-ethynylgona-3,5-dien-17β-ol, acetate and of the progestogen, dl-3-cyclopentyloxy-13-ethyl-17α-ethynylgona-3,5-dien-17β-ol, are substituted for the dl-racemate of the 17-acetate. The tablets are prepared by dissolving the steroids in benzene, mixing the solution with the lactose powder and drying the mix in a current of air, then adding the carboxymethylcellulose and half the starch. With the powder thus obtained is mixed starch paste prepared from the remainder of the starch, the mixture is wet-granulated, the granules dried, the stearate added and the composition compressed into tablets.

Example 3: Formulations for prevention of ovulation are prepared in tablet form consisting of the following ingredients:

	Milligrams						
dl-3-cyclopentyloxy-13-ethyl-17β-ethynylgona-3,5-dien-17α-ol, acetate	5	9.85	2.5	2.	2.0	20.	20.0
dl-3-cyclopentyloxy-13-ethyl-17α-ethynylgona-1,3,5(10)-trien-17β-ol	0.075	0.15	1.0	0.3	5	0.	5.0
microcrystalline cellulose, N.F.	20.0	20.0	20.0	20.0	20.0	20.0	20.0
Magnesium stearate, U.S.P.	0.22	0.22	0.22	0.22	22	0.22	0.22
Lactose, U.S.P., q.s. ad	100.0	100.0	100.0	100.0	100.0	100.0	100.0

Slow Release Polylactide-Hormone Formulations

The formulations disclosed by *G.A. Boswell and R.M. Scribner; U.S. Patent 3,773,919; November 20, 1973; assigned to E.I. du Pont de Nemours and Company* are absorbable, nonirritating pharmaceutical compositions consisting of one or more drugs intimately mixed with or coated by a synthetic polylactide designed to release effective amounts of a drug over a predetermined period of time.

The formulation is of particular value for drugs that require prolonged administration or slow sustained release, for example, certain fertility-control drugs or hormones used for hormone-replacement therapy. The polylactide may be considered as a carrier or matrix for the drug and here the term "polylactide" includes both its generic meaning as a polyester derived from an α-hydroxycarboxylic acid and its specific meaning for the polymer derived from lactic acid (α-hydroxypropionic acid). These formulations permit prolonged release of drugs for a controlled period of time from the sites of parenteral administration and minimize the frequency and thus the discomfort and inconvenience associated with conventional injection formulations. Unlike conventional depot injections, these formulations undergo biodegradation in the body into normal or essentially normal metabolic products, are nonreactive toward body tissue, and can be designed, by controlling molecular weight and composition, to undergo hydrolysis and to release drug from the depot at a desired rate.

The polylactide carrier or matrix is polylactide, polyglycolide (the polylactide derived from hydroxyacetic acid), or a copolymer of lactide or glycolide containing up to 50% by weight of comonomer repeating units of the formula

$$-(R)_m-\overset{R'}{\underset{R''}{\overset{|}{\underset{|}{C}}}}-\overset{O}{\overset{\|}{C}}-O-$$

where R is lower alkylene, preferably methylene ($-CH_2-$) or ethylene ($-CH_2CH_2-$), m is 0 or 1, R' is hydrogen or lower alkyl, R" is hydrogen or alkyl of up to about 22 carbons when m is 0 and hydrogen or lower alkyl when m is 1, and can be the same as R' or different. Preferred, because of availability of starting materials, are comonomer repeating units derived from α-hydroxycarboxylic acids, i.e., units of the above formula in which m is zero.

Illustrative of the comonomers which can be used with lactide or glycolide to form copolymers are β-propiolactone, tetramethylglycolide, β-butyrolactone, γ-butyrolactone, pivalolactone, and intermolecular cyclic esters of α-hydroxybutyric acid, α-hydroxyisobutyric acid, α-hydroxyvaleric acid, α-hydroxyisovaleric acid, α-hydroxycaproic acid, α-hydroxy-α-ethylbutyric acid, α-hydroxyisocaproic acid, α-hydroxy-β-methylvaleric acid, α-hydroxyheptanoic acid, α-hydroxyoctanoic acid, α-hydroxydecanoic acid, α-hydroxymyristic acid, α-hydroxystearic acid, and α-hydroxylignoceric acid.

In addition to being usable as a comonomer, β-butyrolactone can be used as the sole monomer or as the principal monomer along with any of the comonomers recited above, i.e., poly-β-butyrolactone and copolymers thereof can be used as polymers in the formulations. The term polylactide as used is also intended to include poly-β-butyrolactone and copolymers of β-butyrolactone with the comonomers listed in the immediately preceding paragraph.

The drug and the polymer can be mixed, and the intimacy of mixing, particle size, and particle shape of the formulation can be varied, by any of a number of known methods. Intimacy of mixing, particle size, and particle shape of the formulations of the process will depend to some extent on the intended use. High homogeneity can be obtained by mixing the components in the molten state, cooling, and grinding the resulting solid.

A formulation so obtained is suitable for injection as 0.1μ to 1000μ particles suspended in saline solution or a pharmaceutically acceptable oil. In some cases particles with cores of pure drug coated with various thicknesses of polymer can be preferred for delayed and/or sustained release. Relatively large pellets (1 to 10 mm.) may be preferred for reversible implantation in animals by surgery or by injection as projectiles. For this use adequate homogeneity can usually be realized by grinding or milling the drug and the polymer together before forming pellets under pressure.

Known techniques of encapsulation, including micro-encapsulation, can be used to mix the polymer and the drug. The formulations provide a slow steady release of drug in contradistinction to conventional preparations which generally produce a rapid surge followed by a fairly quick decline in drug effect. The following examples illustrate the formation of pellets for implantation.

Example 1: Poly-L-lactide [inherent viscosity 1.26, 0.1% in benzene], 1.90 g. and 17β-estradiol (0.10 g.) were mixed together as a powder and then melted at 230°C. The melt was cooled in Dry Ice, broken into small pieces, and pressed into 50 mg. pellets for implantation in animals.

Example 2: Poly-L-lactide [inherent viscosity 3.97, 0.1% in benzene], 1.90 g. was melted at 250°C., and 2α,17α-diethynyl-A-nor-5α-androstane-2β,17β-diol (0.10 g.) was added to the melt under nitrogen. The melt was cooled, chopped into small pieces, and pressed into pellets at 150°C. Pellets of the product weighing about 80 mg. were implanted in female Holtzman rats and produced an estrogenic response lasting for about one month.

Example 3: L-lactide/glycolide [1/1 by weight] copolymer [inherent viscosity 1.44, 0.1% in benzene], 4.0 g., was melted at 225°C. and 17β-estra-diol, 0.21 g., was mixed into the melt. The homogeneous mixture was poured onto a stainless steel plate, ground into a powder, and pressed into pellets. Pellets of the product weighing about 100 mg. gave a strong estrogenic response over a period of four weeks when implanted in female rats.

TESTOSTERONE DERIVATIVES AS ANABOLIC AGENTS

J.C. Babcock and J.A. Campbell; U.S. Patent 3,313,701; April 11, 1967; assigned to The Upjohn Company have developed therapeutic compositions containing 7α,17α-dimethyltestosterone and a method for their use.

Comparative studies have shown that 7α,17α-dimethyltestosterone [*J. Am. Chem. Soc.,* 81:4069 (1959)] offers an unexpected split between anabolic and androgenic activities at therapeutically effective anabolic dosage levels. With this agent it is possible to provide anabolic therapy which is essentially free of undesirable androgenic side effects. This split in activity provides a sharp departure from related compounds.

For example, the anabolic/androgenic ratio as obtained in controlled, double cross-over studies of anabolic activity in monkeys and androgenic activity in rats is 1.9 for 7α,17α-dimethyltestosterone as compared with 1 for methyltestosterone, a common standard. In humans, the anabolic potency is significantly greater than other commonly used anabolic steroids. A temporary and useful repression of breast tumors is observed on therapy with this compound.

A daily oral dose of 0.25 to 5 mg. per day of 7α,17α-dimethyltestosterone has been found to provide highly effective anabolic therapy essentially free of undesirable androgenic side effects. The same regimen is appropriate for clinical utilization of the antitumor activity described. The exact dosage schedule, of course, must be determined individually according to the subject's age, weight, response to the medication and severity of the condition being treated. In general, however, a regimen of 0.01 to 0.03 mg./kg. bodyweight/day is preferred for children and 0.02 to 0.08 mg./kg. bodyweight/day for adults.

In adapting the active ingredient for use in mammals, including humans, the compositions are administered in unit dosage form as tablets, pills, capsules, powders, wafers, cachets, granules, oral dispersions, and the like.

For preparing solid compositions such as tablets, the active ingredient in crystalline, powdered, or micronized form is mixed with a conventional tabletting component such as lactose, cornstarch, dicalcium phosphate, terra alba (calcium sulfate), talc, stearic acid, calcium stearate, gums, and functionally similar materials constituting pharmaceutical diluents or carriers. The tablets or pills can be laminated or otherwise compounded to provide a dosage form having prolonged or delayed action or of predetermined successive action of the enclosed medication.

For example, the tablet or pill can comprise an inner dosage and outer dosage component, the latter being in the form of an envelope over the former. The two components can be separated by an enteric layer which serves to resist disintegration in the stomach and permits the inner component to pass intact into the duodenum or to be delayed in release. A variety of materials can be used for such enteric layers or coatings, such materials including a number of polymeric acids or mixtures of polymeric acids with such materials as shellac, shellac and cetyl alcohol, cellulose acetate phthalate and the like. A particularly advantageous sustained release coating comprises a styrene maleic acid copolymer.

Example 1: Tablets – A batch of 10,000 compressed tablets, each containing 1 mg. of 7α,17α-dimethyltestosterone, is prepared from the following ingredients: 10 g. of 7α,17α-dimethyltestosterone and 40 g. of lactose. The finely powdered steroid and lactose are thoroughly mixed and granulated with syrup-starch paste. Starch and calcium stearate are used as lubricants, and the tablets are compressed in the usual manner. Administration of these tablets is on a schedule of 1 tablet daily for adults to stimulate weight gain.

Example 2: Tablets – In the formulation of Example 1, 2.5 g. or 50 g. can be substituted for the 10 g. of 7α,17α-dimethyltestosterone to give tablets containing 0.25 mg. or 5 mg., respectively, which can be administered on the same schedule for anabolic therapy.

OTHER THERAPEUTIC AGENTS

MINERAL DIETARY SUPPLEMENTS

Copper Pellets for Ruminants

R.G. Hemingway and N.S Ritchie; U.S. Patent 3,567,818; March 2, 1971; assigned to The University Court of the University of Glasgow, Scotland have developed means particularly useful for supplying copper to ewes shortly before conception or during pregnancy. Copper is then most necessary to them to prevent swayback in the lambs which are subsequently born. The copper is supplied by administering a pellet comprising an alloy containing 40 to 70% by weight Cu, 0 to 15% by weight of Al and a total of 0 to 5% by weight of one or more trace elements selected from Co, Zn and Mn, the balance being Mg. The rate of release of copper can be controlled by varying the proportion of aluminum. A particularly useful pellet is one consisting of an alloy containing 65% by weight of Cu and 35% by weight of Mg and a trace of Co. The pellet should not have sharp edges to injure the ruminant. Suitable shapes are: cylindrical, spherical, spheroidal and ovoid.

For administration to pregnant ewes, the pellet may conveniently be a convex, e.g., hemispherically ended cylinder about ½ to ¾ inch in diameter and 1 to 2 inches long. The density of the pellet is at least 2.25 g./cc to avoid regurgitation. A pellet consisting of an alloy of 65% copper and 35% magnesium has a density of about 4 g./cc. A cylindrical pellet of this alloy, about ½ inch in diameter and about 1 inch long, contains about 7 g. of copper and weighs about 10 to 11 grams.

A pellet suitable for administration to cattle can be similar in composition and density to a pellet for administration to sheep but with a length up to about 3 inches and a diameter about 1 inch. Both types of pellets can be administered by means of an oesophageal balling gun. To reduce loss of pellets by regurgitation or passage in faeces after administration, each pellet may be formed around a high density material (steel, for example), or particles of the high density material (e.g., iron shot of 1/32 to 1/8 inch diameter) may be distributed in a matrix of the alloy.

The pellets may be prepared by any means known in the art. The simplest and most convenient method consists in melting a quantity of magnesium and copper in the desired proportions with a flux in an iron pot. The melt is stirred for 1 minute and then poured into upright cylindrical molds of the desired dimensions.

Example 1: It may be expected that the pellets can be administered to ruminant animals which receive different diets. The results presented in the following table record the mean release of copper (mg. Cu/day) when sheep of several groups were given one pellet each. In each case the individual pellets were weighed prior to administration and again after a known period when the pellets were recovered from the rumeno-reticular sacs of the sheep.

Trial No.	Diet	Number of sheep each given one pellet	Period of test (days)	Mean copper loss from pellet mg. Cu/day.
1	Grass only	15	35	91
2	do	9	42	96
3	do	8	41	15
4	Grass and small amount of concentrates each day.	3	40	47
5	do	4	70	81
6	Concentrates in quantity grass.	8	38	138
7	do	6	42	142

Pellets have also been tested in cattle fitted with permanent fistulas to provide openings into the rumen so that the pellets could be removed at intervals for weighing. Copper was released at rates comparable with those in respect of the sheep referred to in the above table. In practice, to supplement the copper intake of cattle it will normally be necessary either to give more than one pellet or to provide a single pellet of larger dimensions.

Example 2: To confirm the value of the pellet in increasing the blood and liver copper status of sheep one pellet was administered to each of six sheep. Six comparable sheep acted as untreated controls. The sheep grazed together on turnips and grass for four weeks and in addition received some concentrates for a further week. All the sheep were slaughtered five weeks after administration of the pellets.

The mean liver copper concentration of the six treated sheep were 376 parts per million (range, 171 to 576) compared with 24 parts per million (range 14.2 to 52.1) for the six untreated control sheep. The mean blood copper concentration of the treated sheep at slaughter was 0.90 part per million compared with 0.70 part per million for the control sheep.

Magnesium-Containing Pellets

A suitable magnesium-containing pellet for preventing a disease known as hypomagnasaemia caused by magnesium deficiency in the diet of cattle and sheep has been developed by *P. Roebuck and D.J. Whitehead; U.S. Patent 3,577,513; May 4, 1971; assigned to Pfizer Inc.* In order that the pellets, once introduced into the rumeno-reticular sac, remain there for a considerable period it is necessary that the pellet be of a specific gravity not less than 2.2.

A further requirement is that of providing a constant rate of dissolution or emission of the biologically active substance during this extended period. Previously, pellets have been provided comprising mixtures of materials such as copper oxide and clay, or cobaltic oxide and clay, but these were found not to be entirely satisfactory in that after a while the surface of the pellets became partially or completely sealed by an insoluble film from the fluid in the rumeno-reticular sac.

British Patent 1,102,979, provides a pellet having Mg or Mg base alloy as the biologically active substance and a particulate substance of higher specific gravity than the Mg or Mg alloy, in such proportions that the pellet has a specific gravity of at least 2.2.

The particulate material may be from 0.02 mm. to 0.07 mm. average diameter and is preferably iron shot. Experiments have shown that while this is often satisfactory it is found that in a proportion of the animals the pellets dissolve in too short a period to be convenient. This is due at least partly to a close association between the magnesium and the iron shot so that apparently a galvanic action occurs whereby the magnesium is rapidly dissolved.

According to this process the iron (here intended to include steel) is treated to form a refractory coating on it before being incorporated in the magnesium. The preferred method of coating the iron shot is by heating it to 600° to 800°C. or more in air so that it becomes coated with a dark colored iron oxide coating. It is then (while hot or after cooling) mixed with or incorporated in magnesium or magnesium alloy.

For example the iron shot may be mixed with magnesium alloy at a temperature between the liquidus and solidus temperatures of the alloy so that the mixture is in a more or less pasty condition. A quantity of the mixture is ladled out and injected into a closed die to form it to the required shape or it may be introduced into an open die.

The iron shot may be coated with rust but precautions must then be taken to avoid sticking of the shot together as a mass. A still further alternative method is to coat the shot particles with a coating such as a mold wash as used for coating molds before casting magnesium alloy into them. Another treatment could be a phosphate treatment of the iron shot by any known phosphate process. The coating must be sufficiently refractory and/or adherent to withstand the subsequent heat and/or shaping treatment.

A suitable mixture may be 35 to 50% iron shot by weight (e.g., 43 to 44%) remainder magnesium alloy. For sheep a pellet weighing about 30 to 40 grams is desirable, e.g., 35 grams, and for cattle a pellet of 80 to 120 grams is desirable, e.g., 100 grams. The specific gravity of the pellet should be at least 2.2 preferably at least 2.5. The average diameter of the pellets preferably is in the range of 0.02 to 0.07 mm. The pellet may contain other ingredients, for example 10 to 14% aluminum and 1 to 3% copper.

D.J. Whitehead and P.D. Demaine; U.S. Patent 3,594,469; July 20, 1971; assigned to Pfizer Inc. have also developed pellets for supplying magnesium to ruminants. These pellets contain magnesium or magnesium alloy as the biologically active substance and have a particulate substance of higher specific gravity than that of the magnesium or magnesium alloy in such proportions that the pellet has a specific gravity of at least 2.2. The particulate substance may be powdered iron since it is inexpensive.

FIGURE 14.1: MAGNESIUM-CONTAINING PELLETS

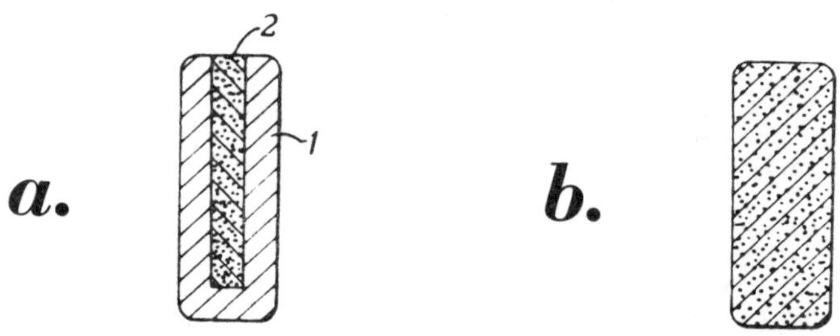

Source: D.J. Whitehead and P.D. Demaine; U.S. Patent 3,594,469; July 20, 1971

Figure 14.1a shows a cylindrical tube **1** closed at one end cast in a magnesium base alloy. The tube is filled with a particulate substance **2** in the form of steel shot held in position by paraffin wax. The shot may be in loose form and plugged at the open end by a disc of magnesium. Instead of steel shot powdered iron or iron oxide may be used as the filler.

In another method, magnesium or magnesium alloy and iron powders are mixed together and then extruded through a die to form a rod which is subsequently cut up into pellets (see Figure 14.1b).

Further magnesium or magnesium alloy and iron powders are mixed together with a binder such as resin, starch based binder, paraffin wax, magnesium oxychloride or waterglass and molded into pellets (see Figure 14.b). In any of the above examples the pellets may be provided with a sheath resistant to corrosion such as a plastics material or a resin lacquer whereby a desired portion of the surface of the pellet may be covered so that the rate of corrosion is controlled.

On introduction into the sac the pellets commence corrosion thus producing magnesium chloride and magnesium oxychloride, which being soluble then enter the bloodstream. The corrosion effect tends to prevent the formation of any sealing film from the contents of the rumenoreticular sac. Furthermore, in the case of the particulate substance being iron powder an electrolytic effect is produced in which hydrogen is given off which assists in the prevention of a sealing film being formed on the pellet surface.

VITAMIN TABLETS

Vitamin-Pancreatin Tablets for Acne

R.N. D'Argento; U.S. Patent 3,322,626; May 30, 1967; assigned to Pannett Products Inc. has disclosed a medical composition useful in the treatment of acne and skin infections. Preferably, this comprises a tablet having an outer shell containing a mixture of vitamin A and vitamin C which are released in the stomach. Pepsin may also be incorporated in the shell formulation. The inner portion of the tablet includes pancreatin and bile salts, and preferably more pancreatin than bile salts, for instance, two parts of pancreatin to one part of bile salts, by weight. They are mixed together, and provided with an enteric outer coating, to form a tablet core or pill, which will remain intact and pass through the stomach unchanged, and into the small intestine.

The pancreatin participates in digestion of protein, fat and starch, acting in the smaller intestine. The bile salts, in the smaller intestine, play a significant role in emulsification of fats, and promoting absorption. The proportions are 250 milligrams of pancreatin and 150 milligrams of bile salts, with an enteric coating.

Since a person suffering from acne is unable to fully dispose of fats that reach the smaller intestine, this composition supplies additional pancreatin and bile, thus enabling the body to complete intestinal funcitions which otherwise would be incompleted.

The shell would contain 15,000 units of vitamin A, 50 milligrams of vitamin C, and 150 milligrams of pepsin. These ingredients, to a substantial extent, are acted upon while in the stomach and ultimately serve to maintain the normal vitality of epithelial tissues.

Silica Gel Stabilizers for Sugar-Coated Multivitamin Tablets

The stability problem caused by addition of vitamin E to multivitamin tablets has been overcome by the process developed by *L. Magid; U.S. Patent 3,646,192; February 29, 1972; assigned to Hoffmann-La Roche Inc.* The sugar-coated multivitamin tablets prepared by direct compression containing vitamin E-active materials are stabilized against cracking of the sugar coat by the inclusion of a small amount of finely divided silica in the outermost sugar coating.

The multivitamin tablets according to this process are prepared by direct compression which is simply the blending of flowable tablet materials into a homogeneous mass which is then compressed into tablets. The success of a direct compression process is dependent on the tabletting characteristics of the active ingredients and excipients of the formula. All ingredients must be in a reasonably flowable and compressible form with a bulk density and particle size suitable for direct compression. Among the vitamin forms suitable for direct compression are dense grade niacinamide, free-flow crystals of thiamine mononitrate and the like.

Recent improvements in tablet excipients have resulted in greatly improved tablets produced by direct compression. In particular, spray dried acacia, direct tablet grade lactose, microcrystalline cellulose, spray dried blends of sugars and acacia and the like have proved very effective in direct compression formulations.

In general, the multivitamin tablets are formed by blending the dry materials in a suitable mixer and compressing the homogeneous mass into tablets. The tablets are sealed and sugar coated in a conventional manner, e.g., the tablets are sealed with a sealant such as shellac, shellac-polyvinylpyrrolidone, shellac-stearic acid or the like by application in a suitable solvent such as, ethyl alcohol and given a subcoating with a mixture such as, gum arabic, sucrose, gelatin and water alternating with a dusting powder, for example, terra alba. The tablet surface is then smoothed by a coating of sugar which is applied as an aqueous syrup.

After application of the smoothing coating, the tablets are polished with a polishing solution or polishing wax composition. The tablets may be colored in a number of ways such as, for example, building up color by having pigment dispersed in the subcoating material or by the use of a special coloring coating prior to the polishing step.

These tablets are stabilized against cracking and bleeding of vitamin E oil by the inclusion of 0.5 to 5.0% and preferably 1.5 to 2.5% weight to volume finely divided silica in the smoothing syrup of the sugar coating. In practice, the finely divided silica is completely dispersed in a smoothing syrup which is in turn applied to the tablets in a conventional manner.

Example: The following formulations were utilized in forming multivitamin tablets.

Ingredient	Parts by weight					
	A	B	C	D	E	F
Thiamine mononitrate, fine granular	2.20	2.20	2.20	11.0	11.0	11.0
Riboflavin	2.75	2.75	2.75	11.0	11.0	11.0
Pyridoxine HCl	1.10	1.10	1.10	5.5	5.5	5.5
Vitamin B_{12} (0.1 percent in gelatin)	1.60	1.60	1.20	6.25	6.25	6.25
Niacinamide, dense	21.00	21.00	21.00	110.00	110.00	110.00
d-Calcium pantothenate	1.50	1.50	1.50	30.00	30.00	30.00
Ascorbic acid (90 percent granulation)	85.60	85.60	85.60			
Sodium ascorbate (95 percent granulation)				257.00	257.00	257.00
Vitamin A acetate powder—500 million units/gm	13.00	12.50	12.50	62.5	6.25	62.5
Vitamin D_2 powder 850 million units/gm	0.50	0.50	0.50	0.60	0.60	0.60
Microcrystalline cellulose	50.00	50.00	50.00			
Dicalcium phosphate, anhydrous, unmilled	60.00	60.00	44.05	68.65	52.85	84.40
Stearic acid	4.00	4.00	4.00	5.25	5.25	5.25
Vitamin E, 50 percent (hydrolyzed gelatin base)	63.00				63.00	31.5
Vitamin E, 60 percent (microfine silica base -Syloid 244)		26.26				
Vitamin E, 33 percent granulation (microfine silica base Syloid 244)			47.70	47.25		
Tablet weight (mg.)	306	269	275	615	615	615

The riboflavin, pyridoxine hydrochloride and calcium pantothenate were passed through a Fitzpatrick mill equipped with a No. 2 screen. The resulting material was then mixed and thoroughly blended with the remaining ingredients listed in the formulations. Then the homogeneous mass was compressed into tablets weighing between 269 and 306 mg. for formulations A, B and C, and between 605 and 620 mg. for formulations D, E and F.

The tablets so formed were sealed with shellac and subcoated with acacia syrup alternating with a terra alba dusting powder. The tablets from each formulation were divided equally into two groups. A first group was smoothed, waxed and polished utilizing conventional procedures. A second group was similarly treated with the exception of the addition of about 2.0% by weight microfine silica gel (Syloid 244) to the smoothing syrup, e.g., USP syrup.

The finished tablets were maintained at 55°C. for 30 days. At the end of this storage period the tablets, from all formulations, which had been finished utilizing a smoothing syrup containing microfine silica, without exception, showed no change in appearance. In contrast, and without exception, the tablets which had been finished with a conventional smoothing syrup exhibited cracking of the sugar-coating and oil seepage.

Stabilized Vitamin C Tablets

L. Magid; U.S. Patent 3,446,894; May 27, 1969; assigned to Hoffman-La Roche Inc. has also disclosed means for stabilizing high potency vitamin C tablets by the use of certain sugars. It has been known that vitamin tablets containing vitamin C are susceptible to discoloration on storage, especially at elevated temperatures. This tendency toward discoloration has assumed special importance due to the recent interest in producing a high potency vitamin C tablet, i.e., a tablet containing vitamin C in an amount of at least 70% and preferably at least 85% as the sole active ingredient.

In producing tablets of this potency it was discovered that granulations and tablets containing such high concentrations of vitamin C and having starch as the principal excipient and/or pregelatinized starch as the principal binder, i.e., where the combined weight of starch and pregelatinized starch comprises at least 50% of the balance of the composition, the granulations and tablets are very susceptible to discoloration on storage, especially at elevated temperatures.

It has been found that sorbose or lactose of their mixture inhibit discoloration in compositions of this nature. The discoloration-inhibiting or stabilizing amount is not narrowly critical, although it should be at least 0.2 weight percent based upon the weight of vitamin C. The preferred stabilizing amount is at least 1%. Obviously higher amounts can be used if desired, but generally no advantage is realized by using amounts greater than 5 weight percent based upon vitamin C.

In addition, the amount should comprise less than 50% of the weight of the composition exclusive of vitamin C, for if present in an amount of greater than 50%, the sorbose, lactose, or mixture would constitute an excipient rather than the stabilizer. In addition to vitamin C, starch, and the sorbose, lactose, or mixture, the compositions can contain other excipients, binders, or coloring agents, flavoring agents, and the like.

Example 1: A mixture (Mixture A) of powdered vitamin C, cornstarch, and pregelatinized starch (Amijel) was granulated with water, dried at 45°C., and then passed through a 12 mesh (U.S. series) screen. The resulting granulation was admixed with a mixture (Mixture B) of stearic acid, talc, and cornstarch, and the resulting granulation was compressed into tablets. Two additional formulations were made containing either sorbose or lactose.

Granulations and tablets of each formulation were then evaluated for color stability by storing for one year at room temperature or for 3 months at 45°C. The formulations and results of these stability tests are summarized in Table 1.

TABLE 1

	Sample Number		
Component, Weight in Milligrams	1	2	3
Mixture A:			
Vitamin C	510	510	510
Sorbose	-	-	50
Lactose	-	70	-
Cornstarch	100	30	50
Amijel	50	50	50
Mixture B:			
Stearic acid	8	8	8
Talc	8	8	8
Cornstarch	10	10	10
Appearance (tablets and granulation):			
3 months/45°C.	*	white	**
1 year/room temperature	***	white	white

*Off-white **Slightly off-white ***Slightly dark

Example 2: Employing techniques similar to those described in Example 1, several additional granulations and tablets were produced containing varying amounts of lactose. The formulations and evaluation of the resulting granulations and tablets are summarized in Table 2.

TABLE 2

Component, Weight in Milligrams	Sample Number 1	2	3	4	5
Mixture A:					
Vitamin C	500	500	500	500	500
Amijel	50	40	40	40	25
Lactose	-	-	5	10	25
Cornstarch	-	10	5	-	-
Mixture B:					
Calcium stearate	5	5	5	5	5
Cornstarch	15	15	15	15	15
Appearance (tablets and granulations)					
3 months/45°C.	*	*	white	white	white
6 months/room temperature	**	**	white	white	white

*Off-white
**Off-white (slightly dark)

Vitamin C Lozenges

A process disclosed by *G.W. Ahrens; U.S. Patent 3,697,641; October 10, 1972* describes a nonhygroscopic nonsugarbase noncariogenic-vitamin C or 1-ascorbic acid releasable base material for use in the preparation of suckable tablets, lozenges and chocolate products. The base material is formed by compounding calcium ascorbate dihydrate alone, or with dibasic magnesium phosphate, with solid glycerides of the self-emulsifying type derived from at least one of the group including edible fats; oils; and edible fat-forming fatty acids. The preferred form of solid, self-emulsifying glycerides are glycerol stearates, glycerol palmitates and mixtures of glycerol stearates with glycerol palmitates containing at least 30 parts by weight percent mono-ester groups.

These products are slowly dispersible in mouth fluids by sucking action causing their contents, including vitamin C (calcium ascorbate dihydrate) and other ingredients that may have been incorporated, as well as dibasic magnesium phosphate a constituent of the base material serving as mineral balancing agent for the calcium liberated from the calcium ascorbate dihydrate constituent to be released.

TABLE 1

In parts by wt. percent:	Base Material Number						
Ingredients:	A	B	C	D	E	F	G
Glycerides:	40.00	41.00	41.00	42.00	43.50	43.50	44.00
Calcium Ascorbate dihydrate:	47.00	56.00	55.00	55.00	55.00	48.00	56.00
Other ingredients:	13.00	3.00	4.00	3.00	1.50	8.00	--.--
Vitamin C activity/per gram in milligrams available:	385	459	451	451	451	393	459

By way of example, Table 1 illustrates some preferred compositions of base materials employing calcium ascorbate dihydrate alone together with the solid glyceride constituents and with or without other ingredients.

By way of example, in addition, Table 2 illustrates some preferred compositions of base materials employing in their formation calcium ascorbate dihydrate in admixture with basic magnesium phosphate together with the selected glyceride constituents, and with or without other ingredients.

TABLE 2

	Base material number												
	H	I	J	K	L	M	N	O	P	Q	R	S	T
Ingredients (in parts by weight percent:													
Glycerides	35.0	35.7	36.0	36.0	36.0	39.0	40.0	45.0	38.0	38.0	34.0	34.0	34.0
Calcium ascorbate	49.0	51.0	44.0	41.0	44.0	50.0	55.0	53.0	40.0	50.0	48.0	42.5	50.0
Dibasic magnesium-phosphate	14.0	13.3	20.0	20.0	18.0	9.0	5.0	2.0	14.0	10.0	15.0	22.0	14.0
Other ingredients	2.0			3 0	2.0	2.0			8 0	2.0	13.0	1.5	2.0
Vitamin C activity/per gram in milligrams available	401	418	360	336	360	410	451	434	369	410	393	348	410

Products prepared by the use of these base materials include, among others, mouth refreshing and flavoring, medical and vitamin tablets and lozenges and chocolates capable of releasing upon being sucked in the mouth, noncariogenic vitamin C or 1-ascorbic acid, anticariogenic effects and effects from other added ingredients as well.

Chewable Vitamin Tablets

The use of nongranulated products has been disclosed by *A. Cavalli and L. Magid; U.S. Patent 3,446,899; May 27, 1969; assigned to Hoffmann-La Roche Inc.* for preparing chewable vitamin tablets.

It was found that when (1) a vitamin, or a mixture of vitamins, is mixed with (2) sorbose or with a mixture of sorbose and a carbohydrate compound selected from dextrose, lactose, sucrose, mannitol, sorbitol or a mixture thereof and (3) a lubricant, in the presence or absence of other conventional tabletting excipients or adjuvants, the dry product can be compressed directly into chewable tablets having outstanding physical and chemical characteristics. Ordinarily, the carbohydrate materials used will be coarse or moderately coarse powders, 60% of the particles passing through a No. 40, 420 micron or a No. 60, 420 micron sieve, as defined in the *USP XVI,* at pages 931 and 932.

The compositions can contain as the active vitamin ingredient a fat-soluble vitamin, a mixture of fat-soluble vitamins, a water-soluble vitamin material, a mixture of water-soluble vitamins, or mixtures of one or more fat-soluble vitamins with one or more water-soluble vitamins.

It was not anticipated that the use of sorbose either alone or in combination with some other carbohydrate or carbohydrates would produce a composition which could be compressed into tablets without first granulating same. With the exception of mixtures containing sorbitol, mixtures containing a single sugar have, at best, been found to be poorly compressible. Sorbitol-containing mixtures are compressible, but the tablets obtained using sorbitol are extremely hygroscopic. This property is, obviously, detrimental to the labile vitamins in the formulation. The tablets which contain sorbose mixed with sorbitol are superior to known tablets which contain only sorbitol.

Example 1: In this example, 7.65 parts of ascorbic acid and 20.05 parts of sodium ascorbate were first intimately mixed. To this mixture there was added 28.74 parts of sorbitol and 27.0 parts of sorbose. Subsequently, there was added to the mixture 1.3 parts of sodium sucaryl, 0.13 part of soluble saccharin, 0.28 part by weight of cherry flavor and 2.6 parts of calcium stearate. The mixture was then compressed directly, i.e., without first granulating same, into tablets weighing 880 mg. The chewable tablets, thus obtained, were characterized by their good stability, chewability, taste and hardness properties.

Example 2: In this example, 6.0 parts of dry vitamin A acetate (500,000 USP units per gram), 40.0 parts of sorbitol, and 33.0 parts of sorbose were intimately admixed. Thereafter, 1.0 part of calcium stearate was added to, and distributed throughout, the mixture. The mixture thus obtained was subsequently compressed directly into tablets weighing 800 mg. The tablets produced in this example exhibited outstanding stability, chewability and hardness characteristics. Furthermore, the vitamin A component of the tablet was stable and the tablet was devoid of any unpleasant taste.

Pyridoxolyl (B_6) Derivatives

Pharmaceutical preparations containing derivatives of vitamin B_6 are disclosed by *G. Schorre; U.S. Patent 3,324,140; June 6, 1967; assigned to E. Merck AG, Germany.* These contain compounds of Formula (1), and their acid addition salts:

(1)

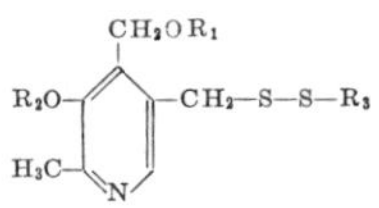

where R_1 and R_2 are hydrogen or acyl; and R_3 is alkyl which can be substituted; alkenyl; alkynyl; aryl or aralkyl, either of which can be substituted.

These compounds can be produced as follows. (a) By reacting a pyridine derivative of Formula (2):

(2)

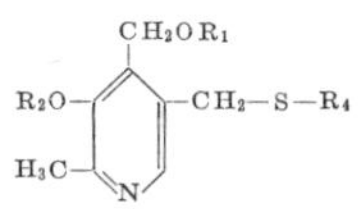

where R_1 and R_2 have the previous meanings, and R_4 is hydrogen, ammonium, or an equivalent of a metallic atom, preferably an alkali metal such as sodium, or its acid addition salt, with a sulfur-containing compound of Formula (3): $Y–S–R_3$ where Y is $–SO_3R_4$, $–SO_2R_3$, $–SOR_3$, Br, Cl, or -S-CN, and R_3 and R_4 have the previous meanings. (b) Or by reacting a sulfur-containing pyridine derivative of Formula (4):

(4)

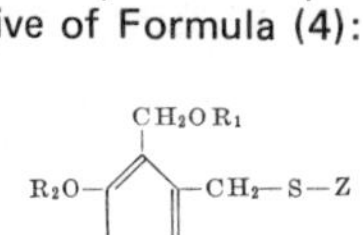

where Z is $–SO_3R_4$, Cl, or Br, and R_1, R_2, and R_4 have the previous meanings, or its acid addition salt, with a mercaptan derivative of Formula (5): $R_4—S—R_3$ where R_3 and R_4 have the previous meanings.

The compounds of Formula (1) and their acid addition salts can be used as therapeutic drugs, particularly in cases where vitamin B_6 therapy is indicated, more particularly for the treatment of cerebral malfunctions. In comparison to the known symmetrical pyridoxolyl disulfide, these compounds exhibit a higher lipoid solubility. For this reason, they penetrate the cellular membranes more readily and thus are better absorbed by the lipoid-rich nerve tissue. These compounds can be employed in a mixture with the conventional pharmaceutical excipients. Carrier substances can be such organic or inorganic substances which are suitable for parenteral or enteral application and which do not react with the compounds, such as, water, vegetable oils, polyethylene glycols, gelatine, lactose, amylose, magnesium stearate, talcum, Vaseline, cholesterol, etc. For parenteral application, solutions are especially used, preferably oily or aqueous solutions, as well as suspensions or emulsions which, if desired, are used in sterilized form or mixed with auxiliary agents, such as preservatives, stabilizers, or wetting agents, or with salts for influencing the osmotic pressure, or with buffer substances. For enteral application, tablets or dragees are particularly suitable.

It is also possible to combine these compounds with other drugs, the concentration being, of course, compatible. Of special importance are polyvitamin combinations. Tablets are prepared having the following formulations.

	Milligrams
Each tablet is formulated to contain:	
Pyridoxolyl-allyl-disulfide	100
Lactose	200
Cornstarch	35
Magnesium stearate	5
Talc	20
The core of coated tablets contains:	
Pyridoxolyl-ether-disulfide	150
Lactose	100
Potato starch	50
Gelatine	4

The core is coated according to standard techniques with a mixture of sugar and arabic gum to make up a coated tablet with a total weight of 500 mg.

GASTROINTESTINAL MEDICINES

Three-Stage Digestive Dragees

A. Hunger and G. Muller; U.S. Patent 3,651,205; March 21, 1972; assigned to Ciba-Geigy Corporation have developed a three-stage dragee, suitable for oral administration containing 4,7-phenanthroline-5,6-quinone together with pancreatin, bromelin, dehydrocholic acid, 5,7-dichloro-8-hydroxyquinoline and a suitable carrier. These preparations are particularly suitable for the treatment of digestive disturbance, and troubles, diarrhea, dyspepsias, obstipations or gastrocardial symptom complex.

Particularly good therapeutic results are obtained with this preparation when it is given in the form of a special three-stage dragee. This three-stage dragee is characterized in that it contains the bromelin in the layer which dissolves in the gastric juices, whereas inside the core the 4,7-phenanthroline-5,6-quinone and the 5,7-dichloro-8-hydroxyquinoline and, isolated therefrom, in a core enevlope, the pancreatin and dehydrocholic acid are contained, the whole core having an envelope which is resistant to the gastric juices but disintegrates in an alkaline medium. This ensures above all the liberation of bromelin whose proteolytic activity leads to optimal protein digestion in the stomach.

After a stomach passage, after the envelope has dissolved, advantageously within 4 to 6 min., the pancreatin and then the dehydrocholic acid are liberated in the alkaline conditions of the duodenum. The fermentative effect of pancreatin considerably promotes the digestion of fats, proteins and carbohydrates. The protein digestion is improved not only directly but also indirectly by induction of the pancreas secretion caused by the protein fission products, the peptones and amino acids. Dehydrocholic acid promotes the resorption of fats and fat-soluble vitamins, emulsifies the ingested food fats and thereby improves the effect of the lipases and develops a choleretic activity. Furthermore, it has a peristaltic effect upon the intestine.

Finally, in the upper portion of the small intestine 4,7-phenanthroline-5,6-quinone and 5,7-dichloro-8-hydroxyquinoline are liberated and distributed in the small intestine. In conjunction these active substances develop an outstanding effect against pathogenic bacteria, fungi and amoebae without affecting the physiological intestinal flora. Dysbioses in the intestines are controlled and a eubiose is restored. The synergistic effect of pancreatin in conjunction with the two active substances mentioned upon abnormal putrefaction and fermentation processes in the small intestine is especially valuable.

Example: A three-stage dragee is prepared in the following manner. Envelope tablets are pressed on a special tabletting machine which consist of a core granulate and an envelope granulate, the envelope tablets being shaped to follow the outline of the dragee and containing in the core 10 mg. of 4,7-phenanthroline-5,6-quinone and 100 mg. of 5,7-dichloro-8-hydroxyquinoline and in the envelope 25 mg. of dehydrocholic acid and 150 mg. of pancreatin as active ingredients. The granulates consist of:

	Mg./Core
Core granulate:	
4,7-phenanthroline-5,6-quinone	10.0
5,7-dichloro-8-hydroxyquinoline	100.0
Wheat starch	15.0
Gelatin	3.0
Arrowroot	11.0
Stearic acid	6.0
Talcum	5.0
Per core	150.0

	Mg./Envelope
Envelope granulate:	
Pancreatin	150.0
Dehydrocholic acid	25.0
Cellulose powder	30.0
Cellulose ether	2.5
Talcum	3.0
Arrowroot	51.5
Aerosil	1.5
Magnesium stearate	1.5
Per envelope	265.0

The core granulate is granulated with water in the usual manner and then dried. Principally, the pancreatin granulate is likewise prepared in the usual manner, but care is needed to ensure that during the granulating operation the ferment content does not drop.

The envelope tablets shaped to follow the dragee outline, having an average gross weight of 415 mg. per tablet, are coated in the usual manner with a cellulose-acetate phthalate lacquer which is resistant to the gastric juices.

The cores coated with the lacquer resistant to the gastric juices are coated with an anhydrous dragee-making suspension which contains the proteolytic ferment bromelin as active ingredient. Of this suspension just so many coats are produced on the core as are needed to give each envelope of the individual dragee core an average content of 50 mg. of bromelin. A suspension for making dragees is composed of the following ingredients.

Bromelin	10.0%
Cellulose ether	5.0%
Talcum	7.5%
Methanol	7.5%
Methylene chloride	70.0%

After having been coated with the bromelin layer the dragees are carefully dried. Finally, the dragees are given a sugar coating consisting, as is usual, of sugar syrup or a dragee-making suspension.

A similar dragee was prepared by *F. Gross, C. Bittner, R. Reipert, G. Mueller and K. Bauer; U.S. Patent 3,574,819; April 13, 1971; assigned to Ciba Corporation* containing as active ingredients 4,7-phenanthroline-5,6-quinone, pancreatin, bromelin, dehydrocholic acid and 7-iodo-5-chloro-8-hydroxyquinoline.

Example: A 3-stage dragee is manufactured according to the method described in the example cited above in U.S. Patent 3,651,205. In this case, however, shell tablets domed in dragee fashion are manufactured on a special tabletting machine from a core granulate and a shell granulate, which contain in the core 10 mg. of 4,7-phenanthrolin-5,6-quinone and 100 mg. of iodo-chlorohydroxyquinoline in place of the 5,7-dichloro-8-hydroxyquinoline used there and in the shell 25 mg. of dehydrocholic acid and 150 mg. of pancreatin as active ingredients.

The coated cores are enveloped with a dragee-making suspension that is free from, or contains only little, water; this suspension contains the proteolytic ferment bromelin as active ingredient. With this suspension a sufficient number of coats but no more is applied to the cores to ensure for each dragee core a mean content of 50 mg. of bromelin. A suspension which contains little water for making dragees is composed of the following ingredients.

	Percent
Bromelin	9.0
Polyvinylpyrrolidone	0.3
Cellulose ether	3.0
Sugar syrup	4.5
Talcum	3.0
Chloroform	28.4
Methanol	11.8
Methylene chloride	40.0

Another, containing no water would be formulated as follows.

	Percent
Bromelin	10.0
Cellulose ether	5.0
Talcum	7.5
Methanol	7.5
Methylene chloride	70.0

After having been coated with the bromelin layer the dragees are carefully dried. Finally, the dragees are coated with sugar which is applied in the usual manner in the form of sugar syrup or a dragee-making suspension.

Silicone Defoamers

A powdered silicone has been developed by *G.M. Grass, Jr. and D.R. MacDonnell; U.S. Patent 3,382,150; May 7, 1968; assigned to Smith Kline & French Laboratories* for use in pharmaceutical and veterinary preparations.

In veterinary practice these compounds are used for treating frothy bloat in ruminants and tympanic colic in horses. In humans the organopolysiloxanes are being used to treat gastrointestinal disturbances.

In prior formulations the silicones were supplied either as an oil or an emulsion. More recently solid forms of silicones have been prepared by adsorbing them on silica gels or other adsorbing agents.

However, none of these forms of silicone are adaptable for the proper dispersion which is necessary to obtain the full effect of the silicone. Not only are these forms of silicone very poorly dispersed in aqueous and solid systems but they are also very difficult to measure and handle in the preparation of pharmaceutical oral dosage forms, particularly tablets.

In this process, an emulsion comprising the organopolysiloxanes, a nontoxic coating material and water is prepared. The emulsion is then spray dried to form dry particles comprising the organopolysiloxane substantially coated with the coating material. The spray dried silicone powder is then tabletted by itself or combined with a medicament, for example, an antacid. The organopolysiloxane will be in liquid form and will be present from 5 to 85%, preferably from 20 to 50% by weight of the total solids comprising the finished products.

The coating material will be present from 15 to 95%, preferably from 50 to 80% by weight of the total solids. The coating material will be a cellulose ester, a natural gum, a gum constituent of a natural gum, sugars such as mannitol, a water-soluble polymer such as polyvinyl alcohol or polyvinylpyrrolidone or a proteinaceous material such as powdered egg whites, casein, milk solids, gelatin and zein or any mixture thereof.

The spray drying is carried out in apparatus conventionally used for spray drying. The drying conditions may vary within wide ranges. It is, however, preferred to use a minimum inlet temperature of about 100°C. and a maximum outlet temperature of about 150°C. Correspondingly the inlet temperature will be higher than the outlet temperature and advantageously will be as high as the limitations will permit. Desirably during the operation, the inlet and outlet temperatures remain substantially constant. The dried silicone is collected in a receiver at the bottom of the main chamber.

Example 1:

Ingredients	Amounts, grams
Methylcellulose, USP 15 cp.	5
Milk solids, nonfat dry	45
Dimethylpolysiloxane	50
Purified water, USP	180

The methylcellulose is dispersed in the dimethylpolysiloxane. The milk solids are dissolved in water and the dispersion is added to the reconstituted milk and agitated to form an emulsion. The mixture is then homogenized to complete emulsification.

This emulsion is then spray dried in a conventional spray dryer using an inlet temperature of 265°C. and an outlet temperature of at least 120°C. The product is then collected as a dry powder.

Example 2: The antacid layer consists of:

Ingredients	Amounts, mg./tablet
Magnesium aluminum oxyhydroxide	500
Glycine	50
Mannitol	350
Methylcellulose	24
Saccharin sodium, USP	3
Polyvinylpyrrolidone (5% in alcohol)	18
Magnesium stearate	14
Cornstarch	12
Flavor, q.s.	

The silicone layer consists of:

Ingredients	Amounts, mg./tablet
Spray dried silicone powder (product of Ex. 1)	50
Mannitol, NF	100
Glycine	50
Polyvinylpyrrolidone	5
Saccharin sodium	1
Magnesium stearate	12
Flavor, q.s.	4

Separate antacid and silicone granulations are prepared. These granulations are made by screening and mixing the magnesium aluminum hydroxide and powdered silicone with the glycine, mannitol and methylcellulose. The mixtures are then separately granulated with the polyvinylpyrrolidone solution. The granulations are then dried, screened and mixed with the flavor, magnesium stearate and cornstarch.

The granulations are compressed into a layered tablet by using a multi-layer rotating tablet press. Either a two or three layered tablet may be formed. Alternatively the antacid and silicone granulations may be intimately mixed and tabletted.

Silicone-antacid compositions having rapid defoaming action and a method of preparing these compositions is also disclosed by *J.K.-C. Yen; U.S. Patent 3,501,571; March 17, 1970; assigned to Smith Kline & French Laboratories*.

The method comprises adsorbing a liquid organopolysiloxane on an inert adsorbent filler compound and granulating this mixture. The antacid material is then separately granulated and the dried granules are mixed together and compressed. Alternatively the granules can be compressed into a layered tablet, filled into hard gelatin capsules or dispersed as the granules per se. The separate granulations are prepared by known methods. For example, the ingredients are wet with a binder in aqueous solution to form a granulation. The granulation is then oven dried and the dried granulation is milled into granules having a size of from 14 mesh to about 100 mesh.

In accordance with this process it was discovered that certain compounds have a tendency to adsorb rather than absorb the silicone. These compounds were found to be excellent carriers for the silicone and produced compositions having rapid defoaming action. The compounds which have this adsorption characteristic with silicone are, for example, carbohydrates such as lactose, mannitol, sorbitol, sucrose, icing sugar (3% starch, 97% sucrose), starch and cellulose compounds; fillers such as, calcium sulfate, sodium phosphate, glycine and starch. Preferably the adsorbent filler used will be lactose, mannitol, sorbitol, sucrose and dextrose. The above adsorbents are present in the total solids from about 5 to 50%.

Example: The first granulation consists of:

Ingredients	Mg./Tablet
Aluminum hydroxide	200
Magnesium hydroxide	200
Mannitol	175
Dextrose	100
Starch, pregelatinized	15

The first four ingredients are mixed together and granulated with 5% pregelatinized starch paste. The granulation is dried overnight at 110°F. The dried granulation is then passed through a No. 20 mesh screen.

The second granulation consists of:

Ingredients	Mg./Tablet
Organopolysiloxane	27.0
Mannitol	125
Dextrose	50
Special icing sugar	150
FD&C Blue No. 1	0.02

The mannitol and silicone are mixed together and passed through a No. 20 mesh screen. The dextrose and icing sugar are then added and this mixture is granulated with just enough colored water to make the granulation wet. The granulation is dried overnight at 110°F. and passed through a No. 14 mesh screen.

Ingredients	Mg./Tablet
Granulation 1	690
Granulation 2	352
Sorbitol powder	30
Talcum	30
Magnesium stearate	7

Granulations 1 and 2 are blended and thoroughly mixed with the other tablet ingredients. The mixture is then compressed into tablets weighing approximately 1.1 grams. Alternatively Granulations 1 and 2 may be compressed into a layered tablet by using a multilayer rotating tablet press. Either a two or three layered tablet may be formed.

Solid Long Acting Antacid

L.L. Kaplan and R.H. Cox; U.S. Patent 3,555,151; January 12, 1971; assigned to Richardson-Merrell Inc. have found an antacid composition and a method for its preparation where the composition, when in contact with acidic aqueous fluids, adheres to the walls of its receptacle over a prolonged period which permits a long acting antacid effect. The composition is prepared by intimately mixing: (a) from 1 to 4 parts of a nontoxic acid counteracting (antacid) compound; (b) about one part of a hydrocolloid; (c) at least 4 parts of water to form an intimate aqueous dispersion of the antacid and hydrocolloid; and (d) finally evaporating the water from the dispersion to form a solid composition where the antacid and hydrocolloid are intimately mixed.

The solid composition is then preferably subdivided and, together with common excipients, formed into quickly disintegratable tablets or placed in water-soluble capsules. The admixture of antacid and hydrocolloid is a physical admixture which, upon contact with aqueous acid fluids, swells to a voluminous gelatinous mass. The gelatinous mass adheres to the receptacle, e.g., stomach, and serves to resist the flow of gastric fluids. Since the antacid is intimately admixed with the swellable hydrocolloid, it also remains in place to perform its antacid function.

The antacid, or acid neutralizing substance can be any antacid such as the various nontoxic antacids used to neutralize gastric fluids. Illustrative of antacids are the oxide, hydroxide or carbonate of magnesium, aluminum hydroxide, magnesium trisiliate, calcium carbonate, combinations of the foregoing, and the like. A preferred antacid is magnesium oxide alone, or in combinations with other antacids.

The hydrocolloid used here is a colloid having affinity of water, e.g., nontoxic materials such as gums, polysaccharides isolated from water plants, various modified cellulose molecules, proteins, clays, colloidal silica and some totally synthetic products. Illustrative of specific hydrocolloids are gum acacia, gum tragacanth; guar gum, locust bean gum; arabinogalactan; sterculia gum; agar; chondrus; algin; methylcellulose; carboxymethylcellulose; hydroxymethylcellulose; and bentonite.

The method of preparation comprises the formation of an intimate aqueous mixture of the antacid and hydrocolloid. A sufficient amount of water, i.e., in a quantity by weight at least 4 times greater than the hydrocolloid, is used to provide an intimate dispersion of the ingredients, where the antacid is entrapped within the macromolecular matrix of the hydrocolloid. The minimum quantity of water, at least 4 times greater than the hydrocolloid is critical to ensure intimate dispersion of the ingredients beyond the standard granulation techniques used in the pharmaceutical art.

The quantity of antacid is less critical provided a sufficient quantity is present to effect neutralization of acid. The water is then evaporated from the mixture, e.g., by pouring the dispersion on trays and drying it at a temperature of about 150°F. The dried dispersion is then preferably passed through a comminutor to reduce the dried material to a 12 mesh or finer particle size. The particles are then preferably formulated into quick-disintegrating tablets or capsules according to known methods.

The maximum quantity of water used is not critical, however, if an excess is employed beyond 6 or 8 parts, it simply means that more water will have to be evaporated from the aqueous dispersion without conferring additional benefit to the process or composition. In order to facilitate dispersion of the materials, both the hydrocolloid and the antacid are preferably in powdered form such as that having a particle size of less than 100 mesh size.

Example: Long-acting antacid tablets were prepared using the process illustrated below.

	Grams
Magnesium oxide (1)	475
Locust bean gum (1)	250
Starch	20
Talcum	10
Magnesium stearate	10
Magnesium oxide (2)	25
Locust bean gum (2)	15

Mix the magnesium oxide (1) and locust bean gum (1) powders in a suitable container. Place 1,500 milliliters of distilled water in a chamber suitable for vigorous agitation, and slowly add the magnesium oxide (1) and locust bean gum (1) powder mix to the distilled water, applying agitation and mixing for one-half hour to completely disperse the powder mix in the water, and ensure the homogeneous admixture of the magnesium oxide with the locust bean gum in the water content. The resultant slurry is poured on trays and dried at 150°F. until solid self-sustaining hard cake-like slabs were formed.

Break up these hard slabs, and reduce to No. 12 mesh size particles through a comminutor. Add the starch, talcum, magnesium stearate, magnesium oxide (2) and locust bean gum (2) to the magnesium oxide (1)-locust bean gum (1) particles previously formed, and compress on suitable tablet punches to a tablet weight of 805 milligrams at a compression hardness of 13 kilograms per square inch as determined with the Stokes Tablet Hardness Tester.

Resin Salts for Diarrhea

J.J. Miskel and W. Schlesinger; U.S. Patent 3,297,664; January 10, 1967; assigned to White Laboratories, Inc. have found that certain swellable resins serve as effective antidiarrheal agents due to their ability to absorb large quantities of fecal fluid within the bowels thereby aiding in the production of firm stools.

The swellable resins which have been found effective for this purpose are irregular granules of very high molecular weight carboxylic type ion-exchange resins, e.g., acrylic acid type polymers which are very loosely cross-linked with 0.01 to 2.0% by weight of a polyunsaturated copolymerizable cross-linking agent and which have only a negligible chain (linear or branched) content. The major component of these swellable resins consists of one or more monomeric materials, capable of both homopolymerization and copolymerization such as acrylic acid, salts of acrylic acid, methacrylic acid, salts of methacrylic acid, fumaric acid, maleic acid, maleic anhydride, itaconic acid, with acrylic acid being preferred. These monomeric materials may be referred to as acrylic type monomeric material or an ethylenically unsaturated carboxylic acid.

The polyunsaturated copolymerizable cross-linking agents which form the minor component of these swellable resins have two or more double bonds subject to crosslinkage with the monomeric materials and may be either aromatic or aliphatic.

Suitable cross-linking agents include: N-N-diallylacrylamide, 3,4-dihydroxy-1,5-hexadiene, 2,5-dimethyl-1,5-hexadiene, divinylbenzene, diallyl sucrose or other diallyl sugar, divinylether or diethylene glycol, trivinyl benzene, 2,7-dimethyl-1,7-octadiene, and the like.

The swellable resins useful as antidiarrheals can contain from 0.01 to 2% of cross-linking agent, with 0.15 to 0.25% constituting a preferred range. The optimum amount of cross-linking agent required will depend to a certain extent on the nature of the cross-linking agent employed.

Where more than 2% of cross-linking agent is employed, the resins do not swell appreciably, and the exchange capacity of the resins is limited due to its dense structure. Where less than about 0.01% of cross-linking agent is employed, chain polymers (linear or branched) result rather than the desired cross-linked copolymers. The following examples show the preparation of tablet forms of the resin.

Example 1: A chewable tablet is made up of the following ingredients.

Resin salt (100% thru 200 mesh)	310.0 g.
Sugar, confectioner's	290.0 g.
Mannitol NF	100.0 g.
Glycine NF	84.0 g.
Sodium cyclamate NF	7.2 g.
Saccharin sodium USP	0.8 g.
Alcohol USP	50.0 ml.
Purified water USP	50.0 ml.
Magnesium stearate USP	10.0 g.
Orange (dry flavor), Flav-o-lox 3X, Polak Frutal Works	8.0 g.

Blend resin salt, confectioner's sugar, mannitol, glycine, sodium cyclamate and saccharin sodium for approximately thirty minutes. Add alcohol and water (as a mixture) and mix until the powders are transferred into small granules. Pass through No. 8 mesh screen and dry at 40°C. Pass dry granulation through No. 12 mesh screen. Add magnesium stearate and orange flavor and mix for about 20 minutes. Compress to target weight of 810.0 g. This mixture will yield 1,000 tablets each delivering 310.0 mg. of resin salt.

Example 2: Coated tablets are prepared using the following procedure.

Tablet core:	
Resin salt	600.0 g.
Sugar syrup (13.3 g. solids)	20.0 g.
Magnesium stearate	2.0 g.
Alcohol USP	20.0 ml.
Purified water	1.8 ml.

Gelatin solution, flour, sugar syrup, shellac, and FD&C Red No. 2 are used to form the tablet coating.

Prepare tablet core by granulating the resin salt with the sugar syrup. Pass granulation through a No. 12 mesh screen. Add magnesium stearate and mix well. Add water and alcohol (as a mixture), mix and compress at a weight of 622.0 grams.

Transfer cores to coating pan. Apply several charges of gelatin solution, dust each charge with flour and dry. Apply several charges of sugar syrup and dry each charge. Apply several charges of shellac and dry each charge. Again apply several charges of gelatin solution, dust each with flour and dry. For smoothing, apply several charges of flour paste and dry each charge. Apply colored sugar syrup to a weight of approximately 1,085.0 mg., dry and polish. This process yields 1,000 tablets each delivering 600.0 grams of resin salt.

The antidiarrheal compositions are administered orally and progress through the digestive tract. The dosage of resin salt is extremely flexible depending primarily upon type, severity and underlying disease. Daily dosages can range from 5 to 10 grams. The usual dosage, however, is from 1 to 4 grams daily with 2 grams representing the average dose.

Emetine-Dehydroemetine Tablets

Pharmaceutical compositions characterized in that the active medicament is released in the lower sections of the small intestine and in the colon, rather than in the stomach or upper sections of the small intestine were developed by *K. Munzel; U.S. Patent 3,431,338; March 4, 1969; assigned to Hoffmann-La Roche Inc.*

The compositions comprise (1) a nucleus, i.e., a tablet, granulate, granule, gelatin capsule, etc. which contains the active drug component and conventional pharmaceutical adjuvants, coated, in the following sequence, with (2) a layer of an acid-soluble coating material which is resistant both to alkalis and intestinal juices, (3) a water-soluble intermediate layer, and (4) a layer of alkali-soluble coating material which is resistant to acid and gastric juices.

This provides compositions which are useful in the oral treatment of intestinal infections, i.e., amoebiasis and schistosomiasis; and it provides a method of treating such infections using the compositions. In a preferred method of treating schistosomiasis, tablets of this structure are administered orally to provide 100 mg. of emetine or dehydroemetine per day for a period of twenty days. Emetine and dehydroemetine can be used in their complexes with bismuth iodide.

To provide the coating which is resistant to intestinal juices, there is used a film-forming, basic amino group-containing polyelectrolyte. Exemplary of such materials are amino group-containing polyacrylates or polymethacrylates, such as polymers or mixtures of polymers of aminoalkyl esters of acrylic acid or methacrylic acid; e.g., the dimethylaminoethyl ester of acrylic acid or methacrylic acid; amino group-containing polysaccharides, especially cellulose derivatives, such as benzylaminomethylcellulose, acetylcellulose-p-aminobenzoate, cellulose acetate diethyl aminoacetate, and the like.

To provide the coating resistant to gastric juices, a film-forming, carboxyl group-containing polyelectrolyte may be used. Exemplary of such materials are natural lacquers, such as keratin, shellac; carboxyl group-containing cellulose esters, such as cellulose acetate phthalate, acetyl-succinyl cellulose; carboxyl group-containing copolymers containing maleic acid as acidic component, such as copolymers of styrene and maleic anhydride, copolymers of the butyl partial ester of maleic acid with styrene and small quantities of acrylic acid, copolymers of maleic anhydride and vinyl methyl ether; carboxyl group-containing copolymers with acrylic acid or methacrylic acid as acidic component, such as copolymers of styrene and methacrylic acid.

Example: In this example, 1,000 coated tablets containing emetine hydrochloride as the active ingredient were prepared. The first step is mixing 70.0 grams of lactose with 25.0 grams of emetine hydrochloride. This mixture was moistened and granulated with a paste of 2.5 grams of swollen maize starch and 17.5 grams of water. Thereafter, there was added to and mixed in, such granulate, 0.5 gram of magnesium stearate and 2 grams of talc. Thereafter, the granulate was pressed into 1,000 biconvex nuclei having a diameter of 7 mm. Subsequently, there was prepared a solution containing 2.0 parts of cellulose acetate N,N-diethyl aminoacetate, 1.0 part of methyl alcohol and 17 parts of methylene chloride. This solution was charged into a conventional rotatable tablet-coating pan containing the above tablet nuclei. A film-coat was applied by rotating the coating pan. Subsequently, the nuclei was dried.

Thereafter, the coating and drying operation was repeated fourteen times. The nuclei which were thus obtained, had been provided with a coating which was resistant both to alkali and intestinal juices. These nuclei were dried for about 12 hours at 40°C.

Thereafter, there was prepared a syrup containing 15.0 parts of white gelatin, 291 parts of water, 564 parts of sugar and 130 parts of gum arabic mucilage. This syrup was introduced into the rotatable tablet coating pan containing the coated nuclei, the nuclei coated with the syrup, until the total weight after drying, was 130 grams. The tablets were then held, for 12 hours, at a temperature of about 40°C.

Subsequently, a lacquer solution containing 1.5 parts of cellulose acetate phthalate, 0.75 part of methyl alcohol and 12.75 parts of methylene chloride was prepared. This solution was applied to the coated nuclei in fifteen separate applications, the nuclei being dried in between each application. Such application was carried out using the rotating tablet coating pan. Subsequently, the coated nuclei were dried for 12 hours at 40°C.

At the end of the drying period, there was applied a coating of 15.0 parts of white gelatin, 291 parts of water, 564 parts of sugar and 130 parts of gum arabic mucilage until a total weight of 170 grams was reached. Then, an additional layer was applied using the same gelatin-sugar syrup, which contained also a coloring material. Such sugar solution was applied in the rotating tablet coating pan, until the total weight of the tablets was 200 grams. The coated preparations, were polished by continuously rotating same in a coating pan containing beeswax.

ANTIDIABETIC PYRAZOLYLPYRIDINIUM SALTS

An oral therapeutic composition for control of hyperglycemia in warm blooded animals has been developed by *E.C. Tocus and V.J. Bauer; U.S. Patent 3,341,413; September 12, 1967; assigned to American Cyanamid Company.* The active ingredient is a pyrazolylpyridinium salt illustrated by the following formula:

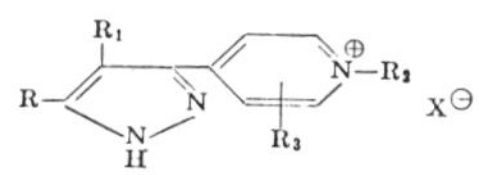

where R is hydrogen, lower alkyl or cyclopropyl; R_1 is hydrogen or lower alkyl; R_2 is lower alkyl, lower alkenyl, cinnamyl, cyclopropyl-methyl or lower alkoxy (lower) alkyl; R_3 is hydrogen or lower alkyl and X is a pharmaceutically acceptable anion such as, chloride, bromide or iodide.

The above compounds may be prepared by a three-stage sequence. Thus, an ester of a pyridine-4-carboxylic acid is reacted with a methyl ketone to provide a 1-(4-pyridyl)-1,3-alkyldione; or ethyl formate is reacted with a pyridyl ketone in the presence of a base such as, for example, sodium methoxide to provide a 1-(4-pyridyl)-1,3-alkyldione salt.

The resulting dione or salt is reacted with hydrazine hydrate or hydrazine dihydrochloride to give a 4-[3(5)-pyrazolyl] pyridine. These latter compounds are quaternized to the active 4-[3(5)-pyrozolyl]-pyridinium salts, with a lower alkyl, lower alkenyl, cinnamyl, cyclopropylmethyl, or lower alkoxy(lower)alkyl halide. The active components have been found, in standard laboratory measurements using chicks and alloxan-diabetic mice, to be orally active hypoglycemic agents. Results obtained from the administration of active components of the compositions compared to standard commercial antidiabetic agents are shown in the table. The amount of active ingredient to be given will depend upon the age, condition, weight and other factors present in the warm-blooded animal. In the instance of a warm-blooded animal of, for example, 75 kg. the dose may vary from 0.075 to 18.75 grams.

	Chicks		Alloxanized Mice			
	Oral Dose, mg./kg.	Avg. Percent Decrease From Control Blood Glucose After 2 Hours	Oral Dose, mg./kg.	Avg. mg. Percent Blood Glucose±S.E. 0 Hour Control	Avg. Percent Decrease in Control Blood Glucose±S.E. 2 Hours	Avg. Percent Decrease in Control Blood Glucose±S.E. 4 Hours
1-methyl-4[5(3)-methyl-3(5)-pyrazolyl]pyridinium iodide	250	73	100	437±38	38± 8	69± 5
1-ethyl-4[5(3)-methyl-3(5)-pyrazolyl]pyridinium iodide	200	55	100	520±18	29± 3	34± 6
1-n-butyl-4[5(3)-methyl-3(5)-pyrazolyl]pyridinium bromide	100	18	100	515±42	62± 3	81± 6
1-methyl-4[5(3)-ethyl-3(5)-pyrazolyl]pyridinium iodide	250	54	100	489±33	55± 9	78± 6
1-methyl-4[3(5)-pyrazolyl]-pyridinium iodide	250	26	100	501±18	14± 8	50±14
1-n-propyl-4[5(3)-methyl-3(5)-pyrazolyl]-pyridinium bromide	250	37	100	450±22	56± 7	40± 8
1-methyl-4[5(3)-isobutyl-3(5)-pyrazolyl]pyridinium iodide	250	30	100	444±33	19± 3	1± 6
1-methyl-4[5(3)-ethyl-3(5)-pyrazolyl]pyridinium chloride	200	38	100	455±18	52± 9	78± 5
1-isopropyl-4[5(3)-methyl-3(5)-pyrazolyl]pyridinium chloride	250	9	100	438±41	15±28	26±39
1-isopropyl-4[5(3)-methyl-3(5)-pyrazolyl]pyridinium bromide	250	12	100	444±27	12± 4	14±14
1-isobutyl-4-[5(3)-methyl-3(5)-pyrazolyl]pryidinium bromide	250	43	100	455±36	41±10	55±13
1-methyl-4[5(3)-methyl-3(5)-pyrazolyl]pyridinium chloride	250	70	100	460±18	36± 8	74± 6
1-methyl-4[3(5)-pyrazolyl]pyridinium chloride	200	22	100	478±32	22±11	73±11
1-n-butyl-4[5(3)-methyl-3(5)-pyrazolyl]pyridinium chloride	200	37	100	436±44	59±15	77±12
1-allyl-4[5(3)-methyl-3(5)-pyrazolyl]pyridinium chloride	100	54	100	446±32	31± 9	34± 9
1-methyl-4[5(3)-cyclopropyl-3(5)-pyrazolyl]pyridinium chloride	100	43	100	455±34	12± 8	38±19
1-methyl-4[4-methyl-3(5)-pyrazolyl]-pyradinium iodide	250	62	100	525±39	8± 3	14± 4
1-methallyl-4[5(3)-methyl-3(5)-pyrazolyl]pyridinium chloride	250	66	100	587±24	49±10	58±11
1,3-dimethyl-4[5(3)-methyl-3(5)-pyrazolyl]pyridinium chloride	100	70	100	615±12	59± 5	78± 8
1-cinnamyl-4[5(3)-methyl-3(5)-pyrazolyl]pyridinium chloride	250	32	100	468±22	19± 8	46±15
1-(3-methyl-2-buten-l-yl)-4[5(3)-methyl-3(5)-pyrazolyl]pyridinium chloride	250	29	100	479±56	60±10	93± 2
-(2-buten-l-yl)-4[5(3)-methyl-3(5)-pyrazolyl]pyridinium chloride	250	66	100	556±36	50± 7	83± 4
1-(2-methoxyethyl)-4[5(3)-methyl-3-(5)pyrazolyl]pyridinium chloride	250	21	100	513±44	14± 6	11± 6
1-cyclopropylmethyl-4[5(3)-methyl-3(5)-pyrazolyl]pyridinium bromide	200	35	100	455±34	50±10	59± 6
0.5% Aqueous Carboxymethylcellulose Solution				406±45	−11± 3	0± 3
Tolbutamide—Standard	50	34	100	478±27	0± 3	−11± 3
β-Phenethylbiguanide Hydrochloride—Standard	50	53	100	452±29	21± 5	17± 3

The active components can be used for oral administration in unit dosage form such as tablets, pills, capsules, powders, granules or oral solutions or suspensions and the like.

Example: 1,000 tablets each containing 100 mg. of 1-methyl-4-[5(3)-methyl-3(5)-pyrazolyl]-pyridinium chloride are prepared from the following ingredients:

1-methyl-4-[5(3)-methyl-3(5)-pyrazolyl]-pyridinium chloride	100 g.
Lactose	50 g.
Starch	50 g.
Calcium stearate	10 g.
Talc	10 g.

The finely powdered ingredients are mixed thoroughly and then tabletted by a slugging procedure.

NONPHARMACEUTICAL TABLETS

PERSONAL PRODUCTS

Soap-Detergent Mixtures

Conventional soap tablets comprise mixtures of alkali-metal soaps from tallow-class fats and nut oils. In general, the lathering properties of nut oil soaps are superior to those of tallow soaps, particularly in lather volume, but as nut oils are more expensive than tallow it is not practical to make soap tablets exclusively from nut oil soaps. It has been suggested to incorporate into a soap tablet a suitable amount of an alkaline earth metal alkyl aryl sulfonate detergent active compound to improve the lathering properties of the soap tablet.

According to *E.H. Evans; U.S. Patent 3,723,329; March 27, 1973; assigned to Lever Brothers Company*, it has been found that if a substantially anhydrous mixture of an alkaline earth metal oxide and an alkyl aryl sulfonic acid is added to a soap base, the production of these soap tablets is considerably facilitated.

By this process, it has also been found that if a soap tablet containing a minor proportion of an alkaline earth metal alkyl aryl sulfonate detergent compound contains in addition a minor proportion of free fatty acid liberated from the soap during the production of the toilet tablet by the use of free alkyl aryl sulfonic acid, the enhanced lather volume characteristics are maintained and also the mushing properties of the resultant soap tablet are considerably improved.

The incorporation of free fatty acid in the soap tablet can conveniently be done by using an excess of alkyl aryl sulfonic acid in a substantially anhydrous mixture of an alkaline earth metal oxide and an alkyl aryl sulfonic acid used to prepare the soap tablet. Hirtherto, an alkaline earth metal alkyl aryl sulfonate detergent compound has been incorporated into an aqueous soap base either by the addition of an aqueous paste of the sulfonate to a sodium soap base, or by the addition of an aqueous paste of a sodium alkyl aryl sulfonate detergent compound to a soap base comprising a mixture of sodium and alkaline earth metal soaps.

These processes have involved the subsequent crutching and drying of the resultant mixture before the milling and stamping can be applied. It has been found that considerable heat energy is required in order to dry such a mixture of soap and synthetic detergent active to an acceptable low water content. In this process an aqueous soap base, preferably dried to a water content of 7 to 13% by weight, is mixed with an anhydrous slurry comprising a mixture of one or more alkaline earth metal oxides together with one or more alkyl aryl sulfonic acids, there being present at least 2 parts by weight of alkyl aryl sulfonic acid per part by weight of alkaline earth metal oxide, the alkyl groups of which contain from 8 to 22 carbon atoms, the soap base and slurry being subsequently formed into tablets.

The free alkyl aryl sulfonic acid is also used to liberate free fatty acids from soap and the soap is used in the production of a soap tablet comprising soap and an alkaline earth metal alkyl aryl sulfonate detergent active compound, the alkyl aryl sulfonic acid being used in an amount from 1 to about 20% by weight of the finished tablet.

Example: A 63% total fatty matter sodium soap base was obtained by the saponification by caustic soda of a 70/30 mixture of tallow-class fats and coconut oil, and this was dried to a water content of 8%. A slurry was prepared comprising powdered anhydrous magnesium oxide and anhydrous dodecyl benzene sulfonic acid (sulfonated DOB 055 from Shell) in a 1:2 molar ratio, the oxide being finely dispersed throughout the sulfonic acid by passage of the slurry through a colloid mill.

As the hot liquid soap base was removed from the drier it was injected with the slurry, passed through an in-line mixer, and then cooled. After the addition of other additives, such as perfumes and colorants, the soap-sulfonate mixture was plodded and stamped into tablets using conventional apparatus. The soap tablets produced by the above method had the following constitution.

	Percent
Sodium tallow soap	56
Sodium coconut soap	24
Magnesium dodecyl benzene sulfonate	10
Perfumes, colorants, etc.	2
Water to 100%	

These soap tablets possessed excellent lathering properties, particularly in regard to the volume of the lather they produced.

Coated Cosmetic Tablets

M.W. Scott and S. Levine; U.S. Patent 3,471,611; October 7, 1969; assigned to Del Laboratories, Inc. have developed a compressed cosmetic powder cake or stick which has a thin film as protective cover. The film is of a material such as polyvinylpyrrolidone which is destroyed on normal use of the cosmetic. The film protects the article, but does not have to be removed before use.

Typical film-forming materials that can be used are a natural film-forming material such as shellac or starch and synthetic film-forming materials such as polyvinylpyrrolidone, polyvinyl acetate, a copolymer of polyvinylpyrrolidone and polyvinyl acetate, polyacrylimides, ethylcellulose, methylcellulose, nitrocellulose, cellulose acetate, cellulose acetate phthalate, methyl methacrylate, polyethylene and polyvinyl chloride.

The film-forming material used is dissolved in a volatile solvent and the resulting solution is applied to the exposed surface or surfaces of the compressed cosmetic powder article to be protected. The ratio of film former to solvent can vary widely. For example, the solid-to-solvent ratio can vary from about ⅒% by weight of solid to about 10% by weight of solid to a remainder of solvent, i.e., the solvent would then vary from about 99.9 to 90% by weight.

The film former solution, i.e., the solution of film former in a volatile solvent, can be applied to the exposed surface of the compressed cosmetic powder article in any fashion used for the application of coatings. For instance, it can be applied as an aerosol spray, as a pressure spray, by brushing, by roller coating, or by dipping. The solvent evaporates leaving a dry (essentially solvent-free) layer.

Any volatile solvent can be used which will dissolve or disperse the film-forming material and which is inert to the film former and to the ingredients of the compressed cosmetic powder cake. Typical volatile solvents useful for this process are ethyl alcohol, a mixture of ethyl alcohol and water, water, acetone, toluene, carbon tetrachloride, methyl alcohol, and isopropyl alcohol.

By way of example, a satisfactorily useful solution of a film former in a volatile solvent constitutes 5% by weight of polyvinylpyrrolidone in 95% by weight of 200 proof ethyl alcohol. This solution can be applied by aerosol spraying, pressure spraying, brushing, roller coating and dipping, to the exposed surface of the compressed cosmetic powder article to be protected. One particular way which has been found to be highly satisfactory is to apply the 5% alcohol solution of polyvinylpyrrolidone by aerosol spraying. For this purpose the 5% solution of polyvinylpyrrolidone in alcohol is packed into an aerosol can in which there is 50% of the polyvinylpyrrolidone-ethyl alcohol solution, and 50% of a liquified Freon gas propellant, e.g., Freon 112 a tetrachlorodifluoroethane.

The quantity of solution applied is such that the amount of film former left after evaporation of the solvent is so thin that the dry film is very fragile, is not readily visible to the naked eye, and is destroyed without noticeable traces on first application by normal use of the article, as by brushing fingers across it, brushing a puff across it, rubbing a brush across it, or rubbing the coated exposed surface of the article on the skin of a user. Thus, the amount of solid film former deposited as a dry adherent film is such that it does not influence the application properties of the compressed cosmetic powder article.

It has been found that a spray time with the foregoing aerosol spray of from about 7 to 15 seconds with the nozzle about 8 inches away from the article yields highly satisfactory results. The process is useful where the amount of film-forming solid deposited as a dry (essentially liquid-carrier-free) coating after evaporation of the solvent ranges from about ½ of a milligram/square inch of exposed surface of the compressed cosmetic powder article to about 50 mg./square inch, and has a thickness of from 0.0001 to 0.005 inch. Generally speaking, an excellent amount of film former to be applied, considered on a dry weight, i.e., after evaporation of the volatile solvent, is an amount not to exceed 0.001 of an inch if applied to a nonporous surface.

Effervescent Mouthwash Tablets

T.L. Welsh, D. Leroy, B.T. Palermo and G.C. Hoss; U.S. Patent 3,518,343; June 30, 1970; assigned to Miles Laboratories, Inc. have produced an effervescent tablet by preparing a powdered tablettable composition comprising an effervescent couple, an antimicrobial substance, a tabletting lubricant, and preferably a flavoring, sweetening and/or coloring agent.

The inclusion of antimicrobial agents in the prior effervescent tablets has been mainly unsuccessful due to incompatibility of such agents with the other materials in compressed form. Also, the liquid state of many of such agents has rendered difficult their inclusion in powdered tablettable compositions.

It has been found that adequate lubrication and antimicrobial properties can be imparted to effervescent tablets by including a lubricant of fumaric acid or particles of a liquid lubricant coated with a water-soluble, oil-insoluble film-forming substance, and by including a solid state antimicrobial agent which is water-soluble. Such tablets can be used for cleaning solid surfaces of all types and can be produced at commercially feasible production rates.

The effervescent couple of the powdered tablet composition consists of at least one solid acid and solid basic material which when dissolved in water react to produce carbon dioxide, which causes effervescence. The acid can be an organic acid such as malic, fumaric, tartaric, itaconic, maleic, citric or mesaconic acid, or a corresponding anhydride such as itaconic anhydride and citraconic anhydride or it can be an inorganic acid, such as sulfamic acid or a phosphonic acid derivative such as disclosed in U.S. Patent 3,325,357. The basic material can be any of the metal carbonate salts such as alkali or alkaline earth carbonates and bicarbonates. Citric acid and sodium bicarbonate constitute a preferred couple due to their rapid reaction and consequent effervescence. As stated above, the tabletting lubricant can be either fumaric acid or particles of a liquid lubricant coated with a water-soluble film-forming substance. The lubricant can also be a mixture of these two materials. When fumaric acid is used at least 5% of the acid based on the total weight of the lubricant and the tablettable composition is employed. If desired, the fumaric acid may be used in larger amounts up to about 14% or even approaching the total tablet weight, since fumaric acid is itself cohesive when compressed.

Mesh sizes of 40 and finer (U.S. Standard) are particularly preferred for use with most powdered compositions. Since fumaric acid is a polycarboxylic acid, it provides the additional effect of taking part in the effervescent action.

The coated particulate lubricant consists of particles of a lubricating oil coated with an oil-insoluble, water-soluble film-forming substance. The amount of the coated lubricant can be varied to suit the desired tabletting speed. It is usually sufficient to use at least about 0.5% of the lubricant based on the total tablet weight including the lubricant. Preferably, less than about 5% of the coated lubricant is employed; however, larger amounts approaching about 50% of the total tablet weight can be used if desired. The lubricating oil in the coated particles can be any of the viscous vegetable, animal, mineral, or synthetic oils, and preferably those having viscosities in about the 100 to 200 cp. range.

A preferred lubricant composition can be formed by including in the tablet about 10 to 40% by weight of a siloxane polymer based on the total weight of the lubricating oil. The siloxane polymer is preferably a polymer of polydimethyl siloxane. This siloxane polymer can be added directly to the powdered composition, or it can be, and is preferably, incorporated with the lubricating oil of the coated particles. The siloxane polymer lends a free-flowing characteristic to the coated lubricant particles when incorporated in the lubricating oil, and it also aids punch face and die wall lubrication during tablet compression. The following example shows the preparation of these tablets.

Example:

Tablet components	Weight, g.	Weight, percent
(1) Sodium bicarbonate	6,780	52.5
(2) Citric acid (anhydrous)	5,712	44.3
(3) Coated oil particles	180	1.4
(4) Flavoring	150	1.2
(5) Sodium cyclohexylsulfamate	60	.5
(6) Sodium saccharin	6	.05
(7) Cetyldimethylbenzylammonium chloride	15	.12
Totals	12,903	100.07

Components (1) and (2) were blended, passed through a screen and dried. The remaining components were blended with this dry mixture and then compressed into tablets on a single punch tabletting machine at a commercial rate. The tablets were 1 inch in diameter and had an average weight of about 4.3 grams. They contained 1.4% of the coated oil particles lubricant based on the tablet weight. The tablets when dissolved in about 135 ml. of tap water produced a pleasant tasting mouthwash solution.

The coated oil particles were formed by spray drying using a refined vegetable oil which had good heat and air stability and which was resistant to microbial attack. The free fatty acids content was 0.05% maximum, the oxygen stability was 450 to 500 hours as measured by the Active Oxygen Method ("Tentative Method Cd" 12 to 57 revised 1959, published in *Official and Tentative Procedures of the American Oil Chemists Society;* 3rd. edition, 1966, Chicago, Ill.), and the Wiley melting point was 22 ± 2°F.

The major fatty acid moieties were: palmitic 8 to 10%; stearic 2 to 4%; oleic 43 to 47%; elaidic 39 to 43%; and linoleic 1 to 3%. A vegetable oil of this description can be obtained under the trade name Durkex 500 (Durkee Famous Foods, Inc.) The film-forming substance was used in a 2:1 weight ratio with respect to the lubricating oil and was a starch gum having the following characteristics: viscosity, 120 to 140 cp.; particle size, 98% of the powder passes through a 40 mesh screen (U.S. Standard); and color, light tan. This starch gum was a stable corn dextrin. A dextrin of this description can be obtained under the trade name Nadex 772 (National Starch and Chemical Co., Inc.) The flavoring was a spray dried flavor oil coated with the same dextrin.

H.P. Andersen; U.S. Patent 3,629,468; December 21, 1971 has also produced an effervescent mouthwash tablet comprising a germicidal agent, chlorophyll, an alkali metal carbonate salt, adipic acid, flavoring ingredients and sweetening agents.

A profound effect on the ability of this product to control breath odors has been shown by the inclusion of a germicidal agent. In theory, any such agent compatible with the other ingredients would be satisfactory, however, those germicidal agents of the cationic surface active class have been found most effective. Examples of these compounds are diisobutylphenoxyethoxyethyl dimethyl benzylammonium chloride, cetylpyridinium chloride, benzethonium chloride and methylbenzethonium chloride. The germicidal agent may be present in amounts preferably from 0.5 to 2.5% by weight. Incorporation of chlorophyll into the composition yields a product which is effective in relieving breath odors due to faulty oral hygiene, halitosis, alcohol, onions, smoking, bad teeth and most other causes. It has been found that the most effective compositions do not contain more than about 1.5 weight percent.

The desired effervescent action is produced upon the liberation of gaseous carbon dioxide by reaction between the gas-liberating salt and organic acid which constitute the tablet base. This reaction is initiated by bringing the acid and salt into aqueous reactive contact with each other in the mouth, e.g., a tablet is placed in contact with the saliva and/or a small quantity of water added to the mouth of the user. The gas-liberating salt used may be any soluble carbonate salt, but is preferably an alkali metal carbonate or bicarbonate or mixtures thereof. Sodium bicarbonate is the most preferred ingredient. An effective product has a sodium bicarbonate content of 35 to 75 weight percent.

The advantageous properties of these tablets are in part attributable to the use of adipic acid as the organic acid constituent of the tablets. In contradistinction to the conventional fruit acids associated with previous effervescent compositions, adipic acid yields a product which is hygroscopically controlled in character. This property solves many of the problems associated with the undesirable hygroscopic behavior of known tablets while still retaining the desirable quality of rapid disintegration in the mouth.

The adipic acid in proportions of 10 to 70% by weight yields a satisfactory product. The preferred range is 20 to 55 weight percent. A possible modification is the substitution of a minor amount, i.e., less than 10% by weight, of adipic acid with a fruit acid such as citric or tartaric acid in order to achieve faster tablet disintegration in the user's mouth without materially affecting the product stability.

A further discovery relates to the use of adipic anhydride as the acidic component of the effervescent couple. Although the rate of disintegration is slowed down by the adipic anhydride a compensating effect is realized by the increased stability. The unexpected effectiveness of adipic anhydride may be a result of its substantial water-solubility or perhaps the fact that it exists in the form of an unstable polymeric-type structure rather than the stable ring structure normally occurring in dibasic anhydrides. Again, substitution of a minor amount of the anhydride with citric or tartaric acid is possible. Also, mixtures of adipic acid and adipic anhydride are contemplated.

Example: The following dry powdered ingredients are prepared in the relative amounts given below, the particle size of the ingredients being from 20 to 250 mesh. The ingredients (shown on the following page) are thoroughly mixed and then subjected to precompression or slugging in a high pressure mold. The resulting slugs are reduced to proper granule size (8 to 20 U.S. Standard mesh) with a Fitz Mill comminuting machine, an oscillating granulator, or other suitable device.

Next, the granules are fed to a rotary tablet machine to produce 550 mg. tablets of about 4 kg. on the Strong-Cobb hardness scale. The resulting 550 mg. tablet has a diameter of ⅝ inch and thickness of ⅛ inch. When placed in the mouth with about 1 ounce of water, effervescence begins immediately, and total dissolution takes place in about 20 to 30 sec. depending upon the acidity of the individual user's mouth and the temperature of the water added.

Ingredients	Parts by Weight
Diisobutylphenoxyethoxyethyl dimethyl benzylammonium chloride	4.0
Chlorophyll	5.0
Peppermint powder	5.0
Sodium saccharin	1.0
Sodium cyclamate	20.0
Sodium bicarbonate	300.0
Adipic acid	210.0
Stearic acid	5.0

SANITATION PRODUCTS

Carboxymethylcellulose Bonded Dichloroisocyanurate

A shaped chlorine-liberating composition which may be efficiently and effectively used with metering devices for disseminating active and/or available chlorine into a marine commode system has been produced by *T.E. Schneider, Jr. and J.L. Halley; U.S. Patent 3,506,764; April 14, 1970; assigned to Tesco Chemicals, Inc.*

The chlorine-liberating composition is initially formulated by uniformly blending the following compounds: a potassium salt of dichloroisocyanuric acid; a blend of microcrystalline cellulose and either methylcellulose or an alkali metal compound of carboxymethylcellulose; and a metallic salt of an aliphatic carboxylic acid having at least 10 carbon atoms. When blending these components it is preferred that they be in substantially dry form. The blending of the various components is accomplished by stirring, tumbling, and the like. It is important, however, that the mixing be carried out in such a manner that the particle size of the various components is not appreciably altered in mixing. Tumbling in a rotating tumbler is the preferred method.

The size of the particles of the various components has a significant effect on the shaped chlorinating composition, specifically the erosion and/or dissolution rate. The dichloroisocyanuric acid and the blend of cellulose and either methylcellulose or carboxymethylcellulose compound should be in a granular form and pass through a No. 10 mesh U.S. Standard Screen and preferably at least 90% of the particles should be retained on a No. 100 mesh U.S. Standard Screen.

The particle size of the particles of the aliphatic carboxylic acid is usually between 1 to 100 microns and preferably between 1 to 50 microns, i.e., powdered material. The powdered material acts not only as a lubricant for the stick while it is being compressed but such material also affects the erosion and/or dissolution rates of the shaped composition when the composition is contacted with an aqueous media.

The mixture of components may then be converted or compressed into a variety of configurations to provide the shaped composition of this process. Forming is usually accomplished by conventional pressure molding in the absence of heat. Satisfactory molding pressures in the range of 400 to 1,500 psi have been used. The typical configuration is commonly referred to as the stick form which is a solid cylindrically shaped or tubular article. These shaped compositions, when contacted with a selected volume of water under conditions conducive to erosion and for a prescribed period of time, will erode rapidly but uniformly to supply a predetermined amount of active and/or available chlorine to a marine commode system.

The composition of this process would normally erode from about 1.5 to 4 ounces with each flush or operation of a system which normally lasts about 15 seconds. It has been found that such an amount of the composition dissolved or dispersed in the amount of flush water is capable of reducing the active Coliform count of the waste material to zero.

Example: A chlorine-liberating composition comprising 90.5 parts by weight potassium dichloroisocyanurate, 7.5 parts of a dried blend of 92 weight percent microcrystalline cellulose and 8 weight percent sodium carboxymethylcellulose (Avicel RC), and 2 parts sodium stearate is intimately blended into a uniform mixture. The blended composition is then molded under 450 psi into 1 lb. cylindrical sticks of approximately 2½ inches in diameter and approximately 5¼ inches in length.

One of the composition sticks is tested in a marine commode system. During several 15 second operations it is found that approximately 4 ounces of the stick composition are eroded with each operation of the system and that each operation effectively reduces the active Coliform count of the waste material to zero. The stick exhibits good stability and uniformity in erosion rate.

Paradichlorobenzene-Encapsulated Dichloroisocyanurate

It is known that the release of chlorine from certain agents such as 1,3-dichloro-5,5-dimethylhydantoin can be controlled by blending this compound with paradichlorobenzene, a dissolution retardant. Initially, when the fused mixture of 1,3-dichloro-5,5-dimethylhydantoin and paradichlorobenzene is poured into the mold and cooled, the 1,3-dichloro-5,5-dimethylhydantoin segregates in the base section of the mold and is not uniformly distributed throughout the cake. This results in the nonuniform release of chlorine as the cake progressively dissolves in use.

J.S. Thompson, R.R. Keast and E.H. Krusius; U.S. Patent 3,496,269; February 17, 1970; assigned to FMC Corporation have found that effective, slow dissolving sanitizing tablets can be produced by blending together a mixture containing from 5 to 25% of a chlorinated cyanuric acid, or salt thereof, and paradichlorobenzene in amounts sufficient to make up the balance of the mixture (normally from about 10 to 95%). The resulting mixture is heated until the paradichlorobenzene melts, and the melted mixture is kept in constant agitation and in a homogeneous condition while allowing the mixture to cool. The mixture is finally divided to form small discrete particles containing chlorinated cyanuric acid or salts thereof coated with paradichlorobenzene, and the discrete particles are pressed into compacted shapes such as tablets.

As a result of the above technique, the individual particles of the chlorinated cyanuric acid or salt reagent are encased in a coating of paradichlorobenzene. When these particles are compressed into a tablet, the resulting tablet has a homogeneous distribution of the chlorine releasing agent throughout the tablet. In addition, the chlorinated cyanuric acid or chlorinated cyanuric acid salt releases free available chlorine in aqueous solution, i.e., HOCl, has good heat stability, and does not lose active chlorine at the temperatures used to melt the paradichlorobenzene and to coat the particles of chlorine releasing agent.

The primary application for these tablets are for use in urinals, latrines or toilets. The tablets are designed for either continuous contact with the water source or intermittent contact with water, as in the case, for example, when the tablets are suspended in a urinal.

Example: Run A – The compositions set forth in the table were placed in a mixing bowl and blended. Thereafter, the mixing bowl was heated until the paradichlorobenzene ingredient melted. Mixing was continued while the paradichlorobenzene was melted so that it was uniformly dispersed throughout the mixture. The mixture was then cooled with agitation and mixing until the paradichlorobenzene solidified. Thereafter, the mixture was placed in a mortar and ground to a fine powder. 10 gram quantities of the formulations were tabletted in a 1³⁄₁₆ inch die using a Carver laboratory press at pressures of between 5,000 and 10,000 lbs. on the ram.

The tablets were then tested for relative dissolving time by means of an accelerated dissolving test. The test was performed by placing a tablet in a ½ inch mesh wire cage which was immersed in a transparent sided Kenmore washer containing 16 gallons of agitated tap water at a temperature of 70°F. The time required for the tablet to be reduced in size sufficiently to permit escape from the cage was designated as the dissolving time. Both the compositions of the tablets and the dissolving times are listed in the table.

Composition (wt. percent)				
Trichloro-isocyanuric acid	"Hexaphos"	Para-dichloro-benzene	Formulation technique	Tablet dissolving time (sec.)
25	25	50	Run A	30,000
25	25	50	Run B	4,400
25	45	30	Run A	18,500
25	53	22	do	5,710
25	53	22	Run B	1,090
25	60	15	Run A	2,970
25	60	15	Run B	870
25	65	10	Run A	2,080
5	0	95	do	Over 50,000
10	0	90	do	Over 50,000

Run B – Several mixtures were made up containing the same proportion of ingredients as in Run A. However, in the makeup of these mixtures, the paradichlorobenzene component was not melted but was merely uniformly mixed with the other ingredients. Thereafter, 10 gram quantities of these mixtures were tabletted in the same manner as in Run A. The formulations which were used and the dissolving time for the resulting tablets was determined in the manner described in Run A. The formulations which were used and the dissolving times of the resulting tablets are reported in the table.

The results shown in the table clearly indicate that the tablet dissolving time increases with increases in the paradichlorobenzene content of the tablet. However, a comparison of the dissolving time for identical mixtures, differing only in the manner in which the ingredients were blended, clearly shows that when the paradichlorobenzene is melted and the resultant mixture is ground and tabletted the dissolving times are much greater than when identical mixtures are merely blended and formulated into tablets.

Encapsulated Halophors

Tablets of encapsulated halophors which release the active halogen gradually over a long period of time have been developed by *P.B. Dalton and L. Katz; U.S. Patent 3,330,885; July 11, 1967; assigned to General Aniline & Film Corporation.*

The prior discovery of compounds which act as carriers for halogens, and particulary such compounds as polymeric-N-vinylpyrrolidone has resulted in the provision of an active bactericide in which the toxic and irritant properties of the halogen are markedly reduced or almost entirely eliminated. At the same time, the effectiveness of the halogen as a killing agent is not diminished and in many instances is actually enhanced by the combination with such carrier agents.

Among the defects, however, of these iodophor combinations is the instability and rapid release of the halogen in most of the applications. Thus, the addition of an iodophor to a large volume of water to be treated to destroy bacteria and the like results in the rapid release of active iodine over a very short period of time.

The general procedure for producing the encapsulated halophor compositions of this process comprises polymerizing a suitable ethylenically unsaturated compound in the presence of the halophor material whereby the latter is obtained in encapsulated form. Any suitable procedure for effecting the polymerization may be used, but it is preferred to carry out the process while maintaining the halophor as a suspension in an inert liquid and in the presence of a suitable catalytic agent contacting the suspended halophor with the monomeric form of the ethylenically unsaturated compound. The latter in the presence of the catalytic agent and under specified conditions of temperature, pressure, and the like, undergoes polymerization in the usual manner on the surfaces of the halophor, and this results in an encapsulated form. The ethylenically unsaturated compounds which are preferred for use in the production of encapsulated halophors are those ethylenically unsaturated compounds which may be polymerized by ionic catalysts and include: olefins such as ethylene, propylene and butylene; styrene and alkyl-substituted styrene; acrylates; methacrylates; acrylonitrile; vinyl esters such as vinyl chloride and vinyl acetate; and vinyl ethers.

These catalyst systems are the preferred ionic polymerization catalyst combinations which are commonly described as Ziegler type catalysts and are more particularly definable as combinations of organometallic compounds on the one hand with a transition metal halide or ester on the other hand. The following example will illustrate the process. Parts are by weight unless otherwise indicated.

Example: 50 grams of substantially anhydrous polyvinylpyrrolidone-iodine complex containing 20% available iodine in finely powdered form is dispersed in 1,000 ml. of dry toluene. The dispersion is placed in a suitable reaction vessel and swept with nitrogen to remove all of the air. There is then added 0.05 mol of titanium tetrachloride and after 5 minutes of stirring, there is further added 0.1 mol of methyl magnesium bromide.

These procedures are carried out at room temperature under atmospheric pressure. The temperature of the reaction vessel is then raised to about 50°C. and ethylene gas is passed through the suspension. The flow of ethylene is continued until the rate of absorption has substantially ceased. This occurs after about 5 hours. The resultant suspension is then cooled to room temperature, filtered and washed with methanol. After drying, the resultant particulate product is found to contain 52.8% polyethylene by weight and an available iodine content of 8.17%. This is equivalent to an available iodine content of 17.3% discounting the polymer indicating only a slight loss of available iodine as a result of the entire polymerization and encapsulating procedure.

The aliquot portion of this product is pressed in a Carver press at 100°C. at 10,000 psi (1.25 in. ram) for 30 seconds between aluminum foil to produce a film. The resultant film is then immersed in distilled water and is found to release about 7.2% iodine (available iodine) at a relatively uniform rate over a period of about 24 hours. The less than 1% decrease in available iodine in the pressed film is indeed remarkable especially since about this quantity is lost in the molding operation itself.

FOOD PRODUCTS

Dried Food Disks

A disk of dried food material is produced by *L.C. Berardi, W.H. Martinez, G.J. Boudreaux, B. Piccolo and V.L. Frampton; U.S. Patent 3,463,641; August 26, 1969; assigned to the U.S. Secretary of Agriculture* having smooth reproducible surfaces for measuring its color objectively. The dry food is prepared in the form of a sandwich comprising outer layers of plastic and an inner layer of dried food product. The system is evacuated at less than 50 mm. Hg for 1 to 5 minutes, then compressed at about 300 to 3,000 psig for 5 to 30 seconds.

The food products include proteins, carbohydrates and lipid-containing (fat) materials. Typical examples of food products include lyophilized egg yolks; lyophilized egg whites; lyophilized peanut butter; precooked, flaked, dehydrated Irish potatoes; dry gelatin dessert mix; instant ground coffee; dried ground sassafras leaves; pancake flour with shortening; dried skim milk; dried whole milk; dehulled, flaked cottonseed meats; dehulled flaked soybean meats; cornmeal; and the like. The disks are prepared by a pressing device as shown in Figure 15.1. In the figure, **1** is a circular housing enclosing removable cylinder **2** which is supported by a circular inset **3** located near the bottom of the housing. This inset provides an open space **4** between cylinder **2** and the bottom of housing **1** which open space

FIGURE 15.1: PRESSING DEVICE

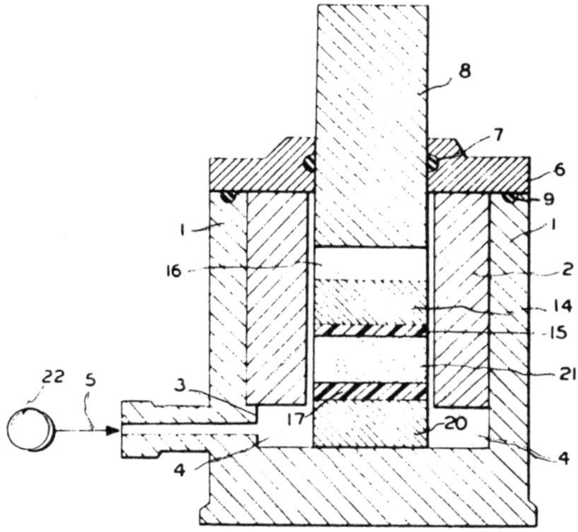

Source: L.C. Berardi, W.H. Martinez, G.J. Boudreaux, B. Piccolo and V.L. Frampton; U.S. Patent 3,463,641; August 26, 1969

is connected to vacuum pump **22** by means of vent **5**. Through this vent open space **4** may be evacuated. Housing **1** also supports a removable top **6** which is recessed to hold flexible circular gasket **7** which fits snugly against plunger **8** and prevents passage of air during the operation of the vacuum system. Housing **1** also has an annular depression holding gasket **9** which serves as a seal between the housing and the removable top when the interior **4** is evacuated. The interior sidewalls of cylinder **2** and removable housing top **6** are in exact alignment and permit unobstructed movement of plunger **8**, which in turn contacts metallic disk **14**.

The metallic disk in turn contacts plastic disk **15**, which forms the upper layer of the sandwich. Metallic disk **20** rests on the bottom of housing **1** and has a thickness greater than the vertical height of open space **4**, thereby sealing the inner opening of bore **16** of cylinder **2**. Plastic disk **17**, which forms the lower layer of the sandwich rests upon metallic disk **20**. Dry food products **21** which form the interior of the sandwich are situated between plastic disks **15** and **17**.

The particular plastic used will depend to some extent upon the dried food product to be pressed. For proteins and/or carbohydrates polyethylene and polypropylene films may be used. For foods containing lipid components, such as egg yolks, disks of polymerized tetrafluoroethylene are preferred. Regardless of the particular plastic employed, it is a critical feature of the process that the plastic disk be shaped to fit into the bore of the press. It should be smooth and free of scratches or nicks which might be detrimental to obtaining smooth surfaces on the pressed food disks.

Example 1: In this example, a 0.7 gram sample of lyophilized egg yolks is placed on the bottom disk which is prepared from polymerized tetrafluoroethylene. The upper tetrafluoroethylene disk is then placed on top of the dried food after the latter had been brushed easily to give a uniform thickness, the two disks and the layer of fried egg yolks forming the ingredients of the sandwich. The upper metallic disk, plunger, and removable top are then inserted as noted above, and the vacuum pump connected to the orifice. When the vacuum has been reduced to about 25 mm. Hg, a period of dwell is held for 2 minutes, after which a pressure of 320 psig is applied for 5 seconds. The pressure is then released, the vacuum released and the sandwich now in disk form is removed from the cylinder.

Example 2: In this example, various dried food products are formed into disks using various periods of dwell after the vacuum has been reduced to less than 5 mm. Hg. The results are shown below.

Dry food	Amount of dry food for disk (grams)	Preliminary evacuation period (minutes)	Pressing conditions	
			Pressing load (pounds per square inch)	Total pressing period (seconds)
Lyophilized egg yolks	0.7	2	320	5
Lyophilized egg whites	0.7	5	640	5
Lyophilized peanut butter	1.8	4	640	15
Precooked, dehydrated sweet potato flakes	1.4	2	1,792	15
Dry gelatin dessert mix	1.0	2	2,048	10
"Instant," ground coffee	1.0	2	2,048	25
Dried, ground sassafras leaves	1.0	2	2,048	5
Pancake flour with added shortening	1.5	2	320	5
Dried skim milk	1.5	1	480	20
Dehulled, flaked cottonseed meats	0.7	4	314	25
Corn meal	1.5	2	1,792	5
Cooked, dried Irish potato flakes	1.5	2	2,560	52

In every instance, a smooth, uniform surface is obtained, and products such as the dried sweet potato disks and dried skim milk disks are easily reconstituted in hot water.

Pelletized Ground Coffee

It has been discovered by *R.A. Hudson, W.J. Richards and G.V. Jones; U.S. Patent 3,511,666; May 12, 1970; assigned to General Foods Corporation,* that filter bags with large pore sizes can be used for extraction of freshly roasted coffee solids if the R&G (roasted and ground) coffee is formed into a pellet prior to being placed in the filter bag.

By pelletizing or tabletting the coffee, filter pores or holes of between 0.01 and 0.1 inch, and preferably 0.03 to 0.07 inch in diameter, can be used to achieve effective extraction during brewing without undergoing loss of grounds through the filter. Dusting is prevented prior to percolation by compression of the R&G coffee pellets. While the pellets break up during brewing, migration of grounds into the brew is prevented due to swelling of the R&G particles upon contact with the hot water.

The pellet is formed of compressed coffee particles under sufficient pressure to hold the coffee in the form of a doughnut-shaped tablet, wafer or other desired shape and being capable of releasing at least 10% more extractable solids than an equivalent charge of fresh R&G coffee. In doing this, the initial volume of R&G coffee is reduced to between 25 and 40%, preferably 30 to 35%, of the initial charge volume. However, the coffee particles should not be disrupted to the extent that coffee lipids are expressed thereby introducing an undesirable oil film or slick in the percolated brew.

More particularly, it has been found that a coffee pellet or tablet essentially free of extruded oil, coffee fines and fissures can be made by roasting the green coffee, grinding, and then sufficiently degassing the coffee for the pelletizing operation. The coffee is then compressed into pellets at a critical pressure of between 8,000 to 10,000 psi, the application of the pressure being controlled to yield a pellet of sufficient hardness to prevent breakage but not so great as to cause pellet capping.

The actual pressure used will vary with the temperature and moisture of the coffee, the blend, the rate or speed of pelletizing and the amount of degassing. However, within this pressure range an R&G pellet can be produced which retains its shape and form during packaging and distribution.

The pellet or pellets of coffee should be packed initially in a manner which assures at least 30%, preferably 50%, void space inside the filter bag material. Where the material is non-stretchable on percolation (cotton), even more void space may be necessary. This is necessary to achieve proper circulation of the water through the bed of coffee during the brewing cycle. If less than 30% void space is present in the filter bag, the pellets on wetting will swell into a compact bed which will not allow proper extraction of coffee solids. In extreme cases, the bag itself may rupture since the coffee particles swell to about twice their size.

In the case of doughnut-shaped percolator packages, it has been found that the filter bag will not achieve good extraction during percolation unless the coffee and filter actually contact the percolator spout. Preferably, the filter material should not only merely touch the spout, but it should form an intimate or tight contact which assures a trapping of the percolating water issuing from the top of the spout and avoids serious bypass of the coffee. Since most spouts are about $\frac{3}{16}$ to $\frac{6}{16}$ inch in diameter, the inner seal should be about ½ to ¾ inch in size and so cut as to allow a snug contact with the spout.

Example: Freshly roasted coffee was ground to a particle size distribution where at least 85% (by weight) of the coffee was between 12 and 30 mesh (U.S. Standard Sieve). In this distribution about 1 to 5% of the coffee was less than 0.01 inch in diameter and at least 30% was less than 0.03 inch in diameter, and no particle of coffee was greater than 0.06 inch in diameter.

The coffee was held under ambient conditions for at least 4 hours to obtain substantial degassing (about 300 cc/lb. of the releasable gas). Then a 34 gram charge of coffee was placed in a doughnut-shaped cylindrical die having an outer diameter of about 2.7 inches and an inner diameter of about 1 inch, and compressed at a pressure of 12,000 psi for 0.1 second. This reduced the charge of coffee from a height of about 1.5 to 0.5 inch. The final tablet did not have any extruded oil or wax visibly present at the surface. No fissures were present in the tablet due to excessive gas release during tabletting.

These tablets were then placed between 2 sheets of polyethylene film having at least 80 perforations of 0.04 inch size diameter for each square inch of film and the film was impulse heat-sealed around the peripheral portions of the doughnut. At least ½ inch was left at these peripheral portions to allow for bean expansion on percolation thus giving a tablet fill corresponding to about 50% of the total void volume prior to bean expansion.

The bag was cut around its outer periphery but merely slit in an X pattern inside the inner periphery to thereby assure good contact and wetting of the cartridge around the stem. The tabletted coffee cartridges were vacuum packed in cellophane packages (in pairs) and placed within suitable cans or packages for shipment and storage. They did not experience any dusting of coffee particles or rupture of the envelopes.

Two cartridges, when taken from the cellophane protective envelope and placed in a suitable stove top percolator and perked for 5 to 9 minutes with 1,333 cc of water gave eight cups of a robust coffee brew similar to that from a corresponding charge of fresh R&G in loose form but which was cleaner, clearer, and had less oil. Solids content and flavor was similar to the conventional brew. No significant migration of coffee through the filter was noted during percolation and the walls of the percolator vessel had less of the typical residual oil film deposited by conventional coffee.

Instant Coffee or Tea

S.-E. Tessmar; U.S. Patent 3,666,483; May 30, 1972 discloses a method of producing unit portions of instant coffee or tea by mixing dry coffee or tea concentrate with a binder substance and forming the resulting coherent composition into unit portions. The binder substance comprises either a mixture of a fat which is solid or semisolid at room temperature and an emulsifier or a mixture of a fatty acid which is solid or semisolid at room temperature and a substance capable of forming a water-soluble salt with the fatty acid.

The proportions of the dry coffee or tea concentrate to the fat or fatty acid should lie in the range from 2:1 to 1:3. The fat or fatty acid serves mainly as a binder for imparting to the powder a consistency which enables it to be given a suitable form, e.g., punched into tablets by a tablet making machine, pressed or molded into slabs, or placed in a tube or portion-containing packet. Suitable fats are cocoa butter and coconut butter, although in principle any edible fat and fat mixture can be used, provided that it can be obtained in a form in which it is free from substances which give rise to secondary flavors.

Suitable fatty acids are oleic acid, stearic acid, ricinoleic acid and the like and mixtures thereof, for example, such which are derived from natural fats. When preparing solid products, such as tablets and slabs, the fat or fatty acid should have a relatively high melting point, e.g., 30° to 50°C., particularly 40° to 45°C., so that the product retains its given form at normal room temperature but which nevertheless is able to melt rapidly and dissolve in hot water (80° to 100°C.). When preparing paste products, fat or fatty compositions or fatty acids are used which have a lower melting point, e.g., 20° to 35°C.

The purpose of the emulsifier is to emulsify the fat in the water when dissolving the product, so that no droplets of fat are visible on the surface of the beverage, which would otherwise render it unappetizing. Suitable emulsifiers include all substances which can form a stable emulsion of fat in water and which, of course, are pharmaceutically acceptable, i.e., have no toxic reactions when taken in the necessary concentration. Anionic, cationic and nonionic emulsifiers of many different known types can be used. Preferred emulsifiers are ethoxylated higher alcohols and alkylphenols, soybean lecithin, sorbitan monolaurate and lauryl sarcosinate. Naturally, mixtures of emulsifiers can be used if so desired.

Example 1: One portion of coffee powder, 2 portions of cocoa butter and 0.2 portion of ethoxylated C_{14} alcohol were mixed whilst heated to about 50°C., whereafter the melt was poured into a mold divided into squares. When the composition had cooled, a slab was obtained in the form of a chocolate bar. A square placed in a cup of hot water rapidly produced good coffee. Owing to the emulsifier present, the fat in the composition is completely emulsified in the water, so as to exclude any droplets of oil on the surface of the coffee.

Example 2: 1 portion of coffee powder was mixed at about 50°C. with 0.5 portion of cocoa butter, 0.5 of a portion of a commercial mixture of C_{18} fatty acids, 0.1 portion of lauryl sarcosinate, 0.25 portion of triethanolamine and 0.01 portion of cetyl pyridinium chloride. The mixture, which was solid when cooling to room temperature, was used for preparing tablets and cubes.

Tea products can be prepared by replacing the coffee powder above with approximately the same quantity of powdered tea. All the products obtained in the examples rapidly dissolved in hot water and quickly gave a beverage ready to drink. No droplets of fat could be seen on the surface. The products had unlimited durability and, with regard to the solid products, showed no tendency to crumble.

Bakery Enrichment Wafers

It is a common practice to add enrichment wafers to bakery doughs and the usual practice is either to add them directly to the dough so that they will be intimately mixed throughout the dough or to add them to an amount of water in a separate container so that the wafer will be dispersed therein and to then add this dispersion to the dough so that it will be distributed more quickly. In either practice, it is important that the wafer disintegrates as soon as possible to thereby hasten its distribution throughout the dough.

M.J. Boroshok; U.S. Patent 3,753,732; August 21, 1973; assigned to Merck & Co., Inc. has found that a hard, shock resistant wafer can be made as a rapidly disintegrating one if the starch used in making it is divided and added at two separate stages. Special advantages are found to occur if the starches which are separately added are of different kinds, namely a pregelatinized starch such as tapioca starch and a nonpregelatinized starch such as ordinary cornstarch. Both of these starches are obtainable commercially. The nutrients which are to be present in the wafer are the usual vitamins and minerals such as riboflavin, thiamine or one of its nutritionally acceptable salts such as the mononitrate, niacin or a derivative such as niacinamide, and iron such as ferrous sulfate. A tabletting lubricant such as calcium stearate is also preferably added.

In practice, the selected vitamins and minerals and the pregelatinized starch are first thoroughly blended together using a conventional mixing or blending machine. A lubricant such as calcium stearate is preferably included in the mix. The product is then directly compressed into wafers and the hardness is immaterial as long as the wafers are fully formed and can be handled without immediate breakage. These wafers are then broken up and are comminuted or reduced through a sieve which can vary from a No. 6 to a No. 30 mesh size. To this granular material is added the nonpregelatinized starch and additional lubricant such as calcium stearate. After thorough blending this preparation is tabletted into wafers.

The total amount of starch to be added is that which is conventionally used in the wafers, i.e., it should add up to about 25 to 60%, preferably 40% of the weight of the wafer. The pregelatinized starch which is added to the vitamin-mineral premix should constitute from 15 to 35% by weight of that premix. The cornstarch added at the final stage should constitute from 10 to 25% of the final granular material to be compressed into the final wafer.

Example:

Ingredients	Mg./Tablet	Quantity/100 Tablets (grams)
(1) Riboflavin	105	10.5
(2) Thiamine mononitrate	155.8	15.58
(3) Ferrous sulfate	2,962.0	296.2
(4) Niacin	1,248.0	124.8
(5) Tapioca starch (pregelatinized)	1,500.0	150.0
(6) Calcium stearate	0.3	0.03
Subtotal	5,971.1	597.11

The following is a step by step description of the process.

(a) In a seven quart Hobart mixer bowl, blend (2), (3), and (4);
(b) Add (1) to above and continue to blend, then add (6);
(c) Pass through a No. 28 mesh screen;
(d) Add (5) to above screened blend, and blend in Hobart mixer;
(e) Compress on a Manesty single punch press equipped with $^{24}/_{32}$ inch set of tooling;
(f) Pass wafers through a No. 12 gauge sieve; and
(g) Combine the following ingredients.

Product (f) blend	542.0 grams
Cornstarch	102.0 grams
Calcium stearate	2.0 grams
Total	646.0 grams

This was thoroughly blended and again compressed as above. There was no evidence of buildup on tablets. They disintegrated in 45 seconds in room temperature water. They had a hardness of 7 kg. on a Strong Cobb hardness tester.

METALLURGICAL PRODUCTS

Iron Ore Pellets

A process for agglomerating moist particulate material has been disclosed by *P.G. Kihlstedt;*

U.S. Patent 3,725,033; April 3, 1973; assigned to AB Cold Bound Pellets, Sweden where the zeta-potential of the material is adjusted to zero. During the initial formation of nodules of moist particulate material, when pelletizing, the capillary forces between the particles and the liquid moistening the particles coact to bring the particles together.

As the moistening substance departs, the agglomerate is held together to an ever decreasing extent by the capillary forces and the particulate material must therefore be bound together instead by atomic forces, i.e., the so-called van der Walls forces, which provide a fully satisfactory binding force only when the interstices of the particles are slight. In order to increase the capillary forces binding the particulate material together, and facilitate the formation of pellets, it has been the practice to grind the materials to very small particle sizes. Such grinding processes are expensive and, furthermore, it is often not desirable to form the pellets solely of very small particles.

The composition of the moist particulate materials is suitably adjusted by adjusting the pH of the liquid moistening the materials so that the particles are at least substantially decharged. Decharging of the particles can be effected by using as a starting material mixtures of particulate material presenting different charging properties in moist condition, so that the electrical charges of the particles neutralize each other.

It is also within the scope of the process to intermix with the particulate starting materials, for the purpose of decharging the same, small quantities of flocculating agents known from sedimentation techniques, for example, flocculating agents of organic type, such as glue, and/or conventional flocculating agents containing, for example, Al^{3+}, Fe^{3+} or Ca^{2+} ions.

It is also possible to combine the three methods, that is adjustment of the pH value, intermixing of particle types which neutralize their respective electric charges and the use of flocculating agents. It is particularly suitable to combine pH adjustment with one or the other of the remaining methods, since the pH can easily be adjusted by adding a small quantity of a suitable acid or base substance. Whether or not the particles in the moist starting material have actually been decharged, can be determined by conventional methods such as by examining the flocculating properties of the starting material and/or by measuring the so-called z-potential and/or by measuring the pH.

Figure 15.2 is a diagram showing the dependency of the z-potential on the pH value of a magnetite-hematite concentrate and a slag obtained from oxygen gas refinement of molten pig iron. The magnetite-hematite concentrate was a mixture (in weight percent) of 52.5% magnetite and 47.5% hematite, the mixture containing 4.20% SiO_2, 0.82% Al_2O_3, 2.66% CaO, 1.08% MgO, 63.4% Fe, 0.08% Mn, 0.67% P, 0.014% S and the remainder essentially chemically bound oxygen.

The slag contained 6.8% SiO_2, 1.14% Al_2O_3, 50.4% CaO, 3.48% MgO, 15.3% Fe, 1.14% Mn, 5.69% P and the remainder essentially chemically bound oxygen. The curve **1** illustrates the variation in z-potential of the magnetite-hematite mixture within the pH range of 8 to approximately 12, weak NaOH being used for varying the pH value.

In a similar manner, the curve **2** shows the variation in z-potential of the slag composition within the pH range 8 to approximately 12, weak H_2SO_4 being used for varying the pH of the slag.

As will be seen from curve **1**, the magnetite-hematite concentrate cannot be decharged and made fully suitable for pelletizing simply by adjusting the pH. Since the magnetite-hematite concentrate and the slag, however, has substantially opposite charging properties they can be intermixed in such proportions and brought to such a pH value that the particles neutralize each other with respect to their electric charges.

Curve **3** in the diagram shows the variation in z-potential with the pH value for a mixture comprising 90% by weight of the magnetite-hematite concentrate and 10% by weight of the slag, and also shows that this mixture of concentrate and slag is well suited for pelletizing purposes when its pH value has been adjusted to approximately 11.5. Weak H_2SO_4 was used for varying the pH of the mixture.

FIGURE 15.2: DEPENDENCY OF ZETA-POTENTIAL ON pH

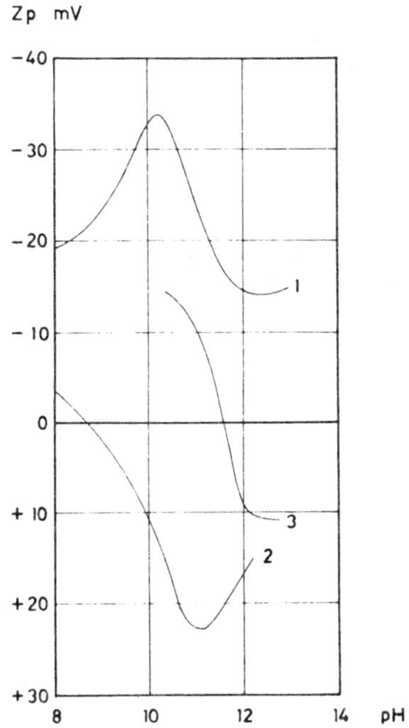

Source: P.G. Kihlstedt; U.S. Patent 3,725,033; April 3, 1973

Baked Ore Pellets

An improved method of making baked ore pellets is disclosed by *A. Van Latenstein; U.S. Patent 3,753,684; August 21, 1973; assigned to Koninklijke Nederlandsche Hoogovens en Staalfabriken NV, Netherlands.* This process comprises the following steps:

(a) grinding the ore;
(b) mixing the ground ore with a binding agent;
(c) moistening the mixture;
(d) forming the moist mixture into green pellets;
(e) then baking the green pellets in a baking zone;
(f) diverting from the flow sequence green ore pellets formed in step (d) which deviate from the prescribed compositional characteristics;
(g) diverting from the flow sequence green pellets and broken green pellets formed in step (d) which deviate from the prescribed dimensional characteristics;
(h) diverting from the flow sequence baked pellets and broken baked pellets formed in step (e) which deviate from the prescribed dimensional characteristics;

(i) forming a combined flow of the green and baked materials diverted in steps (f), (g) and (h); and
(j) mixing the combined flow with fresh ore to constitute the ore being ground in step (a).

The method is characterized in that all the flows of material separated from the main straight-through flow of the ore through the plant are united and combined and are then fed to the grinding plant. This makes it possible to use a simple conveying system for conveying all the return flows. As the return material is collected in storage hoppers of the grinding plant it is thus possible to remove all instability in the process of the forming plant, in which the green pellets are formed.

The following flow diagram (Figure 15.3) will illustrate the process. In the figure, ore is fed from the ore yard to storage hoppers, from which it is fed to a grinding plant. This plant operates according to the principle of dry grinding so that it also includes a drying zone. This drying zone may fully or in part be united structurally with the grinding mills.

A binding agent is then added to the ground ore and mixed in mixers. A binding agent which is often used for fine ore is a sticking type of clay known as bentonite. Mainly during mixing the mixture is also moistened by water so that a kneadable mass is obtained. This mass is fed to the forming plant for the pellets, in which in forming drums or on forming dishes so-called wet or green ore pellets are formed. These green pellets are fed to the baking plant over a screen, formed as a moving roller grid, and in the baking plant they are formed to a bed of pellets on a screen, which is continuously moved through the baking furnace.

FIGURE 15.3: BAKED ORE PELLETS

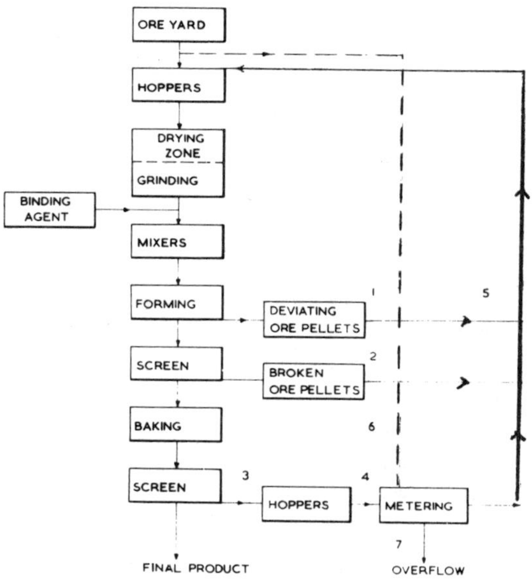

Source: A. Van Latenstein; U.S. Patent 3,753,684; August 21, 1973

After passing the screen behind this machine the burned ore pellets can be discharged to a storage space as the final product. The flow sheet includes grinding mills, mixers, forming apparatus, sieves or screens and baking furnaces, which are known in the art of making ore pellets. So it will not be necessary to give a more detailed description of such apparatus.

Three return flows are indicated by **1, 2** and **3,** relating respectively to green ore pellets of deviating type, dimensions or composition, to broken green ore pellets and to material derived from the baking plant and screened off from the pellets after baking. The return flow **1** of the deviating green ore pellets will occur during starting up and adjusting to optimum conditions of the forming process in a pelletizing device or during switching to another product.

The product of the return flow which is derived from the screen behind the baking machine is first fed to intermediary hoppers. From these hoppers this material is thereupon conveyed as a return flow **4**, accurately metered by metering apparatus. The return flows **1, 2** and **4** are united to a single return flow **5**, which is fed to the storage hoppers into which the ore from the ore yard is first fed at the beginning of the process.

The metering of the return flow **4** takes place dependent on the flow of material from the ore yard to the storage hoppers, for which a signal **6** is used. In this way it is possible to ensure that the so-called baked return is fed back into the flow through the plant in a quantity, which has a constant proportion to the quantity of the ore fed to the manufacturing plant. This minimizes the influence of this baked return on the quality of the final product. Line **7** indicates an overflow, e.g., to a sintering machine, if the quantity of baked return is unexpectedly large.

Fluxed Iron Ore Pellets

The preparation of fluxed iron ore pellets which do not weep a liquid phase on firing has been disclosed by *E. Dominguez, H.W. Hitzrot, Jr. and J.D. Lynn; U.S. Patent 3,754,889; August 28, 1973; assigned to Bethlehem Steel Corporation.* Specifically, an iron ore concentrate, for example, magnetite concentrate, which contains about 85 to 95% iron oxide, not more than 10% silica and not more than 2% alumina is mixed with a binder, moisture and at least one flux. The mix contains about 60 to 95% iron ore concentrate and about 40 to 5% flux materials.

The fluxes added to the iron ore concentrate are limestone ($CaCO_3$) and dolomite [$CaMg(CO_3)_2$]. The fluxes are added to the iron ore concentrate in a ratio of 40 to 60% limestone and 60 to 40% dolomite. The mix is balled in an apparatus, for example, a balling cone or disc or drum. The green balls are charged into a furnace, for example, a traveling furnace.

The green balls are dried at a temperature of between about 212° to 500°F. for about 4 minutes to remove a substantial portion of the moisture in the balls. The dried green balls are then heated to a temperature range of about 2275° to 2400°F. for a time sufficient to harden the dried green balls, about 20 minutes. The effect of the flux mixture is shown in the following example.

Example: Two samples of magnetite concentrate containing 61.2% iron, about 1.93% silica, 0.32% alumina and the remainder incidental impurities were prepared. A flux was added to each sample as follows.

	Concentrate	Limestone	Dolomite
Sample Mix 1	80%	20%	–
Sample Mix 2	80%	10%	10%

The mixes were formed into balls having a diameter of ½ inch on a balling disc. The green balls were dried at 500°F. for about 3 minutes. The dried green balls were then placed in a furnace and were heated to 2300°F. and held at that temperature for about 20 minutes.

The pellets were removed from the furnace and cooled to room temperature. An analysis of the pellets showed the following chemical composition.

	Iron (%)	Silica (%)	Alumina (%)	Lime (%)	Magnesia (%)	Base to Acid Ratio
Sample 1	61.2	1.93	0.32	9.00	0.30	4.13
Sample 2	61.9	1.94	0.32	7.20	1.80	4.00

Visual inspection of the samples after firing showed that excessive weeping occurred in the pellets of sample No. 1. The pellets were fused together and could not be broken apart. However, no weeping occurred in the pellets of sample No. 2. Each pellet remained a discrete particle during firing and cooling. The pellets had a tumble index of about 90% plus 3 mesh.

A microscopic examination of the pellets showed a microstructure of iron oxide bonded together and calcium magnesium ferrites and calcium magnesium spinels and slag products formed by the reaction between the flux added and the gangue material present, substantially uniformly distributed throughout the cross-section of the pellets in sample mix No. 2.

Pellets for Making Sponge Iron

U. Schierloh and P. Heinrich; U.S. Patent 3,765,869; October 16, 1973; assigned to Huttenwerk Oberhausen AG, Germany have developed a process for preparing pellets for use in the direct reduction of iron ore, i.e., the solid/gas reaction of iron ore with a reducing gas to produce metallic iron (generally sponge iron).

Green (nonfired) pellets of iron ore are prepared by pelletizing the iron ore and 2 to 8% by weight of finely divided metallic iron with a particle size below 45 microns in the presence of an aqueous solution, suspension or dispersion of an organic binder, preferably a carbohydrate. Surprisingly, the low-temperature binder, i.e., the starch, dextrine or the like, in combination with the metallic iron powder, affords considerable structural integrity to the pellets during the initial and subsequent stages of the direct reduction in a shaft-type or rotary furnace.

Examples: The following examples are illustrative of the process. It should be noted that an important result is the automatic increase in the compressive strength of the pellets during reduction, as represented by the resistance of the charge within the furnace to the throughflow of gases. When pellets crumble within the charge of a shaft-type furnace, the particles resulting from the deterioration pack the interstices between the unaffected pellets and increase the resistance to throughflow (high pressure drop).

Conversely, when the pellets remain intact because of their high compressive strength, there is little if any reduction in the free cross-section of the charge and the resistance to throughflow rises only slightly (low pressure loss). In both cases, increasing temperatures result in a decrease in the free cross-section which are generally considered by suitable calculation or disregarded, in the event the charges are not at the same temperature. In all of the tests detailed here, the iron ore was hematite of the following sieve analysis.

Weight Percent	Diameter (mm.)
44.84	<0.045
73.34	<0.063
95.45	<0.090
99.05	<0.125
99.46	<0.16
99.67	<0.25
100.00	<0.315

One portion of the pellets, test (A), was prepared by pelletization with 0.35% by weight dextrine (with respect to the iron ore) dissolved in the pelletizing moisture, the pelletizing moisture being the same in all of the cases. In test (B), 0.49% by weight (of the iron ore) of dextrine was used as the binder together with 3% by weight of the pellet of iron powder, at least 96% by weight of which had a particle size below 45 microns. In test (C), the same proportions and characteristics as in test (B) were applied except that the amount of iron powder was raised to 4% by weight. In test (D), the pieces were of similar particle sizes of the same ore, omitting both the organic binder and the iron.

Tests were made with equal piled heights of charge in a direct reduction furnace and the pressure drop in terms of 100% for test (D) was determined. In case (A), a complete collapse of the pellets was observed and the pressure drop was too high to be measurable. In test (B), 85.4% of the pressure drop was observed, in test (C), the pressure drop was 81.3% and in test (D), of course, the pressure drop was 100%, the latter being used as the base.

These results demonstrate that the production of green pellets with low temperature binders alone yield products with no strength at higher temperatures, and only upon the admixture of iron powder and the low temperature binder, do the pellets survive the rigors of the reduction process.

In test (C'), 4% by weight of iron powder containing 96% by weight of particles below 45 microns was used in the pellet with 0.3% by weight dextrine as the low temperature binder. In test (E), a larger size iron powder was employed in the same proportion, 80% by weight having a particle size between 45 and 90 microns while only 20% by weight had a particle size below 20 microns.

The pressure drop in a test similar to that given above, in terms of test (D), showed the pellets of sample (C') with 81.3% and the sample of test (E) with 275%. From this it is apparent that not only the amount of iron in the combination, but also the particle size is critical. When starch was substituted for dextrine, similar results were obtained.

Nuclear Fuel Pellets

Small amounts of barium have been used by *A.J. Flipot and R.E.M. Gilissen; U.S. Patent 3,751,538; August 7, 1973; assigned to Belgonucleaire, SA and Centre d'Etude l'Energie Nucleaire, Belgium* to control the bulk density of nuclear fuel pellets.

Fuel pellets are usually manufactured from ceramic powder, such as for instance, one or more oxides and/or carbides of uranium, plutonium and/or other transuranium elements. After possible addition of a binder, the powder is conventionally granulated, pelletized and sintered to produce pellets having bulk densities within a predetermined range, normally 70 to 98% of the theoretical density of the raw materials.

As each type of fuel pellet generally has an optimum bulk density at which it performs best in a given type of reactor, controlling the bulk density of a batch of pellets undergoing manufacture is a matter of significant importance. Also, the ability to obtain reproducible density from one batch to another and from one pellet to another within the same batch are likewise important. However, production of pellets of a preselected density and the achievement of reproducibility between and within batches of fuel pellets constitutes a difficult problem.

The barium may be introduced into the pellets in the form of a free metal or compounds, including both organic and inorganic compounds. If introduced as compounds, the compounds generally decompose at the temperatures involved in the sintering treatment.

The threshold of effectiveness of the barium, for inhibiting undesired bulk density increase on sintering is at the level of about 30 ppm, calculated as metal, based on the weight of the pellets after sintering. Preferably, about 0.1 to about 1% is used. The exact amount of inhibitor required to produce a given bulk density in a particular pellet-forming mixture may readily be determined by using simple empirical processes. In this connection, attention is directed to the examples in which representative bulk density reduction of values are shown for different amounts of barium utilization.

Example 1: A small amount of barium nitrate is added to uranyl nitrate. The solution is afterwards treated under the usual conditions for UO_2 ceramic manufacturing. The method includes the steps of precipitation using ammonia, drying, calcination at 550°C. and reduction at 450°C. under hydrogen. The obtained product is a uranium dioxide ceramic containing coprecipitated barium impurity.

The comparison of a UO_2 powder containing 370 ppm of barium and a pure UO_2 powder manufactured under the same conditions gives the following results: the two samples of powders are pelletized without addition of any organic or other material, up to a green density of 5.5 grams/cm.^{3} and sintered for 3 hours at 1600°C. under an atmosphere constituted of a mixture of 95% argon and 5% hydrogen. Under these conditions, the pure UO_2 powder provides pellets having a density of 10.35 g./cm.^{3} (or 94.4% of theoretical density) whereas pellets containing 370 ppm of barium reach only a density of 10.07 grams/cm.^{3} (or 91.9% of the theoretical density).

Example 2: A depleted UO_2 ceramic has been mixed with 0.06% of barium carbonate (inhibitor) and 0.3% of zinc stearate (lubricant), then finely ground for 30 minutes in a ball mill. The obtained powder is precompressed at 2,000 kg./cm.^{2}, granulated, pelletized at a green density of 5.6 g./cm.^{3}, and afterwards sintered for 1 hour at 1600°C. under hydrogen. After sintering, the density of the pellets is 9.15 g./cm.^{3} or 83.5% of the theoretical density.

MISCELLANEOUS PRODUCTS

Rodenticide Bait

A rodenticide composition of the metallic phosphide type which can be used on food crops is disclosed by *H.L. Arbauth; U.S. Patent 3,624,198; November 30, 1971; assigned to The AR Chem Corporation*. No rodenticide has previously been approved for use on food crops in view of the toxicity dangers to consumers of food crops treated with the rodenticide. Rodenticide compositions which are capable of completely decomposing to leave no toxic residues on the crops, yet stable enough to remain acceptable to the rodents for a sufficient period of time, have been unheard of.

For example, metallic phosphides, such as zinc phosphide, have been widely used for rat and mouse bait but they have the drawback of rapidly decomposing when wet or under acid conditions. Although zinc phosphide-cereal baits have been formulated for noncrop use, these baits have not been acceptable for oncrop use since in the absence of moisture the zinc phosphide may be latent in its rate of decomposition and may cause an unacceptable toxicity tolerance in food crops.

This improved rodenticide bait is in the form of a unitary body comprising an intimate mixture of particles of metal phosphide, citric acid particles, and a water-insoluble hard wax component, the wax component being uniformly distributed in the unitary body in the form of a protective coating over the metal phosphide and citric acid particles. It has been found that citric acid in the rodenticide bait acts upon absorption of moisture to completely decompose the metal phosphide on a given schedule. In addition, since many rodents such as the Norway, Roof and Polynesian rat are attracted to citrus fruits, the citric acid enhances the value of the bait.

The metal phosphides are any of the metal phosphides capable of being decomposed by moisture to phosphine. These phosphides are well-known in the pesticide art and include, for instance, the phosphides of alkali metals, alkaline earth metals, aluminum and zinc, nickel, iron and other heavy metals. An especially effective and preferred metal phosphide is zinc phosphide which has been widely used for rat and mouse bait. The metal phosphides, particularly zinc phosphide, have an odor characteristic of phosphorus which rodents love. It is preferred, however, to include in the bait composition, in addition to the metal phosphide, rodenticide particles of solid food baits such as are commonly employed in rodenticide compositions. The most popular solid food-type baits are the cereals such as corn, wheat, rye, rice, barley, malt, oat groats, peanut hearts or the like; animal proteins, etc., singly or in admixture. The wax component employed in the bait composition may be any water-insoluble, relatively hard wax or combination of waxes. Illustrative of suitable waxes are paraffin wax, microcrystalline wax, carnauba wax, beeswax, ceresin wax and the like and mixtures thereof. A preferred wax component comprises paraffin wax with up to about 5% by weight of ceresin wax based on the combination of waxes.

It is preferred to employ the metal phosphide and citric acid in substantially equal proportions. The amount of wax employed should be sufficient to uniformly coat and seal the particles of metal phosphide, citric acid and other components which may be included in the bait composition; the actual amount being primarily dependent upon the desired time for decomposition of the metal phosphide. In general, the amount of the wax component will fall in the range of about 30 to 40% by weight of the total composition. In the example, the percentages are based on the total weight of the composition.

Example: To a mixer equipped with heating means is charged cereal grains, stabilized protein particles and 1% technical grade zinc phosphide. After these components are thoroughly mixed, 35% pure microfined table grade paraffin wax and 2% microfined ceresin wax are added and the temperature of the mixture is brought to 180°F. with continuous stirring. 1% anhydrous grade citric acid is then added and after thorough mixing, the entire mixture is extruded under a pressure of 25,000 psi through a two-well shoulder design die having an orifice diameter of ¾ inch, heated to a temperature of 165°F.

The initial well of the die opens into a second well and is of larger diameter than the second well. The second well, in turn, opens into a ¾ inch die channel and is of larger diameter than the channel. The total distance between the entrance to the first well of the die to the orifice is approximately 4 inches. The extrudate is thereby compressed inward and downward in two steps to form a very compact extrudate. The compact extrudate is cut into 1½ inch length to provide a wax bound and impregnated rodenticide bait slug, ¾ inch in diameter and 1½ inches in length.

Pelletizing Carbon Black

Apparatus and method for producing carbon black pellets are disclosed by *P.N. Hare; U.S. Patent 3,751,543; August 7, 1973; assigned to Cities Service Company.* The improvements include increasing rate of pellet formation, production of higher density pellets, reduction in the amount of liquid required to form pellets and increasing the transfer of the work into the wetted powder mass.

The apparatus is shown in Figure 15.4. The pelletizer comprises an elongated pelletizing zone, represented at **1**, which is bounded by a pelletizing conduit **2** having the cross-sectional configuration of two overlapping circles having the overextending segment of each circle removed and thus providing communication between the two partially cylindrical bilateral halves of the pelletizing zone over its full length.

Each side of the pelletizing conduit, i.e., each partial cylinder, is fitted with a rotatable shaft, **3a** and **3b**. Each shaft extends axially through the pelletizing zone along the axis of the partial cylinders. The shafts are supported by bearings **4** mounted on end-closure plates **5** for the pelletizer conduit. Each shaft is provided with a multiplicity of elongated agitating members **6a** and **6b**, hereinafter referred to as pins, which are fixed at spaced intervals along the length of the shaft and which extend radially outward.

The lateral spacing of the parallel shafts and the length of the pins is such that the pins overlap each other upon rotation of the shafts. However, the longitudinal spacing of the pins along one shaft is staggered with respect to the spacing on the other, so that the pins do not collide upon rotation of the shafts but rather clear each other and thus effect interdigitation of the pins of one shaft with the pins of the other. Each shaft is equipped with a variable speed drive unit, generally represented at **7a** and **7b** consisting of an

FIGURE 15.4: PELLETIZING CARBON BLACK

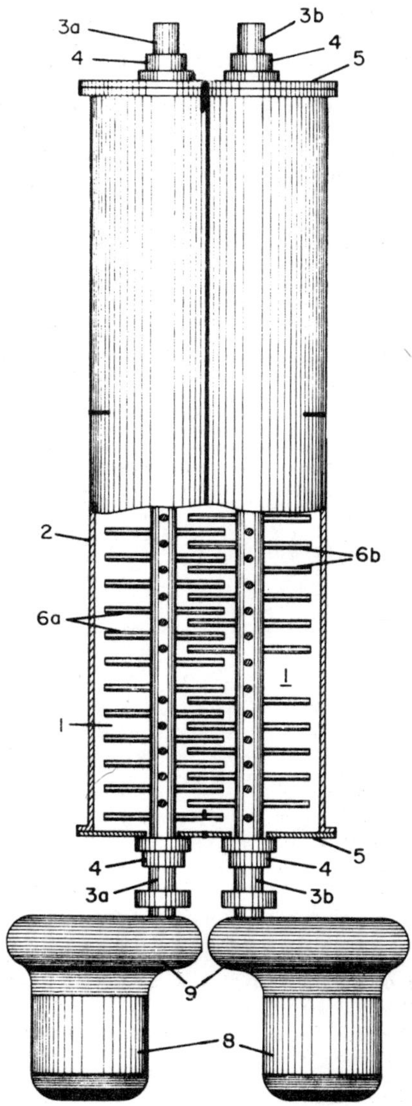

Source: P.N. Hare; U.S. Patent 3,751,543; August 7, 1973

electric motor **8** and a speed reducer **9**. The pelletizing zone has an inlet **10** toward one end for the introduction of powder to be pelletized and an outlet **11** toward the other end for the removal of pellets. A liquid supply conduit **12** extends through the conduit **2** for introducing a liquid pelletizing medium into the pelletizing zone. Two such conduits can be employed for introducing liquid into each partial cylinder of the pelletizing conduit. The method and means described in U.S. Patent 3,535,412 is preferred for injecting the liquid longitudinally into the pelletizing zone and mixing it with the powder therein.

Example: A carbon black having the following properties was pelletized in a pelletizer as shown in U.S. Patent 3,535,412 having a single agitating shaft with radially extending pins. The pins had a length of 7½ inches. The inside diameter of the cylindrical pelletizing conduit was 8 inches and its length was 36 inches.

Surface area (electron microscope), m.²/g.	110
Dibutylphthalate absorption, cc/100 g.	200
Iodine absorption number	290
Transmission, percent	100

The carbon black was fed to the pelletizer at the rate of 90 lbs./hr. while water was being introduced at the rate of 165 lbs./hr. Shaft speed of the pelletizer was 950 rpm. The resulting wet pellets were then dried to a moisture level of 1.2% to provide dry pellets of the carbon black.

In a comparison experiment, this same carbon black was pelletized in accordance with this process. The pelletizer was equipped with two shafts having agitating members 7½ long. Each shaft extended through a partial cylinder having an inside diameter of 8 inches and a length of 32 inches. Carbon black was fed to this twin shaft pelletizer at the rate of 90 lbs./hr. while water was introduced at the rate of 135 lbs./hr. Both shafts were turned at 900 rpm and were rotated in the same direction. The resulting pellets were then dried as before. Properties of the dried pellets produced in the two experiments was as follows.

	Pellet Size, Weight Percent					
	10 Mesh	18 Mesh	35 Mesh	60 Mesh	120 Mesh	Pour Density (lbs./ft.^{3})
Prior art	0.1	41.2	42.2	13.7	1.9	14.4
Process	0.1	29.1	60.1	8.9	1.1	16.8

It can be seen that use of this process provided pellets at a faster rate, pellets having higher density, and use of less liquid pelletizing medium. Reduction of the amount of water required in forming the pellets by 18 weight percent has considerable economic significance in that it results in a substantial reduction of thermal energy need for drying the pellets. Increasing density of the pellets provides the benefit of lower shipping cost.

Catalyst Tablets

Catalyst tablets are prepared according to a process by *W. Rottig and H.-H. Saenger; U.S. Patent 3,755,192; August 28, 1973; assigned to Ruhrchemie AG, Germany,* by mixing the catalyst particles, with or without substrate, with graphite and a polyethylene, polypropylene, polyethylene glycol and/or polypropylene glycol; and then tablettizing the mass.

Preferably 1 to 4% graphite and 0.3 to 1% of the polymeric compound, related to the entire composition weight, are added. Although the total amount of graphite and polymeric compounds may be greater than 5%, such is not considered essential or particularly desirable, since no substantial additional effect is thereby obtained. Graphite is used in its known commercially available form having a carbon content of more than 99% and a grain size distribution such that the amount of particles up to 10 microns amounts to about 50%. Advantageously, the molecular weight of the added polyolefins ranges between 10,000 and 100,000; that of the added polyalkylene glycols is between 5,000 and 20,000. The melting point of the polymeric compounds is preferably about 50° to 150°C. The polymeric compounds are preferably used in as finely divided condition as possible in order to assure a homogenous mixture thereof with the other components. It has been observed that particularly advantageous results are obtained when polymeric compounds with a grain size distribution spectrum containing not more than at most 1% particles of more than 1,000μ and at most 10% particles of more than 500μ are used.

In the following examples the tabletting machine which was used was conventional, commercially available equipment. It consisted of a vertically disposed, exchangeable cylindrical body of stainless steel. Several mold cavities were disposed in the stainless steel body, each of which had two stainless steel ramrods operatively associated therein, and means to drive the ramrods toward each other within the mold cavities. The inside diameter of the mold cavities and the outside diameter of the ramrods, less clearance of course, correspond to the outside diameter of the tablets being produced. The tablet height is determined by the cumulative throw of the ramrods and the clearance left therebetween.

Examples: String-shaped catalyst grains, containing about 37% nickel, about 3% magnesium oxide and about 24% diatomaceous earth, with the remainder being water, carbon dioxide in the form of carbonate, etc., were prepared by precipitating nickel nitrate as well as magnesium nitrate (the latter serving as activator) from a solution thereof with a sodium carbonate solution (both solutions having a temperature of about 100°C.) in the presence of diatomaceous earth.

The precipitate was filtered, washed, dried and molded. The string-shaped particles so obtained were reduced at a temperature of about 500°C. with a hydrogen stream, subsequently stabilized in a known manner, comminuted and separated by sieving so that after sieving no particles of more than 1.5 mm. remained.

1.5% by weight graphite and 0.5% by weight magnesium stearate were added to the product obtained above and intimately mixed in a mixing device. The mixture was molded into tablets, having a diameter of 5 mm. and also a length of 5 mm. in a conventional laboratory preforming press. After a total tablet output of 3.3 kg./mold cavity, the rate of objectionable and/or partly damaged tablets increased rapidly.

At a subsequent inspection of the matrices used, marked stress appearances were observed, which made the further production of unobjectionable tablets difficult if not impossible. Instead of the above noted addition of 0.5% by weight magnesium stearate, the same amount of polyethylene glycol, having a molecular weight of about 10,000 was added to an amount of catalyst as set forth above. The output of tablets was increased to more than 50 kg. per mold cavity.

With a polyethylene glycol having a molecular weight of about 20,000 a substantially identical improved output was obtained. With a polyethylene glycol having a molecular weight of 5,000 the output per mold cavity was improved over the magnesium stearate but was slightly reduced as compared with the higher molecular weight of polyethylene glycol products.

In another example, 0.5% by weight of polyethylene having a molecular weight of about 60,000 obtained by the so-called Ziegler-synthesis in the form of a fine powder was added to the catalyst composition instead of polyethylene glycol, an output per mold cavity was obtained at the subsequent tabletting procedure, which surmounted that obtained with magnesium stearate by more than twenty-fold.

COMPANY INDEX

The company names listed below are given exactly as they appear in the patents, despite name changes, mergers and acquisitions which have, at times, resulted in the revision of a company name.

INVENTOR INDEX

U.S. PATENT NUMBER INDEX

NOTICE

Nothing contained in this Review shall be construed to constitute a permission or recommendation to practice any invention covered by any patent without a license from the patent owners. Further, neither the author nor the publisher assumes any liability with respect to the use of, or for damages resulting from the use of, any information, apparatus, method or process described in this Review.

CAPSULE TECHNOLOGY AND MICROENCAPSULATION 1972

by M. Gutcho

A review of 210 processes collected from recent U.S. patents. The book deals with the manufacture and use of macrocapsules, microcapsules, and other methods of enclosing a liquid or solid in a polymer substance.

The most modern methods are described. These include simple and complex coacervation, physical processes involving centrifugal and electrostatic methods, colloidal wall formation, chemical synthesis in situ, interfacial polycondensation reactions, and many more.

A much abridged table of contents is given here. Numbers in ( ) indicate nos. of processes. Chapter headings are given, followed by examples of important subtitles.

372 pages

CONTROLLED ACTION DRUG FORMS 1974

by J. C. Colbert

Chemical Technology Review No. 24

Speedy antacids and quick-acting analgesics have long been extolled for their fast remedial performance in all forms of advertising. Enteric coatings for specific release along the intestinal tract have been known to pharmacists since the early 1900's. Even the 12-hour cold capsule is now commonplace.

All this is a far cry from today's sophisticated drug design. Hydrophilic polymers and biological binding substances, such as select proteins and polysaccharides, enable the medicinal chemist and pharmacologist to design drug systems by which simple implants will release measured low doses of a hormone or contraceptive continuously for as long as one year. By means of skillful lamination techniques it is possible to withhold release or absorption until a certain poison enters or is generated within the body.

This review covers 211 patents issued since 1956 covering numerous methods of preparing practical dosage forms of human or veterinary drugs having some means of controlling the action or release of the active ingredients. Numbers in parentheses indicate a plurality of processes per topic. Chapter headings and some of the more important subtitles are given in the partial and condensed table of contents that follows here.

ISBN 0-8155-0520-5

340 pages

CONFECTIONS AND CANDY TECHNOLOGY 1974

by M. E. Schwartz

Food Technology Review No. 12

The scope of the technology covered in this volume is generally taken to include products whose major ingredient is sugar. Thus the range of products includes not only candy per se, but also chewing gum, desserts, sweet snacks, icings and whipped toppings, jellies and syrups. Also included are many processes designed to produce some of the basic ingredients of the industry such as sugars, syrups, fats, milk, and whey products. Technology of additives is similarly included, as far as such additives come within the scope of this survey.

Current concerns of the industry with regard to dietetic demands of the consumer have received special attention. Thus candy and confectionery processes geared to the production of low calorie or nonsugar sweets are covered fully.

The technology of the industry is large as evidenced by the appearance of well over 200 U.S. patents in the last ten years. This vast storehouse of information has been organized so that it may be of maximum use to practitioners in the art of candymaking.

A partial and condensed table of contents follows here. Numbers in parentheses indicate a plurality of processes per topic. Chapter headings are given, followed by examples of important subtitles.

ISBN 0-8155-0524-8 **338 pages**

SUGAR SUBSTITUTES AND ENHANCERS 1973

by Roger Daniels

Food Technology Review No. 5

Because of recent restrictions on the use of synthetic sweeteners, there has developed considerable interest and research activity concerning the use of naturally occurring materials to induce or expand the sweetness of natural sugars, so that lower sugar levels can be used for lower caloric content of foods and beverages.

All of these approaches are covered in this volume, as are new synthetic sweeteners with very low toxicity figures, such as chemical modifications of natural amino acids.

The appendix contains important directives by the U.S. Food and Drug Administration on the status, use, and labeling requirements of effective combinations of such sugar substitutes and enhancers.

Except for the appendix, the book is based on 105 recent U.S. patents. Numbers in ( ) indicate the number of processes per topic. Chapter headings are given here, followed by examples of important subtitles.

ISBN 0-8155-0492-6 **275 pages**